*The Bestselling Book
That at Last Puts Beauty and
Health Where They Belong—
Together*

Most writers on beauty concentrate just on the outer you, pouring out reams of often erroneous advice about cosmetics, hairdos and other artificial aids, while ignoring the health that is the essential foundation of beauty. On the other hand, most experts on health and nutrition are so involved in talking about what goes into you, that they fail to make any connection with what happens to your appearance.

Now at last a book shows you how to achieve health and beauty and the dynamic energy that goes with both through the right foods and vitamins, the most natural body, skin and hair care, avoiding the common pitfalls, whether they are harmful commercial products or foolish health-fad gimmicks.

The result is the super simple guide to the super beautiful you.

The Natural Way To
SUPER BEAUTY

Mary Ann Crenshaw

A DELL BOOK

For you, babes,
with all my heart.
And for my perfectly beautiful family.

Published by
DELL PUBLISHING CO., INC.
1 Dag Hammarskjold Plaza
New York, New York 10017

Dell ® TM 681510, Dell Publishing Co., Inc.
Reprinted by arrangement with
David McKay Company, Inc.

ISBN: 0-440-16061-8

First Dell printing—March 1975
Second Dell printing—May 1975
Third Dell printing—May 1975
Fourth Dell printing—June 1975
Fifth Dell printing—July 1975
Sixth Dell printing—November 1975
Seventh Dell printing—December 1975
Eighth Dell printing—May 1976
Ninth Dell printing—July 1976
Tenth Dell printing—September 1976
Eleventh Dell printing—January 1977
Twelfth Dell printing—April 1977
Thirteenth Dell printing—September 1977

Acknowledgments

It is true. There is no way an author can adequately thank all of the people who help an idea become a book. In my case it might involve listing everyone whose life has touched mine within the past two years.

I will try, however, to express my gratitude to all of the very busy people who gave so willingly of their time to answer a lay person's questions (in a lay person's language) on the complicated business of nutrition and beauty. Those who had more than their share of the questions and deserve very special thanks are: Paula Kent, chairman of the board, and Dr. Ron di Salvo, vice president in charge of research at RedKen Laboratories; Dr. Lee Southard of Elizabeth Arden's research department; the entire Estée Lauder research group; Dr. Earle Brauer, research director of Revlon; Dr. Norman Orentreich of the Orentreich Medical Group; Dr. Albert Kligman of the University of Pennsylvania School of Medicine; and Dr. Robert C. Atkins. And, of course, Dr. Jean Mayer of the Harvard School of Nutrition, Dr. Carlton Fredericks, and Linda Clark—all of whom enthusiastically shared with me their immense store of nutritional knowledge.

My very special personal thanks go to my own physician, Dr. Arthur Warren Ludwig, who has coped with keeping me healthy for fifteen years now and always found time to answer the endless barrages of questions, without once losing either his temper or his humor. To him I owe my life, and my gratitude to Dr. Ludwig and his ministering angels—Michelle Okin and Nancy Nitka—is simply inexpressible.

I am grateful to Helen Gurley Brown, editor of *Cosmopolitan* magazine, for setting me on the road to healthy beauty, and to Roberta Ashley and Mallen de Santis, of that publication, for keeping me always on course.

My own pharmacist, Gus Matera, deserves a medal for

knowing his health food just as well as he knows his pharmaceuticals, and for willingly sharing his knowledge with me.

I want to thank all of my friends at *The New York Times* who counseled and/or encouraged—especially Norma Skurka, Barbara Wyden, Marylin Bender, and Joan Cook. And Linda Amster of the *Times'* research department, who knows where to find the answers to all of the questions.

My awed admiration and super-gratitude go to my intrepid researcher, Wendie Owen, who marched bravely in where others (apparently) had feared to tread, and came up with all of the information needed to create the incredible chart at the end of this book. Willowy Wendie, I salute you!

To my editor, Jim Wade, and all the others who worked so valiantly to make this book work—and to all the friends who stood by my side through it all and remained my friends, I can only say, "Here's to your health!" You're already beautiful.

September 26, 1973

Contents

Stop, Look, and Listen

This is not a "reference book." Please, *please* read it from cover to cover. It is meant to deal with all of you, not just pieces of you, so please don't use the index as a quick shopping list. You'll be cheating yourself. Everything in this book relates to everything else and it all leads up to the huge chart at the end which—I hope—will become the one reference item in your beauty and health life.

I am not a doctor.

I am not selling anything.

This book was written from my own (painful) personal experience, out of my years of work as a fashion and beauty writer, and after years of interviews and tons of books, because I wanted to know things that I couldn't find on the back of any bottle labeled "Drink Me." I've tried to put it all together—so that you can get it together.

Good luck. Trust your doctor. Read on.

1. Shape

Finding the Right Path

Remember one thing. I never promised you an herb garden. It's what I thought I'd be giving you when I began this book. Until I discovered that the path through the herb garden is not necessarily the proper route to natural beauty.

Herbs and other wonders of nature are wonderful all right, but sometimes they're more wonderful as herbs than as beautifiers. And here we're only concerned with the things that will bring out the beautiful you.

A lot of home-beauty remedies are simply so much "egg on your face." That's not what you'll get in this book. I don't believe it's what you want. If it is, then I suggest a trip to your local five-and-ten—where such pamphlets abound. And are worth the pennies you'll pay.

No. I don't intend to propagate any beauty myths here, no matter how charming—and natural—they may seem. So, if egg on your face is just that, I will tell you so. And then go on to tell you what you can do with an egg to make it really work for your looks. For your hair. For your skin. And for your shape.

This book won't promise you anything and give you something else. What it will give you is information—often surprising information, always reliable information; information gleaned from the latest research done by experts in the fields of both nutrition and beauty. (And, as far as I'm concerned, the two are synonymous—good nutrition and good looks.) Research done by the brains behind the beauties. The ones who ought to know. And do. And whatever they tell us, we'll tell you.

This book isn't going to be just another healthy food book either, though I believe in healthy food all right, for I grew up in the Old South. Not the antebellum South, but Old South enough so that the vegetables we had were fresh and often picked right out of the garden that very morning. The vitamins were still there. Frozen was not just a nutritionally dirty word—it was an unknown word.

The bread served in our house was made in our house. For even in those days, my mother had her own crusade going against the gumball goo that passed (and unfortunately, still does) for "white bread." And the cornmeal we used in our cornbread (what Southerner is without cornbread?) was the water-ground meal we often drove miles to find.

In those days, no one dreamed of such meal-monstrosities as fake cream for coffee, or imitation butter, or preservatives and more preservatives—all intended to see food past its prime. Who wants food past its prime anyway?

Now, since I am not quite that old, you can see it hasn't been so very long since people ate well.

So what happened? The age of quick food is upon us, and a meal, these days, usually consists of something that any self-respecting animal would reject. (In fact, it has been said that, thanks to the market value of farm animals, their food is healthier than our own.) Gives you food for thought, doesn't it? And it brings to mind recent newspaper stories of a pair of college students who decided to dine on dog foods for a while. And found them tasty.

One problem, though. Dogs, too, are stuck with preservatives. And so they, too, are exposed to the cancer-causing additives just the same way we humans are—the same irresponsible way, it would seem to me.

Today Americans live on such health-horrors as hamburgers, liberally larded with such additives and pre-dosed with the hormones that fattened the beef before it became hamburger. They are loaded with calories and cholesterol and, worse still, slapped between two parts of a gummy textured bun, from which most of the nutrients have been removed. And then that dolloped with a big blob of sugar-loaded catsup. To wash it all down, a cola, perhaps. Cola: the syrupy danger drink that many nutritionists blame for more heart disease in this country than any other single food.

There are other American favorites. There's the hot dog. Loaded with sodium nitrite, one of America's inadvertently most consumed "foods"—a preservative that, under laboratory conditions, has been shown to form a new chemical compound, nitrasomine, which (according to a recent *New York Times* [April 8, 1973] article), once it hits the stomach, it is one of the most powerful cancer-causing agents yet discovered. And yet sodium nitrite hangs right in there. In that hot dog, in you. While the world wonders about cancer cures.

And, of course, the hot dog hasn't been singled out. Most cured meats have been preserved with the stuff. Bacon is one of the most liberally loaded. Just check the labels. In fact, if you check almost any label—as we are going to hammer home to you, over and over again as something you must learn to do—you'll probably be horrified. When you've learned to read labels, you'll have a lot better idea as to what you've been eating.

Fortunately, the U.S. Food and Drug Administration is coming to our rescue. At last. It seems to me—and this is only my own personal opinion—that they have been incredibly lax in keeping America healthy.

For example, did you know that the FDA actually has guidelines on what makes dirty food? And that those guidelines actually permit five pellets of rodent excrement per 1¾ ounces of cornmeal (if they show up in 20 percent of the samples) *before* they consider it polluted.

In peanut butter, you can get up to fifty insect fragments or two rodent hairs (which probably enter via fecal pellets, according to a recent report in *Consumer Reports*) per 3½ ounces of peanut butter before the FDA steps in and yells "dirty."

As *Consumer Reports* puts it, in March 1972 after much prodding from consumers and legislators who thought the public might like to know what comprised "filth" in the eyes of the FDA, they revealed these figures for the first time. Says CU, "The menu all these years, the consumer learned, included a stomach-churning assortment of insect parts and larvae, fish cysts, mold, rot, rodent hair, and excrement." And all this courtesy of the same government agency that is taking steps to restrict the sale of vitamins. To me, it's pretty contradictory.

On the subject of food labeling, however, they are, at last, moving in a positive direction. On January 18, 1973, the FDA announced "sweeping changes in food labeling practices" that, according to a *New York Times* story, would give consumers "a better idea of the nutritional value of about half of what they eat." Why they're only going to tell us about "half"—well, ask them. Still, half a label is better than none at all.

Over the next two years, most of the nation's foodstuffs must be relabeled to show their caloric content, protein content, fats, carbohydrates, vitamins, and minerals. Fresh bakery goods, alas, raw fruits and nonprocessed dairy products would not be subjected to the new rules, unless something had been added, such as Vitamin D in milk, in which case it must be stated.

All about time, we hasten to add—and emphatically. Because perhaps soon such health hazards as "enriched" bread will have labels that say exactly what it is. Not the good staff-of-life-stuff from which your beauty will benefit, but white soft-and-squeezy—and nutritionally empty— slabs of nothing from which practically every valuable nutrient has been removed—to make it whiter, prettier, and deadlier—with only a tiny percentage of these nutrients returned as additives. Would you call that "enriched"? Fortunately, under the new regulations, anything that was called "enriched" previously is *not* exempt from showing its "all," and this means that you will finally find out just how little enrichment you're getting from run-of-the milled white bread.

While they were at it, the FDA has finally given up on their "U.S. recommended daily allowances" of protein, vitamins, and minerals. About time, I'd say, since the amounts they give are generally the amounts needed for survival only, but most decidedly not the amounts that might possibly do something positive for your health and your good looks. That is, after all, what this book is all about. Good looks, beauty, and the natural way to find it.

The FDA allows, contrary to previous policy, a food producer to list the cholesterol content of the product as well as the amounts of unsaturated fatty acids, saturated acids, and other acids. According to the *Times* story, the change was brought about by the concern of physicians that excessive amounts of cholesterol and other fats might be a significant cause of heart disease.

And, finally, if a product is imitation anything, it is going to have to say so. On that I say three cheers for the FDA. You mean that we may, at *last*, know what is going into us?

The Sweet Way to Die

And then there's sugar—the sweet way to die. It must be Americans' favorite food, for they consume 175 pounds per person per year. Sugar is a killer-food—the underworld of the wonder world of healthy food—the culprit in diabetes, heart disease, and obesity, one of the worst diseases in the United States today, as well as one of the most ignored.

According to the U.S. Department of Agriculture, per capita sugar consumption has risen in this country by 40 percent since 1909, the year that department began to keep figures on the stuff. Mothers satisfied kiddies' appetites for the "surprise in the cereal box" by filling them up with empty breakfast cereals that are little more than sugar pasted on top of fluff. Even the United States Senate was horrified enough to act on that when it wasn't even an election year! During a recent five days of hearings before the Senate Select Committee on Nutrition and Human Needs, investigating the television advertising of food for children, four witnesses testified—according to a *New York Times* story of March 6, 1973—that many children's breakfast cereals were nutritionally "hollow," containing over 50 percent sugar. The cry certainly won't be "Look, Mom, no cavities!" if this keeps up.

And yet even so supposedly illustrious a publication as *The Wall Street Journal* in early 1973 covered the cereal scene with an editorial called "The Munchies Menace." So far, so good—except that the editorial goes on to state that sugar is here to stay, so why fight it? They suggest we live with the present awful facts of food life and accept the cavities and other horrors of too sweet living. Frankly, I was shocked. Their attitude (in actual print): "So what?" Mine: Change things! Fortunately, for those with an incurable sweet tooth, there are answers in the works. Artichokes, for example, have been shown to have sweetening properties. A Yale University psychologist, Dr. Linda Bartoshuk (in the *Times* of December 3, 1972) has confirmed the fact. And her work may some day soon (we hope) produce a new way to sweeten the endless drinks Americans seem compelled to consume. The sweetening ability of the artichoke was found to be comparable to two teaspoons of sugar—added to six ounces of liquid . . .

(water, in the case of Dr. Bartoshuk's study). And Dr. Bartoshuk has come up with a new food on me—something called "miracle fruit" which it apparently is. For it has the "miraculous" properties of making foods taste sweet when they aren't. All of this sounds like a boon for those of us who can't have sugar, and for all of us who *shouldn't* have it.

According to these nutritionists, Americans are on a sugar binge, eating more of it annually than flour (which is bad enough) and causing an epidemic of tooth decay and other diseases. Not only that, there is evidence that sugar-rich snack foods may cause nutritional deficiencies of such necessary trace elements as chromium and zinc. During the 1960s, food producers increased their use of sugar in food products by 50 percent. So, if you count on food manufacturers, matters are not going to get any better.

Which brings us to labels. Read them. And read them carefully. *Your life may depend on it.*

But then this is a beauty book, not a crusade, and I am a fashion-and-beauty writer, not a campaigner. Nevertheless, in my wanderings through beauty research I learned enough to be frightened. Frightened of the unseen (and heretofore unlabeled) horrors that lurk in all those easy-does-it foods that contain very little except calories, and do very little but send us on our way to an early, and completely unnecessary—and, I might add, unbeautiful—old age.

One crusader has said it for the American diet. That crusader is Dr. Carlton Fredericks and, so far as I am concerned, he said it all when he pronounced, "If you are what you eat, then God help you!"

We are going to see what we can do to help you change that.

The Deal on Beauty

Whoever said that beauty was no big deal? For it's probably the biggest deal you'll ever make. With yourself. And it's a lifetime contract. And it means work.

Because we can give you the ingredients, but you must bake the cupcake.

Beauty isn't an accident—not even with the born-beautifuls. It requires watchful, never-ending work, and strict attention to what's happening at all times. To your looks, that is. Just one night of being too tired to wash your face, or one bout with boozing, or one day of hitting the candy box can undo all the good derived from months of trying. I have very little patience with people who claim they're trying and then behave in this manner. And, frankly, this book is not written for them.

For I am serious about what I'm writing. If you're not, then don't bother to start reading. If you really want to shape up, prepare to follow the rules to the letter. And if you're not going to then stop talking about how out of shape you are. For don't think everyone isn't onto the difference between talking and doing. If you want clear skin, healthy hair, and nails, the answers, insofar as they are now known, are here. But you must use them and you must use them constantly. Work, work, and more work is what you have facing you for the rest of your beautiful life.

How Do You Know I Know?

How do *I* know? That's what you're probably going to ask. And you'd be quite right in doing so. For beauty, and fashion, is my usual beat. But I care about my looks (that's the fashion part of me at work) and I care to the paranoia point. Bad for me, lucky for you. Because, once I realized that the answer to natural beauty lies in healthy eating and healthful living, then I began to pay a lot more attention to what went in my body as well as to what went on it. And I had trouble finding out. Sure, lots of the information is out there, all right, in some very good books. Lots of the information is out there in some very obscure books. And lots of the information just isn't out there. Or wasn't until we dug it up.

I am not a diet doctor. I am a dieter who wants to know how. I am not a hairdresser. I am an especially exacting hairdresser's client. I am not a skin specialist, but I have made it my business to take the specialized advice of one. (And I got good skin for my troubles.)

Whatever you read in this book will have been tried by me. In fact, one of the very reasons for this book's existence was my own personal need. My need for more information—explicit information like the kind given in our never-before chart; the needs I had when I took my troubles to a diet doctor, or a skin specialist, or a scalp rejuvenator; and so on. For that is usually how a reporter's story evolves. From personal experience. For no matter how hard one tries, it is impossible to be 100 percent impersonal in reporting. By what one puts in or leaves out, one is automatically pre-editing a story.

I would estimate that I have read, and digested, some hundred-odd books—just to get the information that I hope to pass on to you in this single volume. Not only that, I have interviewed and interviewed and interviewed. Doctors, nutritionists, research scientists. I have a low frustration-tolerance. And it's pretty frustrating to have to go through a year's worth of searching just to get the straight, hard line on what it takes to make a more beautiful person out of you. I suffered through it. Now you won't have to. At last my beauty neuroses had some positive effect.

Not only did I search; I have doctors—unusual doctors —who won't stop at the standard academic doctor's answers. Each and every fact in this book has been thoroughly checked with my own private doctors. Check one against the other, I always say. I do it in my private life and in my daily work as a reporter. I most certainly do it in print. So now you've got edited and pre-digested food for beauty. But making it work is up to you. I can't make you do right by yourself. This is the point where your self-discipline must shine through in living, beautiful new you.

Beauty isn't going to drop into your lap, no matter how much you sit and wish. I can give you all the facts. But when it comes to application, you are the only one who must work. Beauty is never accidental. Perhaps good bone structure is a born-with blessing, but even good bone structure can look un-pretty if one's health is not up to snuff, whereas a person with less than perfect bones can be radiantly beautiful with care—painstaking work-at-it care—of all of her. Unhealthy people are simply never beautiful. Period.

Why a Diet Doctor? (I Was a Yo-Yo!)

I have often been asked why I ever went to a diet doctor. The answer is simple. I believe in specialization. If I have an eye infection, I go to an eye specialist. If it's female, I see my gynecologist. But I wouldn't expect that gynecologist to fill a tooth for me. Would you? All of my adult life has been spent on one sort of reducing diet or another. For I am not one of the lucky thinnies of the world . . . the sort of person who can eat, drink and be plenty merry with no fat-hangover. I am the sort of person who may have been born to be fat, for more and more research is being done to find out whether the diets fed to infants set their fat patterns in later life. (Maybe this is one thing I can blame on my mother instead of myself?) The real truth is, nobody knows—yet.

My G.P. diet supervision began at nineteen, when I saw my general physician in Alabama in desperation because of my inability to lose weight. Who wants to be unsightly at nineteen? Or at any other age, for that matter, for fat—unnecessary fat—is simply ugly. And unhealthy, which is far worse. Overweight is the greatest single cause of heart disease. And one-third of this nation is seriously overweight. Put those two together and you have the statistics on why the heart disease rate in this country is so high. Too much good—or perhaps we should say "bad"—living makes for early dying.

At any rate, I was given the usual G.P. diet treatment. First, my "obesity" was not, shall I say, taken very seriously. I was given a standard printed 1,500 calories diet issued by some drug company for doctors to dole to their would-be-thinner patients. Obligingly, I followed it to the letter, and lost nothing. I was, of course, accused by my physician of cheating, which infuriated me, for my stand about cheating has *always* been, "Who on earth would I be cheating except myself?" My doctor, after all, really couldn't care less if I weighed ten to twenty pounds more than *I* think I ought to. (Possibly if it were three hundred pounds too much, any physician might advise precautions.)

But as for cheating? I say again, I have no patience with that. To me, it is the ultimate stupidity. I was the one who wanted to get rid of the fat. And for my doctor to accuse me of lying sent me into a temper tantrum that he probably still hears all the way from New York. So I vowed that I would cut calories until I lost that weight—no matter how calorie-low I had to go. And I did: I lost the weight all right, but I also developed infections and low resistance to any and every germ that wafted by.

Of course—I had depleted my body to the starvation point, and I suffered for it.

I was, however, thin. And so I began to eat again. Not overeat, you understand. I never was, and still am not, a big eater, because I am small, and don't require much food intake to "fill 'er up." But, what is normal eating for a normal person was fat-making eating for me. In, say, five years, I had to make my second foray into practically no-calorie living, meaning foregoing everything I loved, and giving up some things I shouldn't have given up either. I made my twenty-pound-loss goal, all right, but at the expense of my nervous system. This time I had happened, quite accidentally, upon something that saw me through it all a bit more healthily. I discovered the diet delights of melon and cottage cheese. If you're on a low-calorie diet, it's a wonderful combination. The melon acts as a diuretic and the cottage cheese gives you protein. Mind you, at that time I had no idea why things were going well. But they were, and I lost, and, while my nerves may have been shot haywire, my body was not quite in the unhealthy condition it had reached via my previous experiment.

But then melons were out of season, I was down to my desired weight, and bit by bit—and it did, I'll admit, take a few years—that old poundage crept back on. Soon I was back up to that twenty pounds overweight I didn't wish to be, and dieting viciously again.

I was, although I didn't realize it at the time, what is known as a Yo-Yo. The person whose weight goes up, and then down by strenuous dieting. Then, with the return to the kind of eating that might be normal for anyone else, back up again.

Being a Yo-Yo is dangerous. For one thing, that up and down weight seesaw is a tremendous strain on the heart. Some doctors maintain that it is far better to be slightly overweight than to go from one extreme to the other. According to Dr. Neil Solomon, author of *The Truth About Weight Control*, the results of a study on Yo-Yos showed that there were aberrations of metabolism among the overweight. His carbohydrate metabolism tests showed that thirty-seven percent of the obese could not metabolize glucose properly. Twenty-eight percent had protein metabolism problems.

As Dr. Solomon points out, the difference in fat metabolism between the Yo-Yos and the control group of "normals" which were tested with them was dramatic: seventy-three percent of the Yo-Yos had abnormalities in fat metabolism while only fourteen percent of the control group showed them. Now don't go screaming "glands." Even Dr. Solomon points out that glands, and the thyroid above all, have been forever the "whipping boys of obesity." *He found thyroid problems relatively rare among these unfortunate Yo-Yos.* The truth is, as I see it, that very little is known about metabolism. There are, of course, hopes in the world of science for eventual computerized medicine. Some day, just maybe, there will be instant computer printouts that will tell all about each of us. Where some minute part is slightly out of adjustment, the proper diet, or drug, or other treatment can be administered to get it back into alignment. It would be a blessing to us all—if it ever happened—for it would make all our weight problems solved as if by magic (or computer). There are labs right this very moment working on just this sort of thing. But they are very much in the experimental stage, and, until they have declared themselves bug-free, I'm not willing even to mention them. Until that science fiction moment of metabolism truth is actually upon us, we who suffer from the Yo-Yo syndrome will have to cope as we can. I can only say that I hope never to be the Yo-Yo on the end of that diet string again. Now that my weight is where I want it, I intend to keep it that way. And I believe I have the final answer on that. You will, too, very soon.

At any rate, on I went—up and down, losing and then gaining it all back to the detriment of both my looks and my health. The last time I tried dieting with the aid of a general physician was about eight years ago. I guess a reporter's life-style had done its dirty work. In any case, there I was again, at 123 pounds, which for me is like the average woman's 200. At 123, I look bad. And, more important to me than looks, even, I *feel* bad. Logy, sluggish, and uncomfortably bloated. And always overfull.

And so off I hied myself to my doctor. The general physician that I admire so much.

And one of the very reasons I admire him is that he is

the first to admit how little the medical profession really knows about that wonderful mechanism of the human body—the metabolic system. The system that makes everything work as it should to utilize all the energy-making food that goes into your mouth and to make sure it ends up as energy and not as fat.

Now, if the metabolic system is, as we said, slightly out of kilter—well, fat is what it usually makes. Or skinny. Skeletal. I've never had to cope with that. (Only once after an illness, when even *I* found that skeletal is as ugly as corpulent.) The metabolic system involves anything that works on metabolism. And metabolism, according to Cooper's *Nutrition in Health and Disease*, a medical textbook since 1928, is defined as "the process by which the cells convert the nutrients from food into useful energy and at the same time create new molecules for tissue synthesis and other vital compounds."

Metabolism involves glands. What glands? Well, Dr. Neil Solomon is particularly interested in those glands that have an association with obesity. They are: the pituitary, located at the base of the brain; the thyroid—that gland that most fatties blame for all their fat; the adrenals, two small glands that are just above the kidneys; the pancreas, lying behind the stomach and the sex glands. According to Dr. Solomon, the secretions of these glands are "important in relation to each individual's body chemistry."

Then there are the endocrine glands, possessors of their own branch of medicine, "endocrinology"—glands which secrete hormones and which only recently have been thought to have bearings on obesity.

Dr. Solomon says that, in the past, endocrine-glandular problems were thought of in terms of severe disorders only; overactive thyroid gland (hyperthyroidism) and underactive thyroid (hypothyroidism). He goes on to quote Dr. William M. K. Jefferies, a Cleveland endocrinologist and researcher who says: "Now we are realizing that there are very definite milder disorders. Sometimes our usual routine test will not pick up these problems: it is only with some of the more sophisticated techniques that are becoming available today that we can pick up the abnormalities that were formerly missed by the other tests."

Dr. Solomon goes on to say that no two people's metabolisms are identical. How true! For, if they were, then the problem would not be one-zillionth so complicated. The problem, that is, of working out the exactly appropriate diet for each and every individual on this earth. The one to keep that individual healthy and looking his best. Dr. Jefferies is quoted by Dr. Solomon as explaining: "It is extremely difficult to find two people who have exactly the same type of chemistry." Dr. Jefferies goes on to explain that this, apparently, is because we have slight differences in hormone production. And, according to Dr. Jefferies, one of the things that turned up in his research was that "every person has his or her own characteristic pattern of excretion of substances resulting from the metabolism by adrenal hormones." He maintains that they don't know for sure, but they suspect hormones are a factor in body build.

The growth hormone is one that seems to play an important role in the regulation of metabolism. According to Dr. Solomon, obese people often have low levels of growth hormone. But that can be changed by diet alone, as you will soon see. Enzymes, about which you will read more in their very own chapter, are yet one more metabolic factor. They are important catalysts for putting everything into proper action, making sure that your blood chemistry is acting "according to Hoyle," so to speak. And I can personally attest to my own odd, but remarkably and spectacularly beneficial, reaction to enzymes. Still, we will reserve that saga for our chapter on Enzyme Power.

So the metabolic system is still a mysterious setup to practically everyone. Fortunately, my own doctor is wise enough to admit that the medical profession is light-years behind in this subject, partly because there are so few funds available for research in biochemistry. Most philanthropists with money to give are more likely to dole it out to such things as cancer research. Which is all to the good, but where does it leave those of us with biochemical problems?

I, for one, believe (and I'm in good company, for so do many doctors) that biochemistry could well be the answer to some age-old and some not-so-old ills. For if that precise computer print-out of every individual's biochemical makeup were possible, imagine how easy it would be for a physician to locate that possibly small something that is just a bit out of kilter but perhaps causing some truly serious problem.

But watch how my own enlightened doctor goofed on dieting.

Off I went to my G.P. for one more diet. As you may have noticed, I have never ever in my life gone on any kind of fad diet. I do not believe in them. I do not believe that starvation is healthy. I do not believe in—nor could I make it through a hard-working day on—diets that allow the likes of one cup of black coffee for breakfast. I would never make it even to the doctor's office on that meal. And, while I believe the such foods as grapefruit, taken after meals, can be instrumental in weight loss, it's because there's an already-understood reason behind it. And you will discover it by the time you've read this book.

Not only do I not participate in the fad diet of the moment, I never, never go on any diet of any kind without a checkup by my internist on the state of my general health.

For dieting to reduce is, by nature, deprivation of something. Whether it is of carbohydrates or of calories, something must be given up. And that something may be something you need to stay healthy. If your health isn't up to snuff, better just stay overweight until it is—unless that weight is so over that it is your major health problem.

Sometimes the rebuilding of a healthy body can bring fluffy bodies—those that are flabby and generally unhealthy-looking—back into line. Adelle Davis, the grande dame of nutritionists, has been known to advise would-be lose-weighters to look to their general health first and worry about the weight later. Sometimes they never have to look—to their weight, that is. Still, I will say it *over and over again. Check with your doctor first!* Make sure that everything is checked that he has the equipment to check. *Everything.* And then embark on dieting, after discussing a program with him.

My last checkup/pre-dieting visit to my doctor went like this. Cut down on calories . . . not unusual for me, for this is what was always necessary. Again, I was given a pre-printed calorie counter, which, I hasten to add, in no way checked out with the one I'd been given by my general physician back in Alabama. (I have a pretty good memory for the caloric content of, say, one egg. Especially when I've been mentally counting for a lifetime.) And I was sent out in the world to calorie-cut. And I thought I did. But zero. Zilch. Nothing. Six weeks later I had lost three pounds. I was depressed. I had given up alcohol. Even wine with my meals. (Mind you, at that time I had little or no idea of the really detrimental effects of alcohol on everything. I liked the stuff.) And still nothing.

I sat at my desk eating a container of cheese when I'd have much preferred lunch with "the boys." At night, I'd slap a small steak on the grill and have that with a tomato. (Wait until you come to our chart. You'll see just what I was doing.) So I complained to my doctor. I was told to cut down on my multivitamins. Or rather, to eliminate them. Now, even to my layman's medical mind, this seemed odd. If you are cutting down on the nutrients going into your body, shouldn't you be upping your supplemental vitamins rather than cutting them out entirely? So I questioned, as is my custom. And I was told that occasionally vitamins increase the appetite.

As appetite was not, and never has been, my big problem, I decided to ignore this medical advice. I just believe in vitamins and I also have a lot of will power when it comes to eating practically nothing. And I *was* eating practically nothing, while "nothing" kept coming off. Not off my body. Off my nerves perhaps, the ends of which were twanging.

And so I complained again. This time I was told I would be sent a diet pill. "To what purpose?" I inquired. "It isn't my appetite that's the problem. It's what happens inside to what I put there." No dice. I got the diet pill anyway—the first of my life and, I am most happy to say, the last.

For I am militantly anti-amphetamine. With my birth-given set of high-strung nerves, who needs "speed"? If there were ever a person walking this earth who doesn't need speeding up, it is I. But I took the pill anyway, in the hope that perhaps all those years I'd suffered needless self-denial when the answer may have lain in one single little capsule.

Zap! Its effect was potent all right. And terrifying. The sidewalks rolled beneath my feet. My hands shook and were icy. The sweat ran, not only off my brow, but off my body as well. And I was a shrewish, shrieking, screaming, ill-tempered mess. Need I say that there was a fast end to my "speed" run? I coolly informed my doctor "no more" and went back to trying to starve my body into weight-loss submission.

I tried all right, but still nothing happened in terms of pounds removed. And by this time, six weeks had passed and I still had that twenty pounds of overweight to show for it.

And so I screamed, as we are all prone to do, "glands"—specifically, my poor thyroid gland. I had my doctor test. And sure enough, my thyroid was low, 4.0, which is the lowest point on the normal scale. Now low thyroid means, of course, that your body burns its fuel at a much slower rate than it should. Which means that a lot of that fuel may land on you. But the truth is that my PBI, which stands for Protein Bound Iodine and is the way of measuring just what that thyroid gland is doing, was still in normal range and my thyroid didn't need help.

I was convinced, however, that the thyroid was the villain, never dreaming for a moment that, through my own misinformation, I was consuming much more in the way of calories than I believed—and therein hangs a lesson. Always count. Preferably on paper. I demanded, and received, thyroid medication. The PBI went up and so did I. Right up the wall with nerves. And as an added un-attraction, my skin festered with horribly un-lovely pimples. That ended the thyroid medication pronto.

It also ended my general-physician-dictated dieting. Not general-physician-*supervised*, you understand. I've said it before and I'm going to keep on saying it. If you're on any sort of weight-off diet, stay in close touch with your physician. Any diet at all that veers from just plain old eating, no matter how well planned it may be, could, by some fluke, affect your general health. It's up to your doctor to see that it doesn't. It's up to you to diet intelligently, following the ground rules we give you, and to check in with him as often as possible.

My history of dieting with doctors is the reason I believe so positively in the importance, to this overweight culture, of diet specialists. With obesity—and its resultant cardiovascular problems—on record as the number one killer in this country today, doesn't that disease—obesity—deserve a medical branch all its own? Call it "obesology"—whatever. But let's have it.

Because losing weight is individual, watching over diets

is time-consuming, and very few general physicians have
either the knowledge or the time to undertake such diet-
prescribing. Just as Dr. Solomon tells us, no two individ-
uals have identical body chemistries. And, even when you
and a diet specialist think you have it down pat, your
chemistry can change. Not only can, but often does. (Mine
did, as you will see.)

So not even diet specialists are infallible on body chemistry. For it seems to keep outwitting the entire medical
profession. But at least diet specialists spend time and research on obesity alone. Let's hope they will come up with
all the metabolic answers soon.

There are those, of course, and they are "sickies," who
go on dieting until they die. They need psychiatrists. I have
nothing to say on that subject because I can only assume
that the readers of this book are intelligent about such
matters. If a person really wants to diet himself to death,
there is very little any author can do to discourage him . . .
or her. Except to continue to insist that those regular medical checkups be maintained throughout any diet. Your
own doctor will soon notice it if you are starving.

The Shape You're In—And How to Change It

If you're reading about diets, we assume you don't like the
shape you're in. And you want to change it. Well, you can
all right—easily—if you'll stick with me and follow the
instructions to the letter. Losing weight is easy. *Deciding* to
lose weight and having the will power to stick to that
decision is the hardest.

It's a bit like a commitment to Alcoholics Anonymous.
And we will keep pointing out the correlation between
alcoholism and obesity. For learning to think fat, and staying on your diet, day by day, is the equivalent of giving up
that drink day by day when you have, at last, faced the
decision that you can't cope with it.

I have no patience with fat. I have much less patience
with people who are fat and keep on saying they don't
want to be. And then don't do a thing about it. Talking
dieting won't get you thin. Neither will wishing. Neither
will hating *being* fat. Unless you hate it enough to stop
talking and start dieting. Before anything can help you,
you must make the decision that "thin" is where you want

to be and want to stay. For, as we will say over and over again, there is no such thing as a "cured" obese person—only an arrested case.

I often blame misinformation for many a well-meaning person's fat-problems. I have heard too many people say, "I'm watching my weight"—while they survive on fruit salad and cottage cheese (lots of calories) or steak (1300 per small club variety) or a container of yogurt (150 for plain, which very few people choose; 200 for the flavored, and 260 for the preserve-filled kind). It isn't that these folks don't want to be thin. It's that they have been led down the garden path to a non-diet. I intend to correct that, and I have no patience at all with cheaters. It's *you* you're cheating. Because it's you who cares most about the shape you're in. Or out of. And, on one of our diets, cheating will make you fatter than ever while on the other, it will simply mean no loss. So put it out of your mind. Way out.

As for your glands, the chances of the blame going there are slim indeed. Dr. Carlton Fredericks says that all the gland-blame inspired him to compose this doggerel:

> I don't understand women—
> They puzzle most of the males.
> They purchase a diet,
> Refuse to live by it,
> And holler "my glands!" when it fails.

Enough said. More than likely it's your hands that are your problem (if obesity is) as well. The hands that take too much food to your mouth. Or the wrong food. Or both.

We aim to change all that. Without touching your glands. We're going to change your shape by offering you two perfectly simple, perfectly beautiful ways to lose weight. And they're very different, which may be the best part of all. It means that you have a choice. A choice of diets that will let you eat the way you like to eat. And shape up while you're at it. But you have to get on *one* of them first. You have to want those extra pounds gone! There can be no more "I'll stuff tonight and start tomorrow." Tomorrow never *does* come. Especially with will-be dieters!

You'll be doing it without drugs, without shots, without

any single thing that's unnatural. On the contrary, drugs and shots and even diuretics are positively forbidden. They not only won't keep you slim, they may keep you dead. And that's not beautiful.

But you must remember two very important factors:

First, eating naturally good-for-you foods doesn't in any way give you license to overeat. If your mother always told you to consider the starving children, wherever she said they were, forget it. Food is not like Mount Everest. It doesn't have to be eaten just because it is there. No matter which diet you choose as your modus vivendi, stop eating when you feel full. You'll feel a lot better for it. And those starving children will never see the leftovers from your plate, in any case.

Second, think fat! It's your only hope for staying slim. For obesity, like alcoholism, is—I firmly believe—something that can be arrested but apparently never cured. There are plenty of correlations, for that matter, between obesity and alcoholism. Researchers are looking into blood-sugar and metabolic disturbances as possible causes for both problems. So you must remember to behave as if you were an alcoholic. Get through every day *on your diet*. I quite agree with the diet specialist who warned against the phrase "going on a diet" as possibly implying that some day you'll be "going off a diet." Chances are you won't. If you're fat-inclined, you'll probably be watching it for the rest of your life—until those computers and specialists turn up the metabolic solutions. But we're going to make watching it a pleasure, and a torment. And if you'll just keep thinking fat, we promise you won't be.

Diet Choice and Choice Diets

In the past, we dieters had two choices, both torturous. One, we could cut out calories to the bone and suffer the possible health consequences. Or, two, we could hone our appetite to the nothing via the dangerous little "rainbow" pills doled out by the thousands by probably innocent physicians who had other "more important" ailments to cure. Those little rainbows are nothing more than amphetamines —"speed." The same dangerous drug you hear so much about when the drug problem is being discussed. And you've probably got some speed—if you've ever been a dieter—lurking right there in your medicine cabinet.

In December 1972, a news story maintained that, if junior is a junkie, chances are he got started on the stuff by experimenting with the pills from his mother's medicine shelves. It seems that's how it starts in most cases. If your medicine chest is loaded with reducing aids, you are simply setting up drug shop for your child. Learn about drugs at home? Believe me, this is one lesson you *don't* want your children to hear first from their parents!

Amphetamines are among the most addictive of all drugs. Fortunately, moves are being made to have them severely restricted. Possibly that innocent (and it usually is) doctor's hand will be stayed a bit before he freely and haphazardly prescribes amphetamines. Particularly if it goes down on his record, and his patient's, as part of a "drug profile"—something the United States government is considering at this time. That would mean that druggists would, by law, have to record each and every drug prescribed by a doctor for any particular patient and then keep progressive records of each refill of that prescription. That way, if a drug problem is building up, the druggist will see it and notify the physician who prescribed. Sometimes it seems to me that the Federal government's long arm reaches too far. This time, it's got a sound idea. Prevent drug addiction before it begins. For, occasionally, the addiction can begin with that innocent little amphetamine-loaded diet pill. Just remember that "speed" does kill.

Why not forget amphetamines and stick with us for two sensible, safe, and tested diets that will make you lose all right. If, and only if, you have decided to stick with it and lick fat.

The two diets are the high protein–low carbohydrate (notice we said, high protein, *not* high fat) and the low calorie, aided and abetted by four fabulous discoveries for the road to thin. Get with one of them and stay there until you're where you think your body ought to be!

The Low-Carbohydrate Route

Did you know that, if food is your hangup, there is a diet that will let you eat and eat and eat and still remove not only pounds, but inches, as well? And those inches all from the spots where you never wanted them in the first place? It's probably the very simplest method for those who find dieting such an insurmountable problem that they give up before they begin. And, remember, we said you have to begin *sometime*, if you ever want to see the results.

There is such a diet, all right, and it's the high-protein–low-carbohydrate diet—the one espoused by scores of obesity specialists, in one form or another, plus a growing rank of slender aficionados. The high protein is good for you and you'll find out just how good very soon; the low carbohydrate is the key to re-making your shape. After what we've told you about killer-carbohydrates and their role in the average American horror diet, you should have no qualms about cutting down on *them*. Best of all, the high-protein–low-carbohydrate diet is easy. Easy to stick to, since there's no going hungry involved; and, for those who love to eat—or those with enormous, insatiable appetites—this diet is, beyond doubt, the best one for those folks to choose.

Counting carbohydrates is often easier than counting calories. Most of the time you needn't count at all, for the foods you are allowed will come from a very special list of already measured, low-carbohydrate ones. And you'll soon have those down pat in your memory pattern.

If you've got a sweet tooth that can't be pulled, then try our other diet. Because on this one, there'll be no sweets at all. And you'll be shocked at the foods that turn up bearing sugar. Things like catsup, for example, which is loaded with it.

And then there are starches. Those French fries will have to go, and they should anyway. They're a greasy bit of no-good filler that all diets can dispense with. And no breads allowed here.

Vegetable intake is limited to the ones that are low in carbohydrates and usually only one serving per day. Ditto for fruits, which come from the tree already loaded with sugar. Your morning orange juice will just have to be forgotten for the moment.

But that's about the sum of it. Starches and sweets—the two things you'll have to watch on any diet—are the basics to forget on the low-carbohydrate regimen.

You *can*, however, have things you never had before on

a diet. A weight-loss diet, I mean. Like hollandaise sauce. Or butter. Or bacon.

Because the dynamics of this diet are that protein plus fat—which you need on every diet if you're going to keep beautiful—are the fuel that makes the fat sitting on *you* burn. Burn away. In essence, your body is burning its excess fat for fuel. Thus those disappearing inches.

Now, as you probably know, the high-protein–low-carbohydrate diet has come under a barrage of criticism from no less venerable a body than the American Medical Association. I, for one, find it fascinating that they have waited for more than a century to barrage. For not only was this diet formulated back in 1863 by an English surgeon named William Harvey, but it is the same diet that Eskimos have been thriving on for as long as Eskimos have been around. That's long enough to see that they are still with us—and, apparently, thriving on their diet of meat and fat. Those are the principal ingredients of Eskimo meal-planning, for the frozen North isn't the best possible spot for finding fresh fruits and vegetables. And "how do they avoid scurvy?" you're doubtless about to ask. Well, according to one previously cited medical textbook, Cooper's *Nutrition in Health and Disease* (presumably the A.M.A. approves this textbook as knowledgeable), "Eskimos seldom have scurvy on their native diets but they are susceptible to it when they adopt the 'white man's diet.' On their native diets they may include organ meats and mosses that supply some ascorbic acid that might be present." Nutritionist Linda Clark in her book *Stay Young Longer* quotes from an unpublished manuscript by a certain Henry W. Griest and his trained-nurse wife, who spent years among the Eskimos. Mr. Griest maintains that for centuries the Eskimo lived on a totally carnivorous diet, and remained healthy, with rosy cheeks and apparent vigor and brawn. He suffered from neither tuberculosis nor venereal disease and lived to a great age with his teeth intact. That is, until the white man came along and in his inimitable fashion, introduced the killer-diet we all know so well—refined foods and sugar. That was the end of the Eskimo's excellent health.

We "civilized" peoples do have a way with diet, don't we? For explorers have observed that a great many primitives, when left to their own resources in diet—whether it be vegetarian or carnivorous—eat natural and healthy foods and thrive. It is only when hit by civilization and its insidious processed-food villains that their health shows a marked decline.

Explorer Vilhjammur Stefansson, probably the most famous of the Eskimo diet-watchers, traveled to the Arctic early in the twentieth century. He saw that the Eskimos were a healthy and strong people, even though they lived on a diet composed largely of meat and animal fat, the things the A.M.A. insists are deadly. The Eskimos not only did not suffer from obesity; they were, according to Stefansson, "the healthiest people I had ever lived with." Stefansson advocated the general use of this high-protein–high-fat diet but, of course, he was called, among other things, "a fraud." This seems to be the usual attitude with the medical profession toward anything new. Which does not mean that I advocate untested dieting. Never. It simply means that any diet that has been keeping people healthy as long as this one can scarcely be called "untested." Linda Clark goes on to quote Mr. Stefansson as showing that the Eskimos who die young today are mixed-diet-eaters. When they were predominantly meat-eaters, 80 percent of their calories came from fat and that fact, according to Stefansson, made them not high-protein eaters, but high consumers of *fat* . . . the very thing that seems to have the A.M.A. so worried. You know, the cholesterol bogeyman strikes again.

I, personally, have very little faith in the cholesterol-as-prime-cause-of-heart-attacks theory, probably because I have learned, via my own internist, that doctors are beginning to question whether its importance has not been blown up beyond the validity point. Dr. Ernst Reinsh, who is a "weight-reduction specialist" in Southfield, Michigan, a Detroit suburb, comes right out and says it in his book, *Eat, Drink, and Get Thin* (Hart Publishing, 1969): "Americans consume starchy food in excessive quantity. And they mistakenly assume that, bad as starch is for them, fats would be even worse. The cholesterol scare is doubtless responsible for much of this misconception—a scare which has arisen out of fallacious theories. Those of us who minister to fat people know how wrong the 'cholesterol people' have been in their conclusions. We prove their error every day." That's a pretty strong statement, so Dr.

Reinsh obviously is not frightened by fat. As long as it isn't taken with carbohydrates.

Let me just repeat that this kind of eating has been around for a very long time—whether used by men of medical training as an obesity cure, or whether as a natural diet by natives who could obtain no other kind. It's been called the Calories Don't Count diet by Herman Taller, the Drinking Man's Diet, the Canadian Air Force Diet. Even our Navy's nutritionists have done enormous research into this way of dieting. And they proved that eating fat makes you burn fat. And getting rid of carbohydrates is often the answer to a water retention problem. Dr. Carlton Fredericks, in his book, *Eating Right for You*, says that, in his studies of the Navy research, he gradually realized that calories really *don't* count. Not if they come from protein and fat. He goes on to say that this kind of eating, providing you're heavy on unsaturated, as opposed to saturated fat, makes for an unexpected dividend: better regulation of blood cholesterol!

So protein plus fat equals weight-loss—that is the point of the low-carbohydrate shape-making routine. Heaven help you (and that will be all that can) if you mix the high-protein–low-carbohydrate diet with, say, a few candy bars; the fat will go on so fast it will make you reel. It will probably go on with a few pounds (or inches) thrown in for good measure. What is more, it will be twice as hard to get rid of, next time you decide to stick with your diet. And here we are again, hammering home the point. Think fat still, and never for one moment assume you have become permanently thin. As one writer friend of mine wittily put it, "Inside every thin man, there's a fat one fighting to get out!" And how!

Nutritionists, in fact, encourage people to eat fats. And we are going to give you a lot more facts about how fats are an absolute necessity to beauty. But right now you're concerned about the safety of a diet which permits so much animal fat. Remember the Eskimo.

Diet the Low-Carbohydrate Way

My own introduction to the low-carbohydrate weight-loss regimen came about before my weight-loss education. In fact, you might say it *was* my weight-loss education. I was still hanging in there at a firm—well, firmly settled on me, in any case—twenty pounds overweight, seemingly unable to lose so much as an ounce . . . cottage cheese lunches at the desk, or not.

You've seen how I tormented my own doctor, and how I tried, and failed, with the medication method—a method, I hasten to add, that I've always feared. So you can imagine how desperate I must have felt.

Now perhaps twenty pounds may not sound like much to you, but on a small dame like myself it can make all the difference between good looks and dumpy. What is worse, it made me feel ugly. And sluggish. I have already said it, but I'll say it again. It's how *you* feel that counts, as long as you're pronounced all-round healthy by your diet doctor and your very own general physician.

And then, right in the course of my workaday routine, there appeared an answer. It landed me right on the road to the low-carb weight loss. And I lost. At last. It all began—yes, like a fairy tale. Once upon a time I had my usual appointments with public relations people whose job it is to show me the wares of their customers. The particular girl I was to meet that morning was fat, fat, fat. I don't mean plump. I mean obese. So, naturally, I arrived and looked for a fat girl. And, instead, I found a svelte 110-pound beauty, who actually had to reintroduce herself to me. That's how dramatic the change was.

Knowing a good story when it reintroduces itself, I quickly got to the diet point. How on earth had she done it? That was my introduction to the wonder-working ways of Dr. Robert C. Atkins and his low-carbohydrate weight-loss way of life. With Dr. Atkins, it *is* a way of life. For him, it's forever.

This now beautiful young lady sitting before a still-stupefied me told me that Dr. Atkins and his diet (which not only took seventy-five pounds off her body, but twenty years off her looks as well) had literally saved her life. She proceeded to spin out a heartbreaking saga of how, after the stillbirth of her first child, she had, quite inexplicably, begun to gain weight until she had blown up into the unattractive balloon body I had known. And, according to her, she'd tried everything. No food, therefore, no calories (and no health, I might add); amphetamine diet pills; thyroid medication; doctors and more doctors and diets and more diets. And all to no avail. At that point she was, she avows, suicidal. Her marriage was suffering from her miserable self-image and, in point of fact, she simply couldn't find much to live for. Luckily, just at that low-tide moment, her own mother turned up with an answer. Well, at least another alternative—one more kind of diet to try. And this one, it was rumored, was always successful. And so this young woman became a Dr. Atkins patient. And within a few months she was, for the first time in years, back down to size 8.

Best of all, it had all been done without drugs of any sorts. And this was the clincher for me. I fear diet medication, even at the hands of my trusted doctor. But from a stranger? Never. There are a lot of scary types calling themselves doctors, with hypodermic needles filled and ready to shoot you with such things as placenta, urine from pregnant women, and, yes, even "speed"—none of which I'd want shot into me. (Most of these doctors, upon questioning, will admit that dieting works just as well without their "miraculous" injections.) If Dr. Atkins could help me without drugs of any sort, then he was most certainly the man for me.

On the other hand, I learned that his was a form of the high-protein–low-carbohydrate diet. Now I'd had friends who lost enormous amounts of weight on this regimen and who swore by its easy-going weight-loss benefits. But I'd always been afraid to try it. You see, it involves foregoing sugar. And in my pre-Atkins, misinformed, and uneducated dieting days, I didn't see how I could possibly do that. Because I am a hypoglycemic. And just what is that? It's a person whose blood sugar performs peculiar tricks on him. Only recently has hypoglycemia really been studied and isolated as the cause of many ills previously diagnosed as everything from schizophrenia to brain tumor. Hypoglycemia is low blood sugar. And it can make you feel like hell. Sudden attacks of the shakes, even though you may have just eaten an enormous meal. Headaches, dizziness, anxiety, fainting spells, cold sweats, indigestion, allergies. All vague enough to lead most doctors to discount them as "unimportant" or "just nerves." It has only been recently that hypoglycemia has been studied carefully. And found to be the cause of so many patients' "imagined" ills.

It's been studied so carefully, in fact, that it seems to be this year's chic disease. Just like gout was a few years back. Well, that's O.K. with me. Because it means that more and more doctors are going to be learning more and more about hypoglycemia and how to help hypoglycemics. For starters, they've already learned that hypoglycemia is *not* the opposite of diabetes, which involves high blood sugar. On the contrary, it is often simply a prelude to diabetes and, if not properly treated, can lead to that disease.

Hypoglycemia itself can be extremely serious. I know a model who came very close to losing her life from it. And, unfortunately for her, her bout came at a time when very little was known about it. According to Dr. Carlton Fredericks, who has written what is probably the definitive study on hypoglycemia in his book *Low Blood Sugar and You* (and if you have any of the vague, undiagnosed symptoms mentioned, I strongly urge that you get this book and study it carefully) states that, "For one person in every ten, sugar is a deadly food." And we've already shown you that not one in ten, but all Americans—on the average, of course—consume 175 pounds of that deadly substance per person per year.

What happens in hypoglycemia can be blamed on the pancreas—a gland that no one gives much thought to unless he or she happens to be diabetic. (I learned a lot more about my pancreas from what turned out to be an informative, albeit painful, illness. I will tell you all about that in a later chapter.)

The pancreas is the gland that produces insulin. Diabetes is the disease that comes from an underproduction of insulin by that gland, but in hypoglycemia the pancreas overreacts and produces too much insulin. This is called hyperinsulinism. I quote Dr. Fredericks:

A piece of candy or a glass of orange juice (13 percent sugar) will rescue the diabetic from insulin shock. Will it help the person with an overactive pancreas? No—for a very simple reason. The pancreas works *because sugar has been eaten.* (If it didn't, you would be diabetic.) If the pancreas is overactive, sugar isn't going to quiet it down, it will stimulate the gland still more. So it is that the person with low blood sugar makes *himself worse by eating sugar,* and the ironic feature of the disorder is the craving of sweets that accompanies it.

And, I might add, never once in my life's history of low blood sugar did any physician suggest I take a glucose tolerance test. An unpleasant experience, but, then, aren't all diagnostic tests? And the glucose tolerance test is simple. Simple for the doctor. For the hypoglycemic patient, it can produce some terrible headaches and lots of shakes, thanks to the dropping blood sugar. But it also produces answers.

So you can understand, then, my reluctance ever to have tried any diet which excluded sugar. Not under my own care, in any case. Which was lucky.

I'd been suffering from shaky spells all my life—sudden dizzying drops where I felt faint and weak and never could understand why. I *could* understand, though, that tea with cream and sugar could stop the shakes, though I didn't have any idea what the real problem was. Once, when an attack struck while I was at my doctor's, I was finally told, "That's a drop in blood sugar; here, have a honey drop." Knowing what I now know, the thought makes me reel. Repeat: the worst thing one can do for low blood sugar is to eat sugar! Sure, it ups that sugar and stops those shakes all right, but two minutes later, your blood sugar has dropped even lower and you're shakier than ever.

At any rate, I'd gone through a lifetime believing that, with low blood sugar, I couldn't possibly go on any diet that eliminates sugar entirely. And that is exactly what the low-carbohydrate diet does. (Dr. Atkins prefers to call his diet "low carbohydrate" rather than "high protein"—face it, high protein is advisable on virtually any kind of diet!)

However, I decided that Dr. Atkins must know his stuff on the blood sugar level and so I set off on the first of what was to be many, many appointments with Dr. Atkins, the fat doctor.

I was told to arrive without breakfast (and no breakfast is a shaky experience for a hypoglycemic) and to prepare to spend my morning with them, for I was to have, for the first time in my life, that glucose tolerance test. This is routine testing for all Atkins patients. The doctor believes in being careful, which is why I have faith in him.

Now, don't think for a moment that I didn't take full

advantage of the knowledge that very soon I was going to have someone to "watch over me"—or my figure. As it happened, my appointment was for the Monday after Thanksgiving.

You can bet I gorged. I ate everything in sight— Thanksgiving turkey-and-dressing right on through to the pumpkin pie. I was like a condemned woman on her way to who knows where. For, with a lifetime of dieting facing me, why not get as fat as possible? Just to give the doctor something to go on. I am not a big eater, but that weekend I ate for all the rest of my life.

The morning of the appointment with Dr. Atkins arrived. First of all, without breakfast I had, of course, the predictable case of the shakes. And the equally predictable headache that usually came with them. However, I managed to hold body and shakes together until I got into Atkins' office. I was faced with a waiting room full of really fat people—making me feel a bit foolish, but no less determined—and a crew of very nice nurses who ushered me off to an examination room where I was weighed, my urine sampled, and then I was off to the blood tests.

One blood test per hour was the schedule, for five hours running. It seems that the glucose tolerance test is simply not conclusive in less than that amount of time. Fortunately, I am not a person who objects to having my blood taken. And it is lucky, for there was a lot of it spilled, so to speak, on that first visit. There was the first drawing of a blood sample, this one called a "fasting sample," to find out just what the shape of your blood is in after, say, twelve hours of no food. Then comes the surprise.

You are required to down a bottle of what I consider to be the most revolting substance yet dreamed up by medicine. It's really nothing more than glucose, but it's been doctored with cola and given the unlikely name of "Glucola." Even comes in a Coke-shaped bottle—obviously some medical-supply man's idea of wit. At least the Atkins nurses were kind enough to tell you to take your time getting it down. Obviously, they were afraid it might come up.

One-half hour later, another blood test, to see what the effects of the Glucola were, followed by four more blood tests—one per hour.

Now, I wondered why the nurses kept popping into my

examination room to ask how I felt and to know if I felt faint. Sure, I did. I always did if I skipped breakfast. Perhaps that's one fortunate side effect of low blood sugar. It makes breakfast a necessity, and as any nutritionist will quickly tell you, breakfast is the most important meal of any day. "Break fast." Your tummy hasn't had a treat for at least twelve hours. *Think how you'd feel!*

After five hours of blood testing, I faced the doctor, quaking a bit and wondering what it would all be like. I must say, Dr. Atkins did not seem sympathetic to my cause. I'll grant you that his waiting room was full of 300-pounders, or so it seemed to me, so that my 124 pounds of avoirdupois seemed to make him more impatient than worried about my weight problems. His first impression seemed to be that I was intent on becoming a rail-thin jet-setter type. It took a while to convince the doctor that I was serious and that, on my 5′4″ frame, those 124 pounds were too heavy to carry with comfort.

I was given a list of foods that were allowed and asked to read it carefully. O.K., so far, so easy. Then I was asked whether I understood. Thinking, "I'm not a nincompoop, after all," I haughtily replied, "But, of course." Only to find that on being asked to repeat the instructions, I hadn't gotten it quite down pat—yet! Later, it was to become such a way-of-life, way-of-eating, to me that it would take some time before I could change my habits back to the low-calorie life.

This is the way the Atkins low-carbohydrate–high-protein diet works. You are given a small folder that is, in essence, a glucose tolerance test, and this routine is to be used for *one week only*. It is a *no*-carbohydrate list, and any swerving from it can completely wreck your diet. For, you see, in one week you will be tested to see just how your body is reacting to such a regimen.

It involves a complete about-face of all your preconceived notions as to what a diet must be. First, there are absolutely *no* limitations on the amount of food intake, as long as that food intake comes from the list of foods allowed, and those are, of course, the foods that are low in carbohydrates.

Now let me point out that, while fats are among the foods allowed—fats like eggs and butter and mayonnaise—the Atkins instructions state quite clearly and concisely that these may be eaten in *judicious* quantities. Those critics of the Atkins method may consider "judicious" to be synonymous with "enormous." I do not, nor does Webster. So let the critics look to their dictionaries before they condemn.

I do not believe those who claim this is dangerous. I suffered no ill effects other than from that pesky blood sugar, which is *my* body's snafu, not Atkins'!

However, if you believe that you suffer from low blood sugar, *check with your doctor* before you embark on any program that involves omitting sweets.

In the beginning, if you're hypoglycemic, it's going to be rough—there are some sort of withdrawal symptoms, and you'll need expert advice in seeing you through them.

Good will win, however, for the low-carbohydrate diet just happens to be the one that's used in the treatment of hypoglycemia.

At any rate, I was given clear, concise instructions as to what I could eat and what I could not eat. What I could not eat came as a real surprise to me, a lifelong dieter. Organ meats, for one. When you think about it, it's pretty obvious, for things like the liver are the organs that hold the sugar in the body, and sugar is what you must avoid like the plague. Shellfish, of all things—again, high carbohydrates. Tomatoes, onions. It had simply never occurred to me that these two placid little vegetables are loaded with sugar, as are carrots. And alcohol. For the first week, I would have to forego it completely. That hurt. But I reluctantly gave up the alcohol.

I was warned that there were hidden carbohydrates in seemingly innocent products that could completely throw off the accurate results of the test. And this is exactly what the first week's dieting is. A *test*, not a way of life. Nobody, least of all Dr. Atkins, expects you to live on no carbohydrates at all. I doubt that you could—for very long.

Some of the hidden carbohydrates to watch for were chewing gum, tomato products like catsup (one more surprise), diet soft drinks which, it appears, often contain a small amount of sugar—and that small amount of sugar is quite enough to make the test results go haywire. (I might add, it was enough to make me give up diet soft drinks forever, knowing what I now know about sugar.)

I was told to watch out for meats, such as hot dogs, that

might contain starchy fillers (check the labels). In other words, any meat had to be 100 percent *pure meat*.

No fruit or fruit juice, which happened to be no problem for me, as I've never been an orange juice addict. In case it should be an impossibility for you, there is a perfectly terrible substitute on the market . . . terrible to me, but then I don't even like the real stuff. It's called Tropi-Cal Lo and it's simply orange juice that's had all its real sugar removed and fake sweetener substituted. If juice you must, you might be willing to have a go at it. But you would have to be juice-desperate.

I could no longer drink milk. Most especially, I could no longer drink skimmed milk. For it seems that skimmed milk is much higher in carbohydrates than even heavy cream (which was also a first-week no-no). Odd fact, but true, and the world is full of odd nutritional facts, you may find. Fake creamers were most definitely forbidden, as was yogurt and, for the first week, vegetables. None at all. And that was tough. But, then, so is losing weight.

With the Atkins "allowed list" before me, it was not necessary for me to get my hands on a carbohydrate counter. The list was there and I could eat as much of anything on it as my stomach desired. When my stomach didn't desire it, the instructions told me to stop. Stop eating when I wasn't hungry. I was cautioned again, in print, about all the things I could *not* have that first week. And I was warned about such things as sweetened liquid medications, or cough drops—none of which would have ever occurred to me as throwing a wrench into the test, so good thing I was clearly and concisely warned against them.

And then there was a prophetic—it proved—warning, right there at the bottom of those instructions. It said: "We expect you to feel physically improved on this diet. If in some way you do not, please call this office AT THAT TIME rather than waiting until your next visit." Good thing they told me, because I was going to need help.

Right on! I was on my way to becoming a beautiful person. I staggered (literally, from weakness) into the street to begin my new low-carb life-style.

Happily, I had a lunch date waiting with physical and moral support. I needed both. But the problems of that no-carb week were yet to come. Have you ever tried getting a green salad without tomato? Or onion? How to proceed without bread? No organ meats. No sugar.

Somehow I made it through the remainder of that day, but the next was yet to come.

My morning tea, not only without sugar, but no cream! (Remember, as Dr. Atkins strongly states on that little folder, "This is not to be your way of life!") Oh, well, they said all the eggs and bacon and butter, so I absolutely reveled in a gluttonous breakfast of six strips of bacon, three eggs, and used the butter instead of bread. Sounds revolting, doesn't it, but since breakfast is my favorite meal I was happy as a pig in a poke. And behaving like one.

By lunch, I felt a bit shaky. Imagination, I figured. So, for lunch I had an enormous steak and fought with the waiter about no tomatoes or onions and only oil and vinegar and no hard liquor or wine. But I made it. And when I returned to my office, I felt more faint than ever. I felt foolish, but I called Dr. A.—and was put right through to the busy man. I was sure he would tick me off in no uncertain terms about not really wanting to stick—the usual M.D. routine chastisement. Instead, he took a look at my chart once more and came up with the good old hypoglycemia. Seems that my blood sugar, once that bottle of Glucola was administered, *dropped* forty points. Not exactly what you'd expect when you've just drunk a bottle of glucose. Luckily this doctor had the right prescription. I was to take one tablespoon of—get this—*cottage cheese* every two hours.

Picture a desk at *The New York Times* holding one container of cottage cheese and one tablespoon with a maniacal reporter downing her dose every two hours. And just like magic, or just like a shot of insulin (which is, in fact, just what insulin does for the diabetic), that spoonful of cottage cheese stopped the shakes within a matter of minutes.

It was a miracle. I had overcome the power of hypoglycemia to stop me from losing weight. For that *is* one of the problems that keeps you fat. Hypoglycemia causes water retention and, consequently, prevents weight loss. And my doctor knew just the proper dosage to keep my blood sugar at operative level while not disturbing the no-carb message of that first week's diet trial.

I am telling you all this because I am so convinced that

you should not try a low-carbohydrate diet without a glucose tolerance test. There are more hypoglycemics in this country than know it themselves. Thanks to that 175 pounds of sugar we Americans eat per year, our metabolisms are usually pretty wacky. There have been books and books and books written on this problem alone. It's just that either you have your low-carb diet supervised by a physician who specializes in such things (if he tells you to eat candy or pop a honey drop, just run!), or if you don't have such a doctor, and you feel those shakes coming on, then run for that spoonful of cottage cheese. Or a handful (*only* a handful) of nuts—any kind except peanuts—which will do the job and those hypoglycemic shakes will stop. All I know is that for the first week of my reshaping, I headed for the cottage cheese before I put on the morning coffee. That's pretty desperate, if you ask me.

The next week's visit was a decided improvement in my life. We could add some carbohydrates. Meaning I could now have the cream in my coffee and eliminate the cottage cheese (never *did* get to like coffee and cottage cheese!). And I didn't have to wrangle about tomatoes or onions with hostile waiters who thought I was some sort of nut. And I could have some alcohol. Three glasses of wine per week, which seemed like heaven to me. I saved them for truly important dates! And I could eat! All the good things I loved in any—yes, absolutely *any* amount. There were only two forbidden fruits—sugars (I've never had a sweet tooth, except for sugared tea or coffee, so this was not hard) and starches. That part was worse, but not terrible. And think of the rewards.

All the while, at each and every visit, a urine specimen determined whether or not I cheated. For this is how the low-carbohydrate–high-protein diet functions: Once those fat-and-ugly-making carbohydrates are removed from your diet, your body begins to manufacture its own. From the fat you don't want, anyway. And that's the beauty part. *It's the fat you don't want anyway that goes.* Not the fat from your face or the fat from your neck, but the fat from your hips or your thighs or your stomach or wherever it has landed that is where you *don't* want it to be. So that you end up (well, you never end *this* diet really—you go on a maintenance routine) reshaped in your own idealized image.

And remember that I have said that fat is essential on any diet. It is essential to your well-being. It is especially essential to your beauty. But also remember that Atkins said "judicious quantities." As far as I can see, it makes little difference. The Eskimos don't seem to put a limit on their intake of animal fat; and no one has yet proved that such a diet has harmed them. To the contrary—if we Americans were as healthy as the Eskimos before the American diet and civilization's diseases got to them we wouldn't be writing books on obesity. For, apparently, those calories don't count as long as there are very few carbohydrates involved.

. The way I see it, from a reporter's vantage point, is that the fat causes the protein (or fuel) to burn. Then, when there is no more fuel to burn, the body turns to its own available fuel, which is your own body fat. And, of course, it goes first to the spot where the fat exists in over-abundance—namely, those blobs of unattractive fat that are sitting where you don't want them. *That*, as far as I am concerned, is the beauty of this sort of dieting. For I, among many, want to lose weight where I want to lose it. I don't want to end up with a haggard face and stringy neck and sunken bosom. According to one of our other low-carbohydrate diet-espousers, Dr. Ernst Reinsh, "the process induced by the ingestion of fats proceeds at a measured rate which permits the skin to shrink and fit the smaller, firmer body. The patient is not left with the appearance of having recently recovered from some debilitating illness."

It proceeds at a measured rate, all right. So measured, in fact, that by the time I was through—and yes, I finally made my desired weight—I had driven Dr. Atkins half mad with screams of "Why doesn't it work faster?" It doesn't, and that's probably the reason for its beauty-making success in reshape.

Reshape it does. My own shape changed radically. I wasn't once called "Cello-Shape" for nothing. Fate gave me tiny shoulders and rib cage, and hips that get all the fat there is to have. Body fat, I mean. Soon, dramatically, all that changed. I still had my bosom, and my neck wasn't stringy, and my face wasn't drawn, but my too-large hips had disappeared, and so had the fat on my thighs. And that, my friends, is one large accomplishment.

Now I was asked, often, whether I wasn't afraid I was building up to a cholesterol-induced heart attack. I wasn't afraid. I am simply a disbeliever in the whole cholesterol scare. But, and please get this point clearly, *that is just my personal belief*. There are plenty of things I am not afraid of. Such as cranberries during the cranberry scare. And cyclamates. Lots of things that perhaps I ought to fear, but don't. When you live in New York City, you tend to be much more fearful of the tangible threats—like mugging or big-city traffic. So, if you wish, just chalk up that non-fear to a personal quirk of mine. And, if you go on this diet, have your own doctor check your cholesterol level.

Finally, being driven to it by the constant warnings of my friends, I had my internist do a cholesterol check on me. Before he did it, wise man that he is, he told me that, in his experience (and believe me, his experience is vast), a high-protein–low-carbohydrate diet induced lowered cholesterol levels in the blood.

We checked. And, of course, my cholesterol level came up inordinately low. Lower than average, in fact.

What Fat?

There's been so much controversy about fats that I think we should expand on it a bit. I have found *no nutritionist, no doctor* who ever recommended that *anyone* omit fats from his diet. Fats are absolutely essential to health. "Cells," says Dr. Carlton Fredericks, "are built from protein and fats." And he adds that about seventeen percent of those fats are unsaturated.

Now you've no doubt heard, and read, much about saturated as opposed to unsaturated, or polyunsaturated, fats. Unsaturated fats are generally those fats that remain liquid at room temperature, and these include most vegetable oils with the single exception of coconut oil, which a recent *New York Times* article cited as one of the most saturated fats extant.

Saturated fats include the animal fats—lard, fat in meat, milk, eggs, and butter. These are the ones that frighten most people. For they are the fats that have been accused of raising the cholesterol level in the blood and thus, purportedly, setting up their victims for a heart attack via arteriosclerosis.

According to Linda Clark, so many warnings have been issued against the eating of fat that many people have panicked, and are literally afraid to eat so much as an egg. (And you will see, in our chapter on hair, how important those eggs are to that part of you.) Says Mrs. Clark, "Many people are unaware that the body manufactures cholesterol whether you eat it or not. Cholesterol is needed to help your glands." She states flatly that "a fat-free diet is not only out of date, it is actually dangerous." Adelle Davis maintains that cholesterol is concentrated in such vital tissues as the brain and nerves, indicating that it serves valuable unknown functions in maintaining health.

If cholesterol worries you, however, you may bear in mind studies that have been made as to the effect of poly-unsaturated fats on the cholesterol in the blood. An article in the September 17, 1966, issue of *Lancet*, a British medical journal, states quite clearly that "The ability of diets high in polyunsaturated fats to produce sustained reduction of plasma-total-cholesterol in man has been amply confirmed."

So there you have it. Not only are fats essential to your health, certainly to your beauty—without them, you're going to have dried-up everything from skin to hair, and may even go so far as to develop skin diseases such as un-lovely eczema—they are, in the polyunsaturated versions, going to act as cholesterol lowerers, even when the diet remains high in animal-fat intake. So say the medical researchers and we are trusting their work.

Some doctors suggest that the unsaturated fats in your diet represent at least 30 percent of your fat intake. I suggest that you remember that the unsaturated fats are the ones that are liquid at room temperature. It shouldn't be difficult to guess that they'd be the ones least likely to clog up your arteries.

And starting in Australia, and working their way to this country, experiments are going on to lower the saturated fat in meats by feeding the animals a diet high in polyun-saturates. Who knows? Perhaps soon beef can come off of my Bad B list. For, as you will see, the two Bad B's are beef and booze. And booze stays.

The Physiology of It All

There are many other versions of the high-protein–low-carbohydrate diet in use right now. And most of their advocates have written books about them, making it very simple for you to study their individual variations.

I report on the Atkins method because I had personal experience with it. And therefore I am able to give my own accurate version of just how it worked *for me*. How it might work for you, I don't know. The way to find out is to try. And the way to learn more about the Atkins theories is to read his own scientific explanation of its physiology in *Dr. Atkins' Diet Revolution*.

Dr. Maxwell Stillman came up with *The Doctor's Quick Weight Loss Diet* and made quite a splash in dieting circles. He leans more toward the high protein, less toward the low carbohydrate in a diet that is often diametrically opposed to the Atkins one. (For instance, he permits such things as skimmed milk.) And he does not permit fats. Being in the beauty-search business, I don't believe in *that*. I think they're important and have said so. But if you're really in a terrible hurry to lose some poundage, here's what Stillman prescribes:

1. Lean meat with *all* of the fat removed and cooked in *no* fats of any kind. Only broiled, baked, or smoked.
2. Chicken and turkey with all the skin removed (the skin holds the fat here). Again, no cooking with grease!
3. All lean fish and seafood, again broiled, baked, or boiled (or, I assume, smoked) and again without fats. But with Dr. Stillman, you're allowed cocktail sauce or catsup in moderation. And this is where the Stillman and Atkins regimens go in different directions.
4. Eggs, preferably hard boiled. But again cooked with no fat.
5. Cottage cheese, farmer's cheese, or pot cheese or any other cheese made with skim milk and *no whole milk*.
6. Eight glasses of water daily *minimum*.

According to Dr. Stillman, the eight water glasses are an integral part of his regimen in that they wash out any wastes of burnt-up fat. Making them burnt out as well as up.

I have known people who have lost pounds in a hurry. (Just as he claims, it is quick.) I haven't tried it and won't be trying it, for Dr. Stillman insists upon such follies as skinned chicken. And, frankly, I am a career woman and can't be bothered with such time-consuming nonsense if there's any other effective way to weigh less.

Dr. Stillman recommends eight glasses of water a day, which seems to be some sort of startling advice for some people. Don't we all drink eight glasses of water per day? If not, you should. Water is essential to well-being, as it helps wash impurities out of the system. Just remember that the Dr. Stillman method didn't say drink all eight at once.

Dr. Carlton Fredericks, whom I continue to quote, since I believe him to be one of the most solid nutritionists about, as well as one whose books are entertaining (and in the world of nutrition, that's rare), goes into quite a long dissertation about the weird workings of the low-carbohydrate diet in his book, *Eating Right for You*. I strongly recommend that you get a copy and read it all—not just the part on dieting. Every word in it makes good nutritional sense to me. Great food for the mind.

Dr. Ernst Reinsh, whom we've mentioned before, has a book, *Eat, Drink and Get Thin*, that is very different from the Atkins one, but is again based on the same principles of dieting.

When it comes to each of these gentleman's ideas about what works best, I can only suggest that you read them for yourselves. I don't like to be positive about something I haven't tried. That's the point of this book, after all. To try it for you.

Side Effects

Did I get anything on the side? Any unexpected, possibly unpleasant effects from this unorthodox method of weight loss? I did. And I think you ought to know what to expect, although there is nothing in medical knowledge that assures that what happened to me will happen to you.

Remember what I said about individualistic? Whenever you play with your blood chemistry—which is one of the things this sort of unnatural eating does—you are playing with something nobody knows much about. Yes, they are making inroads. Yes, they are coming close. But I don't believe that any doctor can claim to have the definitive answer to individual blood chemistry.

My side effects were minor. They had to be, or I can assure you I wouldn't have remained an Atkins patient for three years. In fact, eating the Atkins way became such second nature to me that, when the time came to graduate, I found I'd so brainwashed myself that I got a good case of the guilts whenever I downed a carbohydrate. But I've told you I'm that sort of person. Once committed to something, I rarely stray. And once committed to this diet, you'd better not stray.

I will never forget the embarrassing evening when I attended a dinner party at which the menu went like this:

Roast pork
Winter squash
Corn on the Cob
Potatoes

Even for a non-dietitian (but, I might add, an occasional hostess) it looked like pretty poor menu-planning to me. I was really stuck. For this was early in my non-carbohydrate training, and I hadn't yet gotten my memory down pat on just what was what when it came to carbohydrates. And, let me add, there wasn't even a salad served, so something had to be chosen from that unbalanced-by-any-diet-standards meal. I knew roast pork was fine. But I opted for the corn. What a mistake I made!

By morning I couldn't zip my skirt, and when I stepped on the scale, I had gained five pounds. Hysterically, I ran screaming to Dr. A., who assured me that I had made the worst possible choice in eating corn, which is super-high in carbohydrates. He patiently explained that, when the body has been cut off from carbohydrates for some time, and then is suddenly hit with some, water retention occurs. He also assured me that, within forty-eight hours, it would be gone. It was, I am relieved to say, but it was experience enough for me to make sure I never cheated, even inadvertently, again. Water retention became my bugaboo, but then water retention had always been my bugaboo. Here again, doctors are still working on the whys and wherefores. Is it the enzymes, the hormones, the glands? As yet, they don't seem to be sure. Or if they're sure, they surely never let me in on the secret.

In the first months of my diet, I suffered from excruciating headaches. That's nothing new. I've had them all my life. And they've usually been premenstrual, at the period when water retention tends to be the highest. This time they came right at the end of my menstrual period. I waited three months to be sure. And each time, they happened. So I rushed to my internist to check on the facts.

They are this: The high-protein–low-carbohydrate diet, just by its being, can affect the growth hormone. And the growth hormone is a nebulous hormone (at least, nebulous to me—I'd never heard of it) that controls water retention. According to Dr. Neil Solomon, it may also hold the key to obesity. Researchers are working on it. However, studies have been made as to the effect of such a diet on the growth hormone. And, it seems that, on a normal breakfast (to take the study example of coffee, toast, orange juice, and cereal), the blood sugar level went up—temporarily— and the growth hormone level remained consistent; whereas on the high-protein–low-carbohydrate diet, if the very same individual had a breakfast of black coffee, eggs, and bacon—all protein, no carbohydrates—the growth hormone went up while the blood sugar level remained steady. Perhaps this is the answer to the machinations of this diet.

Let me say that my headaches ceased when more and more carbohydrate was added to my diet. Ceased as suddenly as they had begun. Except for normal, workaday headaches, and, in my profession, some workaday headaches are pretty big ones. I'll blame those on my profession and not my diet.

I will say that I never felt better in my life. I was bursting with energy and looked it. Never once did I feel faint, nauseous, distracted, or have any of the other side effects the American Medical Association has attributed to the Atkins version of the high-protein–low-carbohydrate diet. And this is the only version, of course, that I can speak about with it-happened-to-me authority. After all, there is only one of me and I have only so much weight to give to research.

I had one side effect that seemed nothing short of a

miracle. My blood sugar seemed to stabilize itself. I no longer had the shakes—ever. This was something new for a lifetime victim of that hypoglycemia. Once I had been on the diet long enough to get my body into the low-carbohydrate groove, I no longer had to rush for the cottage cheese carton. Just as the doctor had predicted, my blood sugar level evened out to a normal condition it had never before known. I call that a positive side effect and one that makes this sort of eating worthwhile, even if you don't need to lose weight.

For there are, of course, modified versions of the diet for people who wish to stabilize their weight. In fact, the moment you reach the weight you've been waiting for, Dr. Atkins puts you on what he terms a "maintenance diet"—a diet which is *still* a low-carbohydrate diet, but not low carbohydrate enough to take off any more weight. It is meant to do just what its name implies. Stabilize your weight at the point where you want it.

Friends who have tried this diet on their own have reported such things as menstrual abnormalities. When they questioned me, I advised them to see their doctors at once and to tell that doctor that they were on the diet. For hormonal changes are not to be taken lightly and, if one is on the birth control pill (as one of these young ladies was) it makes the going doubly difficult. It's up to a physician to decide the course to take there. But there's little doubt in my mind that a diet that is, by Dr. Atkins' description, "deliberately unnatural" can do some pretty unnatural tricks. What you and your doctor must decide is whether the benefits (and there are many) outweigh the oddities. And proceed, always medically supervised, from that point.

Can It Be Dangerous?

Can it be dangerous—the high-protein–low-carbohydrate diet? After all you've doubtless heard of late, you'd be abnormal not to wonder.

I was never afraid for a moment, as I have told you. For this was the very first diet in my life that I'd been able to live with for over a period of three years without a single illness as a result. I've shown you what starvation diets did to my health. They left it wide open for colds, streptococci infections (boils, to us), and anything else germy that happened my way. Whenever I decided to go the starvation road to thin, I steeled myself for the inevitable ill health that was sure to follow.

On the low-carbohydrate diet, as I have told you, I simply never felt better, both in body and in spirit. I was thrilled with my new shape, better than any I'd ever had before; thrilled with the non-haggard-making effects of the diet. I felt peppy and cheerful, and a troublesome stomach ailment (and I'll tell you all about *that* later) simply, for the moment, ceased to exist—or at least gave me less trouble than it ever had before.

Now, as for danger, let me give you my own opinions on the dangers of any sort of dieting. They exist *because* of dieting. I do not believe that any human being should be expected to stay on any sort of reducing diet forever. I don't even think he or she should stay on the same *kind* of diet forever. Because deprivation of anything is eventually going to cause some odd things to happen.

Balanced eating—wholesome, natural food balanced eating—is always the best answer to health, once you've gotten your weight where you want it. After that, what you have to do is watch. The scales, your waistline, and then the minute anything starts to move on the upward direction, get on one of our two diets immediately and stick there until things are back to your ideal.

There are many different theories about the amounts of carbohydrates needed each day to keep one in perfect health. Even Dr. Atkins maintains that all this varies with the individual. And that's the thing. Individualism again. For me, his guideline was "Never eat anything that's over ten carbohydrate grams." I never counted what that added up to per day, but that basic guideline—10 grams and no more—kept me on a low enough carbohydrate level to keep me in good-looking shape.

But as for dangerous, let me just say practically every doctor I know or know of has been on one version or another of this diet. They know it works, and they obviously don't feel it's dangerous or they wouldn't be doing it. That, at least, has answered the question to my satisfaction.

The Ketosis Question

Ketosis seems to be the fright-word for the American Medical Association where the high-protein–low-carbohydrate diet is concerned.

What is ketosis? It is the state your body is in when it is putting out ketones and *they* are "little carbon fragments that are the by-products of the incomplete burning of fat." According to Dr. Robert Atkins, ketosis is what makes his diet work, for it means that your body is burning its fuel as it should.

When I was under this doctor's care, I simply never questioned *what* was burning. I could see that my own body fat was disappearing, and I knew that my internist had declared me healthy. So that was about all I chose to know, as I have never been much for the more complicated chemistry of such things. My question has always been simple. "Does it work?"

Since there has been such a to-do in the ranks of the medical profession on the subject of ketosis and its possible dangers—both to adults and to the fetuses of yet-unborn children of pregnant mothers on the diet—I did a bit of research of my own. And came up with some interesting data.

According to one medical textbook, ketogenic diets have long been used in the treatment of children with *petit mal* epilepsy who did not respond properly to drug treatment of that disease. These children were hospitalized and carefully controlled during their diet-treatment. It was found that such a diet was successful in controlling attacks of epilepsy and had a favorable effect on the restlessness, hypermobility, and irritability usually found among children with this disease. Not only that, there was no mental depression such as may occur with drugs! In fact, some children, who had previously been considered dull or mentally retarded became alert, bright and sociable. That doesn't sound like the things we've heard leveled at the low-carbohydrate diet of late. These children remained on theirs for one to three years.

But then I came up with yet another, even more fascinating bit of medical research on the ketosis question. This one is again from the medical journal *Lancet* and is a paper by R. H. Johnson and J. S. Walton from the University of Glasgow and H. A. Krebs and D. H. Williamson, Department of Clinical Medicine, Radcliffe Infirmary, Oxford.

The title of their paper is "Post-Exercise Ketosis." And what it proves is that "An abnormal glucose-tolerance curve after strenuous exercise was first observed by Courtice et al. (in 1936). The shape of the curve after exercise is very similar to that after prolonged fasting or in subjects given a low-carbohydrate diet."

In other words, strenuous exercise can put you in ketosis. So does the American Medical Association suggest that we give up strenuous exercise? Does it not recommend jogging, for example, or stair-climbing as beneficial not only to the body but to the heart as well? And are not pregnant mothers often sent off to exercise classes designed especially for mothers-to-be? Are the doctors who recommend such classes then endangering these pregnant women's fetuses? I, for one, would love to know the answer.

Back to the Low-Cal Life

Then one day a funny thing happened on my way to the diet doctor. I got fat, overnight and inexplicably. Without changing one element of my diet. I was more than just horrified, I was frightened. And panicked. And furious.

Stepping on the scales for my daily weight-watching, I had gained seven—yes, *seven*—pounds in my sleep. How could it be possible? I don't have to tell you, I'm sure, that I rushed to Dr. Atkins' office screaming with outraged indignation. And was told it was only water retention, all over again—this time probably caused by an attack of nerves. You can bet I was nervous all right. And I was surprised to learn that nerves *can* be responsible for a certain amount of that water-holding that's every dieter's *bête noire*. I was told to go off to a movie and that it would all be gone in another forty-eight hours. It wasn't. On the contrary. Within forty-eight hours, I had gained five more pounds, putting me almost back to my starting poundage three years previously. Think how discouraging *that* was for me, a super-aware, super-sincere dieter. And those pounds just wouldn't budge—to anywhere.

I shouted, shrieked, and temper-tantrumed while I kept

the hot-lines going between my office and Atkins'. My diet was cut back to the first week no-carbohydrates version. Nothing. No loss of weight, but a lot more loss of temper.

I was given more urine tests, which proved that I was *not* cheating. According to those urine tests, my body was burning what should have been body fat. (Later on, I found out just what it was burning—and what that was was *me*.)

My thyroid was tested once more and found to be at its same old 4.0 level. Low, but still normal. Atkins, however, elected to try the thyroid route one more time. I balked, remembering my pimply face from the last thyroid fool-around. But I tried, and still no weight-off. Just more frazzled nerves and less and less patience with the whole idea.

I was asked to list every single food that went into my mouth for a period of three weeks. And I did. And, try as he would, the doctor couldn't find a single point on which I'd gone awry. Of course I hadn't. I was the one who was furious. I was the one demanding to lose. Why, after all those years of low-carb eating, would I start to cheat on myself?

I remained on this no-carbohydrate routine for close to three months, and now I believe that strenuous dieting like that can be dangerous indeed. For right at that moment my nails began to go. Right to the quick. And, while they have never been particularly long, thanks to my quick-draw-on-the-typewriter kind of job, they'd never in my life been in such condition. They peeled and they became infected and I was miserable.

Then my hair began to break and look lousy—and was lousy. For, just before the Christmas holidays, a time when every woman likes to look her best, I was looking my worst. I thought, in a moment of fashion-consciousness, that I would get my hair permed. And I was told in no uncertain terms by the man in charge of such things that he would do it only if I would sign a release, relieving him of all responsibility in case it all disappeared. You can imagine how that affected a hair-freak like me. And, of course, I remained a straight-hair, a very unhappy one, and set off to enjoy the holidays as best I could under the stringent-dieting circumstances.

Now, in the course of my perm-thinking, I got a clue. I was told my hair hadn't enough protein. And I scoffed at the very suggestion, for, since I was eating nothing else, how could it possibly be? Soon I would know.

I sought help for my nails. I saw skin specialists and insisted that I must have a fungal disease. I was dismissed (summarily, I think, as being nothing more than another neurotic, hysterical woman—standard operating procedure for doctors who don't know the answers) and I was sent away with the suggestion that I drink gelatin. But I *was* told that it was obvious I wasn't getting enough protein. I dismissed that as nonsense. I was probably getting more protein than almost anyone. After all, on the no-carbohydrate diet (which I was still on three months after this horror story began) what else was there? Protein, usually in the form of meat, fish, or eggs, and salad. And that was my life.

As for my health? I'd like to forget that.

And so the Christmas holidays arrived, and I told my diet doctor, "The hell with it. I'm going home and I'm going to eat everything in sight!" Which is precisely what I did.

And, hard as it may be for you to believe it, I lost weight. Let me tell you, it was just as hard for me to believe it, and even harder for the doctor.

But it was a fact. Within one week of doing the biscuit-and-grits diet route, I lost. Furthermore, my nails began to grow. And visibly so. Now I've been told by researchers and specialists in the fingernails field—if, indeed, there really *is* such a field—that this kind of growth is not possible. I can only report, once again, what happened to me. And that is what happened, I'll swear to it.

After a week of luxury eating, it was back to New York and my disciplined way of eating. I returned to the low-carbohydrate dieting—and lost all the fingernails I'd grown, while putting back all the poundage I'd lost. Are you confused? I was, but I was beginning to put things together, and to ask a reporter's kind of questions. And I finally began to get some answers.

What was happening to the protein I was eating? I checked in with my internist, as is my wont when things aren't going quite suitably, and I learned a fascinating fact. My body was actually taking the protein from my nails, from my hair, and from the protein I was eating, and *using it to produce carbohydrates.*

Because, you see, your body is a much smarter machine than you may think. After three years of low-carbohydrate, deliberately-unnatural dieting, my body had figured out just what I had tried to do to it. Just how I'd tried to fool it into burning up itself—its extra self, in any case.

Needing some carbohydrates (and mind you, I'd been on a *no*-carbohydrate routine for three months by now— and this is one place where I'll come right out and say, "Yes, I think no-carbohydrate eating *is* dangerous for longer than a week at a clip") my body had learned to pass the extremely unnatural regime that had been imposed on it. It simply made its own carbohydrates. That is why man has survived for so many centuries, in so many environments, and with so many different variations of natural diet available to him. His body simply adapts to whatever is at hand. And makes the most of it.

In my case, the most it was making was fat.

Now Dr. Atkins tells me that he *has* what he terms a "reversal diet" for just such situations. But the chances of your ever needing such a diet are slim, indeed. I just happened to be the one-in-a-million freak to whom this sort of thing happened. Ah, well, I'm not the norm in anything else, so why expect to be the norm in dieting, either? Once again, unlucky for me, but lucky for you. For you can profit from my un-luck. And should this kind of thing ever happen to you on a low-carbohydrate regimen, you will know how to handle it.

When I asked Dr. Atkins in an interview why he hadn't used the reversal diet on me at once, rather than keep me on such a long and restrictive no-carbohydrate regimen, he replied that he simply hadn't realized that I was that desperate.

The moral here is that even your own diet doctor doesn't take you too seriously if you weigh 112 and you think it ought to be 102.

Should you ever need it—and I hope you never let your dieting come to that—the reversal diet does just what its name implies. And *is* what its name implies. A complete switch-about in your way of eating. A switch to an *all*-carbohydrate diet. The theory is that this is going to throw your smarter-than-diet-doctors body off base once again. It will be confused enough, after a week of this kind of eating, to respond, once again, to the low-carbohydrate routine. And even Dr. Atkins insists that *no one* should consider this kind of diet for more than one week. Ever!

But never mind. By this time, I simply wanted out. I'd had enough of experimentation and deliberately unnatural eating. Though the results, originally, had been ideal, they were—at that moment—far from it. And I was ready to take over my body myself. I was going to hit the low-cal life, just one more time. But not without that omni-present checkup from my internist as a go-ahead. And not without a warning to him that I might, as in the past, get sick. But there were happy diet surprises ahead of me.

Diet Director, Self-Employed

My education as my own diet director was, in fact, my re-education into healthy eating. After all, if I was going to dip into those supposedly deadly carbohydrates (I had been thoroughly brainwashed about carbohydrates, by now, and probably all to the good—good for my health, that is), I had to make sure I was at least getting the sort that would do me some good. The kind like healthful whole grains and fresh vegetables and fruits. The forbidden pleasures I'd foregone for the past three years.

For I was convinced that something in that Alabama homecooking was responsible for the sudden return of my hair and the equally sudden loss of that poundage—whether it was water *or* fat. At least it was, at last, gone. And I intended to see that it stayed that way. Gone.

I decided to cut my caloric intake to 1,000 per day. For a person of my size and bone structure, this allows for three perfectly normal meals a day. A big man would require many more, even for weight loss.

The answer to determining that amount of calories required by *you* is the weigh-in method. And that means that you must weigh each and every day of your life. Without fail. Begin by cutting to 1,500 calories per day, which is usually enough to make weight come off of most metabolically sound people. I am not so metabolically sound, as you have already seen by my hypoglycemia. Better still, ask your doctor—for you will have had a thorough physical by now—what he considers to be the best starting point for you.

And then just go right on weighing in. If the needle goes

down, you're on. If it doesn't, cut more, bit by bit, until it does. And keeps moving in that happy downward direction. Then you'll know what is required to get the poundage moving.

Now I can't possibly stress enough the importance of daily weigh-ins, regardless of the diet route you choose to take.

With Atkins, I was told to weigh, without fail, every day of my life. And that weigh-in should be at the same time of day, and in the same kind of clothes. While I was with Atkins, I had to set my own bathroom scale up four pounds so that it would jibe with his. I mean, why kid myself into thinking I'd lost more, when I'd get to his office and be four pounds heavier? That scale is still set up four pounds. So if it's wrong, then I'm really four pounds lighter, which is fine with me.

The weigh-in at the same time every day is to assure that any water retention you have acquired will probably be consistent. That is why I prefer to weigh in the morning. It seems that the body does acquire a bit of water during the day—from liquid intake, et al.—and I would just as soon not see that on the scale. I don't like being unnecessarily depressed. So keep a beady eye on the needle. If it starts going up, you start cutting down on the calories.

I embarked on my own low-calorie diet—with a lot of help from the nutrition knowledgeables of the world. People like Adelle Davis, Linda Clark, and Carlton Fredericks. And I learned. Plenty. Plenty about all the things I had been doing wrong, plenty about all the things I still hadn't learned to do right.

I learned about health foods—which to go for, which to avoid, for you can be fooled just as easily in health-food shops as you can in any other shop. I had, however, learned one lifetime valuable lesson from low-carb life. I had learned to watch labels carefully. I will hammer this home to you again in a moment, for your health and your shape will depend on this one lesson. I learned that some so-called health foods are pretty meaningless. Take granola, for one, the favorite cereal of the long-hair set. Earthy, they think it is. Recent stories in newspapers across this country brand granola as just one more commercial cereal —no better, no worse for you. Dr. Carlton Fredericks devotes an entire chapter in *Eating Right for You* to shopping in health-food stores. I think it would be wise for you to read it before you head for the commercially healthful life.

As far as I'm concerned, one of the most important beauty lessons you will ever learn is the reading-the-label lesson. It's something that must always be done. And don't think you won't find it confusing. I told you in the beginning I would hammer on this point over and over again, for it is that important. Just for kickers, a friend told me today that he couldn't imagine why he seemed unable to lose weight. And then went on to tell proudly how he'd given up booze, but had spent the previous evening with a friend drinking magnums of diet soft drink, instead. (I *know* this gentleman, and he meant magnums.) Of course, the diet drink in question contains sugar, so that by the time he downed all that, he might as well have gone out for a piece of pie.

So often would-be dieters are well-meaning but simply misinformed or uninformed. I, before my re-education, was most certainly misinformed. The things I thought were low in calories turned out to be among the highest-caloric items on the counter scale. That's the reason, of course, for that super-accurate chart I have compiled. Narcissistic needs—my narcissistic needs that, I hope, will keep you from making all the mistakes I needn't have. If I had only been informed, the way I'm going to inform you. For not only am I giving you a chart that will tell you everything you need to know about the nutrients needed to make you beautiful, I am going to give you a chart that lists both calories and carbohydrates. Just to make things easy for you.

As for those labels: read every single word on them. You're going to find, until that new labeling law gets into action, that most of them are confusing. They will say such mysterious things as "eighty-five percent carbohydrates." What does that mean to you—eighty-five percent of the jar? Of a spoonful? What? I was never able to find out until I set a researcher off to sink her teeth into the mathematical problem and come up with the answers on our chart.

So, on labels, you won't find out much about calories and carbohydrates. Or vitamins. Yet.

But you will be able to spot hidden sugar—anything that

might make it dangerous for your kind of dieting. And you'll most certainly spot all those additives, should you be choosing from cans, or other prepared foods. You may just decide you'd rather not have it after all. Labels are instructive and important, not only to your dieting, but to your health, as well. It won't take long to see the difference between pure-and-natural food and synthetic food.

Bye-Bye Beef—So Long, Booze

It didn't take very long for me to discover that, in my new low-calorie life, there were two foods I simply couldn't do *with*. They were just too calorie costly.

One was alcohol, which came as no surprise to me. After many years of on-and-off low-calorie living, I'd known that alcohol would have to go. And go entirely. Perhaps you may prefer liquid lunches. My blood sugar won't permit it, so alcohol went instead.

But beef? Well, that was part of my diet education, and what a shocker it was! Remember those little steaks I'd thought I was low-cal dieting with, back when I was begging for thyroid pills? Do you think I realized at the time that beef is one of the most fattening foods you will find anywhere? Shocked? I was, too. I think that this sort of misinformation is probably responsible for much of the American obesity problem. As well as the heart attack figures.

If you will look carefully at our chart, you will find that there are approximately 100 calories in every ounce of steak. I say "approximately" here. The chart gives it all to you exactly. And in that chart I've gone one step beyond in trying to give you sizes as well as weights, so that you will be able to determine at a glance (should you be caught at a restaurant without your food scale) just exactly what these weights look like.

But—and prepare yourself here—one ounce of steak (or that 100 calories you read about in most calories counters) equals approximately a forkful! That's correct. Check your weights and you will soon see. Now, I am not a beef lover, especially knowing what I now know about the additives that go into it, so I am not a big beef eater. But even I could never subsist on one forkful of beef per meal. So put it quickly out of your head that steak and salad makes for the ideal diet meal. If you are eating a small shell steak, it could mean your entire day's budget of calories. For me, it meant a day and a half. And, once again, it's tough to get by on one meal every day-and-a-half.

So you can see that the standard businessman's lunch of a steak and a martini is death to your waistline and could be death to your heart. Think about it before you order next time.

Now beef is good protein, all right, and you need plenty of that. The figures on just how much you *do* need seem to be variables with different nutrition-and-medical authorities. Some say a minimum of fifty-six grams per day. Others place the number at eighty.

But there are many other equally good ways to get at protein other than through beef. For starters, even wheat germ contains, gram for gram, more protein than meat.

One ecologically inclined woman, Frances Moore Lappé, who feels that we are rapidly using up our natural protein resources (animal protein, that is), has written a fascinating book called *Diet for a Small Planet*. It is in paperback, and will give the real lowdown on substituting vegetable protein for animal. Not that you will necessarily become a vegetarian, but you should be aware of all the protein facts. And you should never be misled into equating them with beef alone. Fish is excellent protein, and it's hard to get fat on fish. Measure for measure, with few exceptions, it is usually extremely low in calories and has no carbohydrates.

You may as well face the unpleasant facts and learn to re-educate your food thinking. Beef is the fat of the land, any way you slice it. And it could be the fat on you, if you don't watch out.

For even on a low-carbohydrate diet, which supposedly allows all the meat one longs for, beef is the first thing to go—if your diet is supervised by a doctor experienced in such things, the way mine was—should your weight loss stop. That's right, beef. Who's to explain that? But it's a fact of diet life you'll have to learn.

So I cut beef out of my life entirely, once and for always. And now I sit back on my not-so-big-now backsides and laugh while the rest of the world worries about the prices of beef. Well, not really laugh, for the prices are disgraceful. There's an easy answer, though, and a lot of housewives, at this writing, have apparently discovered it. And that is to just forget beef. Without it, you'll probably be healthier and certainly richer. Not a bad combination, is it? You see—sometimes lots of good discoveries come out of dieting.

As for that other great weight-maker, alcohol, I simply cut it out of my life as well. That was a lot harder than beef, because I like it better. The hard-drinking newspaperman (or -woman) isn't just a movie myth. Those deadline pressures can be just as tough whether you're writing about hemlines or politics. And I thought that alcohol took the pressure off. Later, after I'd given it all up, I found out just what bad things it had been doing not only to my looks, but to my well-being.

First of all, alcohol is, plainly and simply, fattening. Here again is something that can manage to fatten you up no matter *which* diet you've opted for. Now, I'll grant you that alcohol is allowed on the low-carbohydrate diet. But, here again, is one thing that will go in a flash, assuming you've an aware diet-doctor watching over you, the minute you stop losing weight. Alcohol, it seems, has an uncanny ability to produce carbohydrates within the body—even though distilled alcohol such as gin, or vodka, or scotch, contains no carbohydrates at all. Never mind. We're concerned about what it does to your weight. And it can make it go up, even when you're watching carbohydrates. So be forewarned.

As for calories, check out the chart and you'll see. If you really want to drink all your meals, you can try it, of course, but I doubt that your health would hold out for long. I'll absolutely promise you one gift from alcohol: it will wreck your looks, and not necessarily just in the long run. It will dry your hair, break your nails, ruin your digestion, eat up your beauty-making vitamins, harm your vital organs, rob you of sleep, slow down your sex life and wreck your shape. Do you still really want it that much? Well, if you do, then for goodness' sake, take nutritionist Linda Clark's beautiful advice and do as she does. Limit yourself to one glass of wine per day. With that, you've had enough.

And, while you're on the low-cal life, don't forget to add it to your calorie list for the day. It's a very big part of your diet.

Just one more not-so-good word about alcohol. It's the all-time water retainer. If you just happen to have low blood sugar, it's even worse. *Both* cause water retention. And water, as you know, shows up just as fat as fat. Just watch out for booze. I personally don't think it's worth it.

After I first launched into my own low-calorie routine, I felt absolutely sinful. For I could eat such hitherto forbidden favorites as *bread*, which just happens to be my weakness. Now I've told you I was, fortunately, trained from childhood to avoid that refined white goo that passes in this country for white bread. Dr. Jean Mayer of Harvard's School of Nutrition calls it "the edible napkin"—just something to put food *on*. (For you world-travelers, Dr. Mayer came up with another shocker. It seems that French bread, the delicious kind that you get in France, may taste better, but is actually less nutritious than our own tasteless kind. *Quel désillusionnement!*) No, the bread I ate was the kind made without preservatives—yes, I keep my bread in my refrigerator and always have. It's the safest way to avoid spoilage. The whole grain kind, often with crunchy beads of sprouted wheat or wheat germ added. I'll never forget the taste of my first sandwich in three years. It was positively ambrosial and made me feel sensuously wicked. Sounds pretty silly, I know, but, boy! I'd forgotten how much I loved certain foods I'd given up in the search for shape.

As for soft drinks? Well, I'd learned my lesson about sugar when my own low blood sugar was test-confirmed. I simply can't have soft drinks because of their sugar content. That content is high—high enough to make soft drinks one of the primary villains in the cavities problem, along with those sugary breakfast cereals that are being investigated.

But I ate all right. Ate all the good fresh vegetables I could get my hands on. And I must say here that getting my hands on them wasn't so easy in New York City. I can never understand why, with all the Long Island farmland around us, fresh vegetables seem to be limited to relatively common ones. And they get boring. Fresh and boring is always better than canned and nutritionally empty, however, so they were a treat.

And I ate fruits, though not the ones that came in cans

and were heavily sugared. Here again is where you watch the labels. Or check the chart. Be aware that you're loading up on deadly sugar and wrecking your diet at the same time.

And, while I ate these hitherto forbidden fruits, I studied. Every single nutritional book I could find. For getting my diet-doctorate, so to speak, was a serious business with me. As serious as getting rid of my weight.

Count to 1,000

I learned plenty. I learned to count, for starters, and so must you. One of the solutions to the diet problem is learning to be honest with yourself. I have found that the easiest possible way to be sure no calories slip by my lips uncounted is to write everything down on paper. When you see it that way, you're in for some real surprises. Get a notebook and date it. And, for that date, write in your weight *and* your measurements for that day.

As you watch them both go down, you're going to be more and more proud of that little record book. It may sound like a bore at first, but it will turn out to be the literary treasure of your diet life.

If you work, as I do, then don't forget to write down your lunch—right to the last forkful. So your companions think you're nuts. So what? You'll be thinner and more beautiful than they are soon, and you'll get the last laugh then. Take a sheet of paper with you or commit that meal to memory and jot it down the moment you get back to your desk. Then, when working day is through, transfer it to the "lunch" counter on that day's page.

Do not forget to add in the calories spent on the cream in your coffee, if it was cream rather than milk. Check out the chart and see that even *black* coffee with not a single element added comes up to 2.3 calories per cup. (It has to do with the natural oils in coffee, but those calories are there nonetheless.) And if you're a heavy coffee-drinker which, for the sake of your health, I hope you're not, then those 2.3 calories definitely add up.

At the end of the day, tote up the columns and you'll see exactly what you're getting and know how to adjust your eating habits accordingly. There will, no doubt, be plenty of things that *could* be eliminated, and when everything's down in print it's easy to see which ones you prefer to dispense with.

Tonic water, without any alcohol, adds up to 71 calories per glass; plain club soda, which has 0 calories and carbohydrates, is said by many nutritionists to cause that to-be-avoided water retention. The bubbles in it cause bubbles of fat in you. Skip it and stick to water. It's full of good minerals.

Just don't ever skip your daily count. It's every bit as important as your daily weigh-in. And it's going to tell you a lot about why you're in the shape you want out of!

With a Lot of Help from My Friends

While I was counting my daily thousand, I still studied every health food book in sight. And I came up with what were, for me, four little friends that—guess what?—made me skinny!

I didn't discover them all at once, you understand. One at a time, I tried them. And when I had counted all four, I seemed to have come up with a formula that was, for me, seemingly infallible for making *my* weight come off with a sudden rush that surprised even ever-doubting me.

The four were lecithin, cider vinegar, kelp, and vitamin B-6. And we're going to give them to you one at a time—more digestible that way.

I can only say that I put them all together and came out thin! In two weeks, I lost twelve pounds—all the pounds I had gathered before my diet about-face from low-carbohydrate to low-calorie living. I found it difficult to believe. Dr. Atkins had to be shown before he would believe it, and it seemed pretty ludicrous for *him* to be asking *me* how I did it. But there I was: thin again and still healthy.

Now, since this fortuitous accidental fat-off formula fell into my lap by sheer luck, I have tried the same recipe on innumerable willing guinea-pig friends. You'd be surprised how many guinea pigs one can come up with when the carrot at the end of the stick is a brand new, thinner shape. It should tell you how many people weigh more than they really want to. So far, the mysterious mixture of these four ingredients has never failed to take off pounds, as long as a low-calorie regimen was strictly adhered to. For I wouldn't dream of suggesting that these four, together with unlimited food intake, would make you lose weight. If you ever come up with a formula like that, you've no doubt got a ready million waiting for you. That's a beautiful dream for now. And, for now, those of us who wish to get our weight down and keep it there will have to diet in one form or another. But my four little friends sure did make things easier. And quicker, which is the best part of all.

Now I wish I could tell you that I had vast numbers of control subjects, and laboratory tests on the usefulness of these four seemingly magic weight-offers. I can't. But I have tried them. My friends have tried them. We have all lost weight, rapidly. And since each of them is nothing more than a food—with the single exception of B-6, which is just what it says it is, a vitamin—I don't see how it could hurt you to try.

Check with your own doctor anyway. I did.

Lecithin

Pronounce it "less-i-thin" and call it a miracle. For lecithin is a substance that, while not exactly misunderstood, is perhaps not understood. We know where it comes from. It is found in egg yolks, and in some vegetable oils. But mostly lecithin is simply a little soybean stuff that you may take as you like—in oil, in capsules, in granules. But take it if you want to watch your shape change.

And here's one spot where you might as well not ask your doctor. According to Linda Clark, most of them never heard of the stuff. My own wise physician has a crew of weight-lifters for patients (seems they come to him to straighten them out when they've inflicted weird-diet ills on themselves). He tells me that they eat great quantities of lecithin to tighten up those sinewy muscles. Let me point out that there's nothing wrong with having *your* muscles tightened, either.

But since lecithin is a food, not a drug, I feel totally safe in recommending it without qualification.

I learned about lecithin from the experts—experts like Adelle Davis, Linda Clark, and Edward R. Hewitt, who is the author of a pamphlet called "Lecithin and Health." (Probably available in your health-food store tract-rack.)

Lecithin is found in every single cell of the human body, and its concentration in the brain is 17 to 20 percent.

According to Linda Clark, that's important, because lecithin has a high phosphorus content. And, says Miss Clark, "No phosphorus, no brains." Not stopping with brains, Miss Clark goes on to say that lecithin is essential for the proper function of all glands, including the sex glands.

But what you're interested in is what lecithin can do for your body. Lots, for lecithin is an emulsifier, used in the manufacture of chocolate. (Remember, you *do not* eat chocolate on the grounds that it contains lecithin. You eat lecithin.) It keeps that chocolate liquid and thus keeps it moving. And lecithin does the same for your fat—keeps it moving, moving right off you.

Lecithin tends to be a natural diuretic as well. And remember that, for as long as you diet *my* way, no unnatural diuretics are permitted. *Ever.* The reason is simple. Diuretics tend to wash away the body's potassium salts. And the most ironic part of all is that potassium is the very thing that prevents water retention in the first place. And to me, water retention—for all that doctors may reassure me "it's only water"—looks like fat. It also makes you feel fat, which is just as bad. Keep the potassium, lose the water—without dangerous diuretic drugs. Anyway, without potassium, you're dead.

With all the fat-moving it does, there is some evidence that lecithin can also be an effective cholesterol-reducer. According to *Lecithin and Health*, Dr. Lester M. Morrison of Crenshaw Hospital (wish I could claim kinship, but I can't—kindred in spirit only) in Los Angeles has published observations he made as director of a research project at the Los Angeles County Hospital.

Dr. Morrison selected a group of fifteen patients who previously had not responded to treatments with low-fat diets, nor to a number of agents reputedly effective against cholesterol. These fifteen patients were given six tablespoons of lecithin daily without any other added prescriptions, and blood tests were taken once a month to establish the content of serum cholesterol. The experiment lasted three months, during which time the patients commented that they were feeling better and had more energy for both physical and mental work. And it was noted that the patients, on the whole, *did not eat more, nor put on weight.* At the end of the three months, twelve patients showed a 30 percent decrease in cholesterol, on an average basis.

But not only does lecithin do all these seemingly impossible fat-moving tricks, it is also the best source of two of the hardest-to-get B vitamins. Those are choline and inositol, and they are two of the B vitamins that, as you will soon see, are two of the most important to hair health and beauty. Thus while you're making your body lithe with lecithin, you're doing the same for your hair.

Not bad for a soybean, I'd say.

And we won't stop at that. Lecithin doesn't. It's full of vitamin E, the sexy shaper-upper. The one that seems to be the panacea for practically everything, including your love life. (Perhaps that's why lecithin has its sex-gland effect ... it's the old chicken-or-the-egg question.)

I happen to *like* lecithin. Other still-faithful lecithin-eaters swear it tastes like soap. But there are any number of ways to make sure you get your daily ration. And as far as I am concerned, one to two tablespoons a day should do it.

If you must disguise it, then you can mix it with your morning orange juice (assuming the low-carbohydrate diet hasn't been your choice; then you can mix it with that Tropi-Cal Lo). Or milk. Or broth. I sprinkle a tablespoon of lecithin granules over the wheat germ I eat each and every morning of my life.

I think when you see lecithin's effects in the mirror, you'll learn to love it. For, to me, almost anything tastes delicious if it's getting me skinny!

You won't get much information off a lecithin label. And even the health-food folk who sell it can't help much. So I've dug up all the data available and put it into my chart under Fats and Oils. For, even in its granular form, lecithin is still a fat—which drives the point home one more time that eating fat can make you skinny and healthy into the bargain.

There's one more thing to mention about lecithin. After all, those weight-lifters that take it so regularly aren't out to *lose* weight. They need it. So it isn't that lecithin *reduces* you (your low-calorie or low-carbohydrate dieting does that). On the contrary, it simply shifts your weight around to where you want it. And if, perchance, you are skinny, but have lumps on your hips or thighs, as did one of my wonderful guinea-pig friends, it seems to remove them. This particular guinea pig is thrilled and vows that it is the first time in her ever-thin life that she was able to be thigh-less. Not thinner—just not lumpy. Pretty miraculous, isn't it?

As for which form of lecithin to take, take your choice. But they tell me that the granular form of lecithin is the most potent kind (by "they" I mean a quantity of lecithin manufacturers, who really haven't done much research into their product's values), and the capsules, the least potent. I go for granules myself.

One last word on this miracle. You will be, of course, happy to see that there are O carbohydrate grams in lecithin, sixty-eight calories in a tablespoon of the granules, and twenty-five calories in a tablespoon of the oil. Keep that in your calorie-count notebook.

The Cider Vinegar Brew

The second do-gooder to come into my new low-calorie life was cider vinegar. And you heard it right. Vinegar! You see, I *had* been doing my health food homework, and I kept coming up against that vinegar brew, which was touted as a cure-all for everything from rheumatism to high blood pressure. You name the disease, "they" said cider vinegar could cure it.

Now the kind of cider vinegar I'm talking about is the kind you'll find in your health-food store, not the white stuff seen on the supermarket shelf. The pure kind, made from apples, and from apples especially grown for cider—that's what we need.

Because this kind of vinegar retains all the good things that apples had to begin with. Such as potassium. Remember how important we told you potassium was? So important that you can't live without it. Literally.

So, I decided, what harm? I experimented with that old folk-remedy of one teaspoonful of cider vinegar in a glass of water, to be guzzled after each and every meal, by me. It seemed theoretically sound enough. After all, oil and vinegar don't really mix. Maybe oil and my fat wouldn't, either, and vinegar just might win out.

Now don't think I took the heady plunge into vinegar without checking with my internist. I'd heard dreadful things about how it could burn a hole in your gut, turn your bones into jelly—all that nonsense. I didn't want any ulcers in the name of skinny.

I was summarily reassured. In no way could it harm me. When you think about it, that's pretty obvious. For a teaspoonful of vinegar is just about what goes into a salad dressing, isn't it? And here we were diluting even more. So I began to drink vinegar brew, every day, after every meal. And inches is what I lost.

Now there is one super-important word of warning about vinegar. You must remember to brush your teeth after every brew. Or drink it through a straw (which I find too much bother to consider). Or even just rinse your mouth thoroughly after every dose. Because vinegar, if it stays in your mouth, does *not* work wonders on your teeth and your teeth are not what we want you to lose.

You should be brushing your teeth after every meal, in any case. Or, if you can't carry around a toothbrush, do as my dentist instructed and rinse vigorously. It has the same cleaning effect and will get rid of that furry-tooth feeling that's so distasteful.

Don't be fearful. Vinegar is harmless, indeed, as long as you rinse. I haven't had a cavity in years.

Help from Kelp

Then came help from kelp. I was taking my lecithin and drinking my vinegar and still reading and learning all the while.

I learned a lot about kelp. For kelp is loaded with iodine and iodine is what makes that mysterious metabolic system burn up the fuel the way it should. I have already told you, perhaps too often, that my metabolic system burns everything too slowly, so that the fat tends to pile up. I'm just unlucky, I guess. Some have it—a perfect metabolism—and some, like myself, just don't.

But, at this point, I wasn't thinking thyroid. I wanted to see whether my low-normal metabolism could be turned up by iodine the way one could turn up the flame in an oven.

And so I checked out kelp.

Kelp is seaweed, pure and simple, although it goes by some other rather spectacular aliases. "Badderwrack, bladder fucus, and kelpward" are just a few of the more unattractive ones. It's still seaweed to me. And, fortunately, in its food form, it's available in easy-to-swallow, compressed-seaweed tablets. Thank heavens.

Now, for all of my life, I'd been listening to lore about the un-fat Orientals and how they got, and stayed, that way by eating loads of food from the sea. Not only fish, but seaweed and other nutritional gifts from the sea.

For the Orientals are traditionally slim (in spite of the rice), relatively heart-attack free—or at least they were until cola drinks hit that culture, along with the Western world's overprocessed horror-diet—with much lower blood-pressure rates than our country's. And along with all that, they have, as you have surely noticed, lots of lustrous, strong, and healthy hair. Mind you, I'm speaking generally, of course. But just look around.

So I decided to add kelp to my helpers—all the while reading every word I could find on the subject—and I discovered that this is a real wonder food. For it *is* a food, which means that it would be awfully difficult to overdose on kelp. And yet it acts, in some mysterious way, as a thyroid normalizer. It makes the fat grow thin and the thin not get any thinner. In short, it works on your metabolism *only* if that metabolism was faulty already. Who can ask for anything more from seaweed?

On top of that, if you *do* have really faulty metabolism, and must take medication for it—doctor-authenticated thyroid problems, not just "glands" that are used as an excuse for being too lazy to diet—kelp doesn't interfere with that medication. It isn't a drug so there's no conflict of medical interests.

On my "help me, kelp" program, I swallowed five or six tablets of kelp every time I downed my vinegar brew. And I kept getting thinner. But I kept thinking fat!

B-6

Right about the three-quarter mark in my great weight-moving race, I came across a mind-blower—right in a book by nutritionist Linda Clark. It was the story of a general physician in Texas, a Dr. John M. Ellis, who happened upon the thin-making effects of vitamin B-6 quite by accident.

He was, it seems, treating patients who complained of

tingling and numbness in fingers and toes, as well as leg cramps. Dr. Ellis treated these symptoms by prescribing for his patients dosages of fifty milligrams of vitamin B-6 daily.

He found that their tingly symptoms disappeared within three weeks, but he also found something he hadn't expected. These same patients began to lose both weight and inches, especially around their waistlines—up to three inches in many cases—and this without changing one element in their diets. Except for the B-6, of course. And when that B-6 was stopped, apparently the good results stopped, as well.

According to Mrs. Clark, Dr. Ellis finally learned the reason: B-6 works together with the minerals sodium and potassium to set up a body balance of the two—and both minerals are ones which work to regulate body fluids. Meaning that vitamin B-6 helped regulate the curse of every dieter—water retention.

Now I rarely approve of separating the B-complex vitamins, for the simple reason that the B vitamins are not simple. They are complex indeed. You will see in our "Vitamin Vitality" chapter that the B vitamins should not be separated—particularly by a vitamin-novice. For they are put together in such delicate balance that an overdose of one will cause a deficiency of another. As I said, I will explain this more fully in a later chapter.

But with B-6, I decided to make a single exception. I was already taking a potent B-complex formula every day. I decided to add the fifty milligrams of B-6—just to see.

I saw all right. I saw my body getting skinnier by the day. Now mind you, all this while, I was still counting to 1,000 on my daily calories. But I was having the time of my life using those calories in the foods I loved. Foods like that whole-grain bread—my particular weakness—and I was probably doing the healthiest eating I'd done in years, thanks to all that diet self-education.

I ate raw wheat germ for breakfast each morning. I'd eaten wheat germ in place of cereal for years, mostly because I like it. But when I read that even the little bit of toasting in the wheat germ one ordinarily finds in the supermarkets could destroy some of the vitamin E content, I hopped over to the raw variety. At first, it tasted like green weeds. Then I grew to love it. And I topped it off with that necessary daily dose, one tablespoonful of lecithin, and a bit of cream (all, I might add, added up at the day's end. And carefully added, too.).

Every meal was ended with that cider vinegar brew that washed down the kelp. And now the B-6.

Then soon, very suddenly, miraculous things began to happen to my shape. My clothes actually hung on me. (Perhaps I should say, *off* me, for at this point there was trouble keeping them from falling off. I never thought I'd come to the point of complaining about nothing to wear because I couldn't keep things *on*. Usually the complaint comes the other way around—when you find you can't fit *into* your clothes. Or, at least, it always had with me.)

All of the weight that caught up with my low-carbohydrate act, and learned to bypass it, went off, and then some. And the inches went off as well.

I wasn't content to accept my own experience as the fact, for I know that I am not the norm. I do have abnormal blood sugar, and I did have that very low-normal metabolism, so I decided to try this particular formula on someone else—everyone else I could find. The first trial run was on a lush young thing who was summer-jobbing at the *Times*. She couldn't have been more pleased at the chance to play guinea pig for me. (I told you—guinea pigs are all over the place when it comes to diet-trials.)

This young lady swore she couldn't lose weight. Sound like an old story to you? It did to me, and I swore she could lose that much-too-extra weight that kept her just short of being a ravishing beauty. For here was a girl, a very young girl—nineteen—who had the beautiful bone structure all right, all hidden by lots of unnecessary, and unbeautiful, fat.

Needless to say, she screamed "glands." And, of course, I declared nonsense. For I do believe, with Carlton Fredericks, that the chances of the glands being the culprits are slim, indeed.

This girl went on the prescribed 1,000 calorie diet and learned to count to precisely that amount and not one calorie more. She took lecithin, she drank vinegar, she swallowed kelp and vitamin B-6 . . . and, since she wasn't taking a B-complex before, I suggested one for her.

Within one month, she had to buy a completely new back-to-school wardrobe. What nineteen-year-old wouldn't be delighted with that! Not only was she delighted with her new clothes, but with her new body and those beautiful bones that had finally begun to emerge from beneath the layers of fluffy fat that had hidden them all of her life. Her father, who paid for the new wardrobe, was nevertheless so delighted with *her* results that he went on the diet himself.

My last report from this heretofore fat young lady was that she weighed in at 112 pounds and was looking glorious.

And that's not the only trial-without-error in this low-calorie-plus routine. One of the characters in *The New York Times* art department (all art departments seem to have characters, ours has more than most) wondered aloud, and to me, how I could eat my lunch in the same Greek restaurant that he did and keep on getting thinner while he grew fatter. For, though the Greeks are good cooks, their cuisine is not noted for its slimming effects. My fast answer—and I have lots of them now—was a mini-course in calorie counting, plus the suggestions he forget beef-and-booze, switch to fish (a Greek favorite, and something they do particularly well), plus a recommendation to the four friends of the low-calorie routine—lecithin, vinegar, kelp, and B-6. There is a marvelous caricature that hangs over my desk. It shows this arty character pulling in his belt by three notches. And all done in three weeks.

As for myself, when my low-calorie life had taken me as low as ninety-eight pounds, I stopped. After all, no man wants no woman.

But I continue to *think fat!* I always will.

The View from the Plateau

Let us stop for a moment to consider the plateaus that you will inevitably reach during your low-cal diet life. (I have never seen—or perhaps I should say, *rarely* seen—such plateaus on a low-carbohydrate regimen. For there the weight loss seems to be agonizingly slow, but steady all the way.)

You *will* hit plateaus—points where your weight seems to hit "stop" and the needle on the scale refuses to go any lower, no matter how conscientiously you stick to your calorie count.

So you might as well expect them and be prepared for

them. For they will disappear just as suddenly as they came. The pattern is a dieting classic. The point is that you not be discouraged by such inexplicable slowdowns in your weight loss and *never* be tempted to give up and go back to eating. If you do, you could blow the whole diet, and all the time you've spent on it.

Just believe me when I say that the plateau days—and they can stretch to days and days and days—*will* go away just as suddenly as they came, and you will, one fine day, find yourself three, four, or as much as five pounds lighter than the day before.

Occasionally you can nudge yourself off the plateau by a few little tricks, such as limiting your "meat" to fish for a few days. I know of a doctor who puts his patients on "shrimp days" to combat the plateau periods. Shrimp seems inordinately able to get things moving off again.

I have my own method, and that is done with mushrooms. I broil them in polyunsaturated margarine and eat them on a slice of thin toast as that day's "meat course." My mind is fooled into thinking it's had meat, but my body knows it's had practically nothing in the way of calories, and the dip begins again.

You must remember to keep counting, carefully, using my chart and your notebook, and never to be disheartened. That weight will go away. It has to.

Your Weight—Normal or Ideal

Dr. Robert Atkins taught me something about weight I'd never heard before—nor since—but it certainly stuck in my mind. It is that your normal weight is not necessarily the same thing as your *ideal* weight.

When a patient makes his or her first visit to Dr. Atkins, he carefully takes a history. "Was your mother overweight? Your father? Brothers or sisters?" Ad infinitum. "Have you ever had to diet in your adult life?" (And the word "adult" is seemingly very significant.) "How much did you lose? How many times? When?"

It seems that what all this means—or rather, what it tells the doctor—is just what your *normal* weight is, as opposed to what you would like it to be.

If you have been on a reducing diet more than three times in your adult life, then the high point from which you started is your normal weight. And in my case, at 124, it was far from ideal. Twenty pounds over ideal, in fact. And, according to Dr. Atkins, whatever your *normal* weight is, that's the point your body will head for, should you ever be un-wise enough to stop thinking fat!

Now some people are lucky. Their normal and ideal weights are the same. Must be nice. But from the number of people on reducing diets these days, I would think these lucky folk are the rarity, not the norm. My only advice is to remember there is no such thing as a *cured* fat person— only arrested cases. *So keep on thinking fat!* All through your, by now, skinny life.

Vitamin E—The Reshape Vitamin

Vitamin E has been called almost everything. The vitamin of the seventies, the vitamin in search of a disease, the sex vitamin, the heart vitamin. Some call it fad, some say it's fabulous. I happen to believe it's one of the greatest shape-changers ever to come along in the shape of one small capsule. Sort of a sex symbol of the vitamin world.

For the E-addicts claim that vitamin E can make your bosom bosomier, your hips curvier, your skin smoother, your hair shinier, and *you* sexier. It's a lot to expect from a vitamin. But I personally know of one young lady who swears that her bosom went from flat-chest to sexpot by vitamin E alone. She swears that it is the only element in her diet that had changed.

Adelle Davis claims that research indicates that vitamin E plays some role in the production of normal sex hormones. And she goes on to explain that a number of physicians have pointed out that young people these days seem to be losing their secondary sex characteristics. "The hips of boys and men are often too large, whereas girls and women frequently have flat chests and slender hips," says Miss Davis and adds, "It has been my experience that when the diet is made completely adequate and vitamin E is increased temporarily to perhaps 100 units after each meal, these children develop normal sex characteristics quite rapidly. . . . I have seen a few cases where normal breasts have developed after flat-chested women from twenty to thirty-five years old have conscientiously followed an excellent nutrition program." When Adelle Davis confirms it, it's time to take notice of the shape-making aspects of E. And isn't it convenient that it makes women out of girls and men out of boys?

I believe in large doses of vitamin E for the best possible beauty-making effects. But here, it's trial and error for you. For, as I keep repeating, individuality is the name of the game—and in beauty, thank goodness for individuality! Some doctors recommend dosages of 800 I.U.s (international units) per day. I know beautiful women who take 1200.

You will probably notice, throughout your vitamin dosage tryouts, that you, individually, may need more or less than the dosages I will give as recommended by the experts. And, if you check the chart, you will probably find a good reason for that. It should be obvious that if you find you are heavy on a food high in a particular vitamin, then you are going to need less of that vitamin supplementally. The vitamin power of food seems without chemical peer. But I still believe it must be supplemented.

The point is that you take the amount that makes *you* look and feel your very best.

There is one thing about E, however, that you'd better watch out for. It has true aphrodisiac properties. Or at least it has them in my estimation and the estimation of some other knowledgeable nutritionists such as our friend Dr. Carlton Fredericks, who swears he had to give it up for a while to get his work done. Seems he had too much E on his mind.

By the same token, vitamin E works for those who claim they are too exhausted to have any interest in matters sexual. I have suggested the 800 I.U. dosage for these people and they say it's a phenomenon. Whether it's a case of suggesting the positive, I do not know. I only know it works ... somehow.

Chew It Up

There are plenty of basic ground rules of dieting. Counting is the first one we've pointed out. Thinking fat is another. Thinking fat—for always—is probably the most important. But there's another that's little considered and probably has much more to do with the success (or not) of your dieting than you would imagine. And that one is "Chew it up."

Whenever you eat, whatever you eat, and however you're dieting, chew, chew, and then chew some more. But *never* gulp it down.

Remember how I told you what a sneaky creature your body can turn out to be? Well, I will show you how to sneak one by on your body. Dieting fair play, I say.

Now, if you gulp your food, your body is somehow convinced it hasn't gotten any. So you go on feeling hungry—and cheated—and probably go right on eating. And that's disastrous to your diet, all right.

You see, if you down whatever food you're allowing yourself *too* fast, your gastric juices don't have time to get out there and get ready to work, and your stomach doesn't know what hit it. So it hits back by making you go on being hungry.

Now . . . if you chew, just as slowly as you possibly can . . . dawdle over your food, in fact, whenever you can . . . you will find that you are less and less hungry and are, in fact, soon eating less and less.

I believe it's a simple question of boredom. Too long working at the same plate makes me want to give it up reasonably quickly.

Linda Clark tells the story of Elizabeth Keyes, a lifelong overweight sufferer who finally learned how *she* could get thin and passed her theory on to other would-be thinnies in a book called *How to Win the Losing Fight*, which Mrs. Clark tells us can be ordered from Gentle Living Publications in Denver, Colorado. (I must admit to not having read Mrs. Keyes' book for the simple reason that I had discovered the secret long ago, on my own. Here, however, are her ground rules.)

According to Mrs. Keyes, all overweight people, in general, are gulpers. And, just as we predicted, their appetites are not satisfied, and so they go on eating, taking one more helping after another. Mrs. Keyes suggests that you take a bite that is nothing more than pea-sized. Then put down your fork and chew awhile. Only when that bit has literally disappeared from your mouth may you reach for another.

According to Linda Clark, Mrs. Keyes tells of an overweight woman who tried this method. She ordered an enormous meal—obviously her custom—and then tried to eat it pea-bite by pea-bite, according to Mrs. Keyes' directions. Soon she shoved the plate back, maintaining that she would be sick if she had to eat any more. She had eaten about half the food on her plate. In short, she was full up with chewing!

Weight Watchers is only one of the weight-losing organizations that recommend careful, slow chewing of whatever you eat. You'll find that doctors do the same. Dwell on it, savor it, and you'll enjoy it more, your body can use it better and you'll eat less. And have less body to show for it!

Don't Just Sit There!

Do something. Anything as long as it means moving. For one thing is sure. A sedentary life makes for sedentary fat . . . fat that just sits there, usually on your bottom, where you most certainly don't want it to remain. You sit and the fat sits, too.

I have found to my amazement that, whenever I go on holiday, even to a place like my Alabama home, where life moves on four wheels and a walk just might get you arrested (Try it in California: I've *known* people who were stopped for walking and termed "suspicious characters") I still lose both pounds and inches.

For these days walking isn't the norm in most places outside of the big cities. Never mind. When I hit my Southern country *and* that Southern cooking, I tend to lose both weight and inches, no matter how much fried chicken, black-eyed peas, and biscuits, gravy, and grits I may consume.

Dr. Robert Atkins admits that even he, the paragon of no-carbohydrate diet virtue, cheats (those are his very words, but don't *you* try it) when he goes on vacation. He vacates his diet theory as well and even goes over the hill to the point of soft drinks. Knowing what he has taught me, no vacation will ever get me to that low a diet life again.

The fact remains that, no matter how motionful your day to day routine may be (and believe me, the pace of a newspaper reporter can get fast, indeed), there's still a certain amount of sitting down involved.

And for some reason, sitting down in a car is a more fat-moving experience than sitting at a desk. Perhaps all that jostling has the same effect as an exercise machine? (Have you ever noticed that car, plane, or train trips can bring on the same hungers as exercise?)

The point I want you to remember is that when your life is sedentary, watch that diet—and that scale—even more closely. When you're on vacation, still watch it. But if you're sitting at home (*or* sitting down on the job), just watch out!

Exercise

While I'm talking about moving, let me say a word about the most important sort of motion to get yourself into— and that's exercise.

I can't imagine any would-be beauty, or any would-be shapely woman, who thinks she can get there without exercise. I have been a denizen of Nicholas Kounovsky's Studio for Physical Fitness for longer than either I or Nick care to think about. To me, it was a beautiful place to be long before it became the Beautiful People's place to be.

I go through my gymnastics workout twice a week (at 9:00 A.M.), and it is what makes me lithe instead of dried-twig stiff. For at one point I had a six-day-a-week, nine-hour-a-day job that simply left me neither time nor energy for anything. Once out of that, I just got lazy. Then one fine spring morning I leapt out of bed and found that I was, by now, less than a gazelle. I called Kounovksy's that red-hot moment and made an appointment for that very day and I haven't, unless really bed-ridden, missed one session since.

Recently I was fortunate enough to attend the Madison Square Garden performance of the Russian Women's Olympics Gymnastics Team. To say that it was phenomenal is an understatement. Not only were the performances hard to see-and-believe, but the sellout audience was a phenomenon as well: 19,700 people—the first time in the Garden's history that a sellout crowd had ever turned out for a gymnastics performance.

And they were 19,700 enthusiastic people, I might add, bearing banners with such legends as "Right On, Olga"— referring, of course, to the mighty-mite Olympics gold medal winner Olga Korbut, who, I have heard, has her own fan club on the West Coast, and sporting Olga T-shirts and all.

I found it encouraging. For the audience here was not just into spectator sports. Many of the ones seated near me were from high-school gymnastics teams, or were instructors of gymnastics. All seemed well-informed on their subject. It gives one hope that perhaps the next generation will be less into getting out of life via the drug route and more into getting a whole lot more out of life.

Exercise is more than just a way to lose weight. In fact, I have never lost one pound by exercise alone. On the contrary, you might just find your weight a couple of pounds more with regular, controlled, and muscle-building exercise for, you see, muscle weighs in at more than flabby fat. But what do you care, if the body is leaner and more lithe-ly? That, after all, is the object. And your diet, plus your thinking fat, will keep your weight well in control.

In New York City, there are scores of beautifully controlled and beautifully equipped ladies' gymnasiums, where they put you through such things as trapeze and rings and (almost) promise not to let you fall on your pretty head.

If you don't have such a gym setup in your town, then look up your local Y, and find out about exercise classes. Or see whether your town's dancing teacher gives ballet classes. (If she doesn't, perhaps you can be the incentive for one.)

I feel that real, serious ballet is probably the very best exercise of all, for all of you. I found, years ago back when I studied ballet, that my muscles really told me just how much work they were doing—they were good and sore most of the time, which meant they were tightening up with every class. Flamenco dancing (now that discotheques aren't around so much any more) is another thing that will soon let you know where your weak muscles are. When I first came to New York as a fashion student, I was gung-ho to do everything this fabulous city had to offer. I took my gym classes *five* times a week (my father paid the bills in those days—I'd still take them five times if I could) and flamenco dancing twice. And my body certainly showed the results.

But I will never forget one particularly strenuous dance class session—one in which we had to leap in the air and then down from one knee with a whirl to the other. Let me tell you that the next day I had to lift my legs with my hands to get up and down my fashion-school steps. It was serious exercise but, with the beautiful arm work (think of those castanets), the emphasis on straight backs, and terrific posture, it really turned out a classful of better-shaped bodies.

It's too bad about those discotheques. Back in the swinging sixties era, they were a delight. For I love to dance (as you might have guessed), and my favorite partner and I used to do the discos on an average of four nights per week. (I was not going against my own advice and burning the beauty candle at both ends. I used to go to bed until 11 P.M., *then* get up and go out. I still got the sleep required, and no booze to boot. Bad for balance.)

I still dance, to records and radio, around my own apartment, alone or no. So it looks silly. Who's to see me? Only the muscles remain as my silent witnesses.

There are a great many good books on the subject of exercises. Some I have read, some I haven't. Most of the time I am more occupied with exercising than with reading about it, so that is the reason. And, as for books on yoga, which are multitudinous, I have read not one. I regret it, too, because yoga is, indeed, a centuries' old, time-tested method of exercise that can scarcely be discounted. If there is a chance for you to join a yoga exercise class in your community, then I'd certainly give it a whirl.

Here we go again. It's a question of personal, individual preference. You have to pick the method you *like* best, and that you will be most likely to stick with! Stick-with-it-iveness is important in exercising as well.

Once-in-a-while exercising not only won't do your body much good, it could cause a lot of trouble to an unaccustomed-to-such-work heart.

You'll notice I haven't mentioned the obvious exercises such as swimming, horseback riding, golf, tennis. Surely if these things are your bag, you're already into them, and need no reminders from me. But walking, while it's beautiful to do, is simply no substitute for some of the more muscle-controlled methods. If you try something as all-muscle-using as gymnastics, I think your next-day soreness will soon show you that.

My own gym instructor, Russian-born Nicholas Kounovsky, has written two books. The first was my reason for coming to him. Unfortunately, it is out of print and available only in schools and, probably, libraries. It is called *Six*

Factors of Physical Fitness, and the photographs are explicit enough for anyone to follow—as far as she can. His second book, which is relatively new, is called *The Joy of Feeling Fit* (and isn't it?). It will provide safe, easy-to-follow exercises to do at home, without benefit of that instructor by your side. Elizabeth Arden's famous "exercise lady," Miss Craig, has done several books of exercises to do at home.

My favorite book of ballet exercises is called, simply, *The Classic Ballet*, published some time ago by Alfred Knopf. I don't know if it is still around, but if you can possibly get hold of a copy, just try to follow the exercises within, starting at the very beginning (no need to show off here with how much you may know—it could hurt), and you will soon find out which muscles are calling for help.

One word of warning about exercise—do not leap into it too quickly if you haven't had any for a while. Don't get lazy and be misled into thinking you can let machines do it for you. They can be dangerous. Now I am not talking about the kind of machines that create a tension you use your own muscles to work against. This method is used with the greatest possible success by possibly one of the greatest gyms in New York City—Pilates Gym on 56th Street, another favorite Beautiful People place.

I am talking about the electric-whizzer where you do absolutely nothing and they shake you up. That's just the trouble with them. They shake you up. And while they don't shake off the fat, insofar as I can see, they can do serious harm to your innards—or so my doctor has warned me. I had an experience too terrible to go into in any beauty book. Let us just say that machines of this sort once did a beautiful job of shaking up my healthy kidneys. Fortunately, my doctor caught them, and me, in time. And let me tell you, he was not in the least sympathetic, saying he thought I ought to know better and that I'd better never let myself be so shook up again. Don't say you haven't been warned. Anyway, exercise isn't a lazy matter.

Sexy and Slim—Synonymous

I didn't write the book, but I wish I had. It's Dr. Abraham Friedman's *How Sex Can Keep You Slim*. Because I believe it, all right—passionately!

Sexual exercise is about the only kind I know of that isn't work and still works on your shape. Dr. Friedman's peg is "Reach for your mate, instead of your plate." Pretty great advice, it seems to me. For Dr. Friedman goes on to advise his patients to use sex as an effective weapon against overeating and to increase their sexual activity as much as possible. I can't imagine any would-be-thinnie rebelling against that sort of medical counseling.

Remember that compulsive eating has long been equated by psychiatrists as a sex-substitute. Now, this is an over-simplication of the psychological facts, of course, but I'm sure you get the message. According to Dr. Friedman, the increased sexual activity enables you to lose weight by substituting one emotional need for another—in other words, the substitution of sex for excess food. (Conversely, they say that lean and hungry makes for sexier, so there's something to be said for keeping that stomach not quite filled.)

Dr. Friedman goes on to put it in more scientific terms, and quotes Dr. Alfred Kinsey (yes, that one) as stating that the pulse rate of a sexually aroused person increases from a normal rate of about 70 per minute to as much as 150 per minute or more. And, according to Dr. Kinsey, this is equal to the pulse rate of an athlete during his maximum effort, or of a man involved in heavy labor. In addition, there are, says Dr. Friedman, "multiple contractions of the muscles of the buttocks and pelvis, thighs, abdomen, thorax, arms, legs and neck, sometimes of great intensity." Think of those muscles you're using! (As long as you don't bother to think about it *while* you're using them. Could ruin your performance.) And Dr. Friedman adds, "It has been estimated that about two hundred calories are expended during the average act of sexual intercourse." Beats a walk in the park any day.

As Dr. Friedman puts it, "The best prescription for emotional over-eating is sex, taken as directed." Okay, Doctor, that's one I'll buy.

When the Menu's Not Your Plan

One of the most embarrassing moments in my dieting life occurred during the first week of my Atkins regimen—the one where *no* carbohydrates are allowed and any slip can ruin the whole test, putting you back to "start" on the diet game board. And I can assure you I wasn't about to go back there, for the whole first week got complicated as you have seen.

But I got invited to dinner at the house of a friend who prides herself on her gourmet cooking and exotic menus.

And this is what was served:

Drinks
Quiche Lorraine
Argentine meat stew—made with tomatoes,
    corn, catsup, potatoes
Vegetables
Green salad with tomatoes and onions
Chocolate mousse

I stared. And I was horrified. For, as you can clearly see, there was not one item—well, there was one, but I was too new in the game to spot it—that I could eat. I sat there stupefied and wondering how to get out of it all. To further complicate matters, this friend lived in a suburb of New York, so I couldn't even plead a headache and call a cab, and head for home and no-carbohydrate tranquility in my own kitchen.

Would you like to know what I did? I asked for two hard-boiled eggs. I am sure you can imagine the embarrassment of such a situation, not only to me, but to my hostess. But wasn't it lucky that she is one of my oldest and dearest friends, as were all the other dinner guests? Never mind. I was forgiven, though I got a lot of merciless ribbing just the same. But I got my eggs and my diet-trial was saved. On my next visit, Dr. Atkins informed me that I *could* have eaten the Quiche Lorraine and left the crust. I suppose I was not, at that point, cook or carbohydrate knowledgeable enough to know. Better luck next time.

There is a moral to this story. If you are on the first week of your absolutely *no*-carbohydrate regimen, it is perhaps best to avoid at-home dinner invitations. (In restaurants, *you* have the choice.)

During your entire low-carbohydrate life, it is often wise to level with the hostess. It will save you both the kind of situation I so unwittingly got myself into. If she plans to serve a one-course meal of spaghetti and meatballs, then you can arrive *after* dinner. (Even the meatballs will be tomato paste-covered and you can't have that.)

Most friends—if they're friends enough to have invited you to dinner in the first place—are understanding on such matters. Usually they're interested in how you're losing weight anyway and are not only eager to help but anxious to learn how you're doing it.

At any well-planned dinner party, there's a meat course and a salad you can eat if all else turns out to be sweet or starch. But beware of hostesses who have reputations for serving Chinese food that is loaded with sugar or one-course dinners consisting of such things as tuna-noodle casseroles, or hostesses who simply don't plan well and offer potatoes, corn, etc., all in one meal. When in doubt, explain your problem to your hostess and let her tell you what's for dinner.

Cocktail Circuit

Your first diet-jolt, if you've chosen the low-carbohydrate diet, is going to come at a cocktail party . . . I'm reasonably sure of that. First of all, gin and tonic or Bloody Marys are just plain *out*. You'll have to learn to stick to Bull Shot, instead—vodka with consommé—if you *must* have that drink. I think that booze is the big beauty killer, but I'm sure I can't convert every one of you on the first try. Soon you'll give it a whirl, and, once you discover how much better you look without booze, you'll probably give it up for good. Meanwhile, beware of mixed drinks bearing carbohydrates. Make yours pure, with water or club soda. As for wine, check the chart and you'll see it has more carbohydrates than hard liquors (especially my one-time favorite, champagne). And, of course, all sweetened drinks are definitely out.

But what to do about all those crackery hors d'oeuvres? There's a trick to that. You'll learn to eat the cheese *off* the cracker (remembering Jean Mayer's bit about American breadstuff being little more than a napkin, in any case) and deposit the uneaten cracker in the nearest waste basket. You will opt for celery filled with cheese. You will go for the little sausages. You may have anything that you have, by now, learned isn't carbohydrate-loaded.

But at the first cocktail party of your diet look to your carbohydrates.

What If You're the Only Fattie in the Family?

Now somebody's surely going to ask me the question, "How can I possibly diet when the rest of my family is thin?" Or even too thin, and trying to fatten up. (Remember the Jack Sprats. *They* worked it out, so I'm sure you will, too.)

The answers are easy but they'll provide no easy-diet way out for you. I'm not going to let you get away with either glands or a thin family—not if you really *want* to slim down. It can be done, and your family and your friends simply don't become involved. If, for example, you have chosen the low-carbohydrate route, the fact that you are even dieting will be almost undetectable to anyone besides yourself. You will have to forego all the starches, so you simply won't eat the potatoes and bread and desserts (and I'd rather not see your family eat them either).

I have a feeling that, after your diet education, you may just do some family-educating on your own. For once you know the horrors of what we Americans are usually eating, you may want to change your menus for the sake of your family's health, most particularly where children are involved. You may, for example, no longer permit them calories and cavities via endless amounts of sugared soft drinks and desserts. You will, I am sure, find a child-appetite–adequate substitute for such nutritionally empty nonsense, but that may come later.

First, let us assume that your family eats breakfast. If they don't, it is the first thing they should learn to do. Check in with your physician if you're a doubter and he will, assuredly, tell you as much. About the only things you'll forego for breakfast on low-carb—assuming your breakfast is the usual one of juice, coffee, cereal, eggs, bacon, toast—is the juice, the toast, and the sugar in your coffee. For sugar, you'll substitute a no-calorie sweetener like saccharin or you'll have it black. You can put the cream in your coffee and still get slender.

You'll give up your juice, or use an artificially sweetened one. You will forego the toast, or muffin, or grits (if you're from my land), or anything that smacks of starch. The rest of your family will eat everything they want. You will eat your bacon and/or ham and eggs. Even sausages, as long as they're pure meat and don't have any cereal fillers. And, as for cereal, you and, we hope, the rest of the family, will start learning to love wheat germ. And top it off with lecithin. It's good for every one of you. If your family refuses wheat germ, pity them. You eat it anyway and let them learn to feed themselves healthily on something like real oatmeal. (Sneak in wheat germ—they'll never know!)

So you'll have a menu that goes like this:

BREAKFAST:

Family:
Orange juice
Coffee, tea, milk for the kids (none for you)
Cereal (something wholesome, never empty, and preferably wheat germ)
Eggs
Bacon, ham, sausages
Toast with butter or polyunsaturated margarine (good for everyone)

You:
Wheat germ and lecithin with cream on top
Coffee, tea, with sweetener (no sugar) and/or heavy cream
Eggs, with polyunsaturated margarine (to hurry the fat off) or butter
Bacon, ham, or sausages

(You see how little you have to give up?)

Forr LUNCH, you can eat something like this:

Broth (never any cream soups on this diet!)
Fish or fowl, broiled or baked, or any other meat as long as it's pure meat
Salad
Cheese
Coffee with or without cream, definitely without sugar

DINNER:

Try this: Give your family any meal they'd like, but don't plan one that's all starch such as the one that almost wrecked my diet. Remember? Allow yourself, the dieter, some room to move. Your family can eat the potatoes while you simply omit them. And the bread. And the desserts.

How about—

Family:
Soup
Lamb chops
Rice and French string beans with almonds
Broccoli with hollandaise
Green salad
Coffee or tea and milk for the kids
Homemade applesauce (unsweetened for health's sake)

You:
Lamb chops
French string beans with almonds *or* broccoli with hollandaise sauce
Green salad
Coffee or tea with or without cream, no sugar
Unsweetened homemade applesauce (stay under the 10-gram amount!)

Now you see how easy it really is? And how very little your low-carbohydrate diet will differ from your family's? You can, of course, all have giant steaks if your budget will allow it. With beef at $3 per pound, I am happy to see that more and more American housewives are doing without beef. For, until we improve the polyunsaturated diets being tried on our cattle, I'd prefer to see us *all* eliminate the stuff from our diets. I do believe, however, that once you learn to love such lighthearted meats as fish and fowl, you'll find how much lighter *you* feel—less stuffed, less heavy—and you'll stick with them. I have never found a soul who returned to the heavy beefeating life, once they'd learned to love another meat.

Now there are a great many books to be read if you're into meal planning for a family and don't want to stray from your regimen (you'd better not, or I'll be worse than disturbed!). *Dr. Atkins' Diet Revolution* contains recipes plus meals. *The Low Carbohydrate Diet Cookbook* by Roy Ald is a paperback aid to good recipes with little carbohydrates.

One of the best books in the cookbook field for any dieter to consider is Yvonne Tarr Young's *The New York Times Natural Foods Dieting Book*. It hasn't really received the attention it deserves, in my opinion. For this diet-bright lady has gotten together recipes for both of our diets—low-carb and low-cal—and, at the end of each recipe, she has toted up the carbohydrates and calories for you. Makes life a lot easier for me!

If you're on a low-calorie diet, your eating's easy. You can eat anything your family can *if*—and this is the biggest *if* in your life—you count to 1,000 calories and stop. Or 1,200, if that's your point. Or even 1,500, although I doubt very seriously if your weight is going to come off at that. Still, we work downward with calories, as we've shown you, and you simply start *somewhere* below 1,500 and remove calories until you begin to remove pounds and that removal *shows* in the numbers on your scale.

What you will do in your menu-planning is try to avoid beef, the Bad B. Everyone is trying to avoid it these days, thanks (and I mean thanks) to the prices. So you've got double blessings by giving up the stuff. If you want to serve, for example, lamb chops, and your family likes them thick-cut, then get your butcher to thin-cut one for you. And eat just *one*. It may sound small, but if you eat it slowly, your body won't realize that fact.

On a low calorie diet you can even go the tuna-noodle casserole route . . . as long as you *keep my chart in hand* and watch over every single mouthful that goes into your mouth.

Count and keep counting. And keep that notebook up to date and up to weight, and that weight should go steadily down. If it doesn't, you're not counting right—or counting everything, one or the other.

To make that counting easier, I am going to give you a swift-reference list of the things that help to make you shape-up faster. Then, when you want the precise amounts for your notebook, you may check the precise chart at the end of this book.

You will find, when you check the chart, that such excellent shape-makers as vitamin B-6 are not so prevalent in foods—or at least not properly measured. I am including, however, a list of the foods that are high in B-6, and still suggest that you never forget to take your fifty milligrams of B-6 daily—calorie diet or low-carb. (Along with all the other Beautiful B vitamins, of course.)

The unsaturated fatty acids—the ones that seemingly make the fat on you slip off to somewhere else—are listed here as well, and although you will find, via the chart, that they may, and usually do, have the same caloric content as the saturated ones, they have a weight-off way about them. Try them and see.

I've listed foods high in iodine as well, although no matter how much of these foods you may eat—*never* forget about kelp.

FOODS HIGH IN
UNSATURATED FATTY ACIDS

Sour cream	Sunflower oil
Whipping cream	Chinook salmon
Condensed milk	Tuna, canned in oil
Dry, whole milk	Avocados
Cooking fats (lard and vegetable)	Beef pot pie
	Dry, country-style ham
Margarine	Almonds
Corn oil	Cashew nuts
Cottonseed oil	Peanuts
Olive oil	Pecans
Peanut oil	Mature, dry, raw soybeans
Safflower oil	Full-fat soybean flour
Soybean oil	Walnuts

FOODS HIGH IN IODINE
(A HELP TO KELP)

Fish	Light pearl barley
Shellfish	Oatmeal or rolled oats
Seafood	Desiccated liver
Apples with skin	Fresh common red beets
Cranberries, raw, fresh	Raw carrots
Figs, raw, fresh	Raw cauliflower
Oranges, raw, fresh	Raw green peas

FOODS HIGH IN B-6

Yogurt
Crab
Haddock
Atlantic salmon
Sardines (Pacific)
Shrimp
Tuna
Apricots
Avocados
Bananas
Cantaloupe
Dates
American-type grapes
Raw, fresh oranges
Dried peaches
Pineapple
Raisins
Watermelon
Light pearl barley
Bran and bran flakes
Cornmeal
Brown rice
Enriched long-grain
   white rice
Whole-grain wheat
Wholewheat flour
Raw wheat germ
Beef (all cuts)
Chicken (all cuts)
Heart
Lamb (all cuts)
Liver (all types)

Ham
Veal (all cuts)
Almonds
Pecans
Mature dry peas (raw)
Mature dry soybeans
Soybean flour
Walnuts
Common beans
Lima beans
Mung beans
Broccoli
Brussels sprouts
Cabbage, common varieties
Cauliflower
Sweet corn
Cowpeas and black-eyed
   peas
Kale
Lentils
Mustard greens
Parsnips
Green peas
Bell peppers
Pumpkins
Sauerkraut
Spinach
Sweet potatoes
Tomatoes and tomato
   products
Turnips

2. Skin

For radiant skin you need lots of things—not the least of which are *joie de vivre* and the will to work at it—and, of course, the knowledge about *how* to work at it, which is what I plan to give you here. That *joie* is going to show up in glowing, translucent, happy skin, whereas tension, worry, and unhappiness will make for a sallow, drawn, unmistakably unlovely complexion.

For happiness is radiance-power, all right, and it shows up, right there on your face. (So do your thoughts, for that matter, so I would suggest here that you try to keep them beautiful, as well!)

The will to work at it is something else, and it's something *I* can't give you. Nobody else can. But here's where your *joie de vivre* will see you through. It will keep you from giving up. And giving up is what you must never do. For, with skin, as with every other beauty part, it's work, work, and more work, and that's the big secret behind being beautiful, whether you like it or not.

Beautiful skin is something that doesn't just happen by itself. It requires your dedication. And keeping your skin in top shape is simply not a matter that will bear putting off or sloughing off. You can never say, "Oh, just this once I won't bother." You might get away with it just once, but soon your skin will show its displeasure.

So keep your *joie* and remember a little anecdote told me by a friend. Seems that when she was a child she complained to her mother how she hated to brush her teeth. Her mother told her in no uncertain manner, "Well, get used to it. You'll be doing it for the rest of your life."

Consider me as stern as she was, and get used to it. All beauty regimens must be kept up *always and forever*. If you're not looking great, need I tell you to work harder?

Clear, Don't Cover

I maintain that everyone, without exception, can have beautiful skin, assuming she (or he—for it's just as important to a man, and pimples on any gender do not "attractive" make) is willing to work on it. Endlessly. Now I know that someone is going to attack me for that statement, but it won't change my opinion one iota. For I've seen too many seemingly miraculous skin re-makes in my day *not* to believe.

I am, of course, assuming basic good health, for good health is basic to beauty, and I hope that I've given you (and you'll be getting more) enough information to assure *that* for you. But then basic good health is basic to much more than beauty—it's basic to life, so obviously you start with health. You train yourself always to think about what you're doing to your body to keep it in great shape—in every sense of that word.

As for skin—years ago I did a story for *The New York Times* in which I predicted transparent makeup as the coming face fashion. My leadoff sentence was, "If you don't have great skin, you'd better get to work on it—fast—since soon there'll be nowhere to hide." That little sentence was killed pronto by my copy-editor, who called it a "scare lead" and could not be moved from his opinion that, since everyone doesn't have good skin, we shouldn't frighten the ones who didn't. *My* argument was (and still is) that everyone *can*. No dice. That lead was killed anyway, which is too bad, since it simply meant I've had to put off saying it in print until now.

But I believe my point was clear. And it was that even the commercial cosmetics companies, whose job it is to sell and sell and sell some more, have caught on to what good skin specialists have known all along. And that is that it's far better to fix whatever is wrong than to cover up a bad situation with layers of gooey makeup. Goo that's bound to make that bad situation worse. In point of fact, many cosmetics companies—along with most of the female population—are more concerned with maintaining a healthy skin than with good cover-ups. Thank goodness. For what I want you to do is work at getting the kind of skin no woman would want to hide. And then keep it glowing and showing.

How Did I Find the Right Road?

My introduction into the wonderful world of wonderful skin came about much as did my diet-education. I lucked up and landed in the lap (figuratively) of one of the most famous skin specialists in the land—a man who probably nurtured more to-be-envied complexions than any other skin specialist in the world.

He was Dr. Erno Laszlo, Transylvania-born (I've always believed there was a secret there!), educated in Hungary, and beauty-maker par excellence to some of the world's most famous faces. Faces like Greta Garbo, Gloria Vanderbilt, the Duchess of Windsor, and a long list of lovelies rightly dubbed by *Women's Wear Daily* as "the Laszlo girls."

Dr. Laszlo taught me a lot—all of which I intend to pass on to you. For with my Laszlo life came the realization that most of the myths about what makes beautiful skin are just that. They're often propagated to—what else?—sell cosmetics you probably don't need in the first place. Who really gives a hoot about what happens to your skin?

Well, *I* care. So here are but a few of the beauty myths that you ought to see for what they are—nonbeautiful nonsense.

Myth No. 1: Always splash your face with cold water after washing it. Sure. Go ahead, if you want to lock in all the impurities that today's polluted air can dish out and onto your skin.

The simple fact is that you should *never* use cold water on your face. You may skinny-dip in any icy ocean, if the spirit moves you, but when you wash, wash hot. For hot is the only way your skin can receive the benefits of the good things you put on it (and we'll tell you what they are). And, equally important, when your skin is hot, it can catch its breath. So kill Myth No. 1.

Myth No. 2: Never wash your face with soap and water—particularly if you're over twenty.

Nonsense! As Dr. Laszlo once remarked in an interview, "If God had not given us water, I would have had to create it." There was plenty of flak from *that* remark, but the doctor was right. Soap and water are the basic and essential ingredients for making clean skin. And clean skin is the basic ingredient for beautiful skin.

So don't let Myth No. 2 get you. You won't end up a wrinkled old crone, just from washing your face. In fact, an unwashed face seems as unsavory as an unwashed body, now doesn't it? Forget Myth No. 2.

Myth No. 3: The older you get, the more you need

creams—moisturizing creams, hormone creams, night creams, cold creams, slathered and lathered on in a horribly creamy mess.

No! You may need some cream all right, but probably a lot less than you believe. For some inexplicable reason, most women—unless their skins are unmistakably oily—insist they have dry skin. It has become almost a status symbol to say so. I thought so, too, until Dr. Laszlo educated me to think differently. How happy I am that I was informed in time. For the cream-need myth is possibly one of the most dangerous to your skin's beauty. So dangerous that I'm going to devote a chapter to avoiding it. Avoid Myth No. 3.

Tighten Up

Have you ever noticed a once-beautiful complexion that has been obviously overtanned and then slathered with cream, in hopes of repairing the overburn? Check out any beach or beach community and you'll find one. Sags, doesn't it?

Well, that's just exactly what the cream-need Myth No. 3 will do for your skin. In short, it will soften it so much that it will run down your face like ice cream thrown against a wall. Ugly analogy, all right, and your skin may be just as ugly if you go with Myth No. 3.

The real answer to truly beautiful skin lies in tightening it up. It's the theory behind many a famous beauty's famous face. Sort of an instant facelift, done cosmetically, rather than surgically.

Not only do you not need as much cream as you probably believed, but your skin doesn't even want it. It can't handle the stuff—at least, not in large quantities. (In fact, ten minutes of just about any cream is just about all any skin can handle.)

RedKen Laboratories sent me an educating little booklet which says that dermatologists and biochemists know that the skin contains only a minute quantity of any oil. "The belief," say they, "that oils are going to have some miraculous effect, that cosmetic creams (all containing oils) will feed the skin is in error of the scientific facts. The assertion that creams penetrate the skin is not literally true, but the term, 'penetrate', has become a part of all cosmetic advertising since it best expresses the public's conception of a cosmetic cream."

There we go again, with our preconceived notions about creams—actually influencing the cosmetics companies, who ought to know better and probably do—to give us things we not only don't need and can't use, but things which just might do us harm.

If anyone had told me twenty years ago (and I was worried about wrinkles *then*) that *now* I'd be washing my face with soap and water twice, sometimes thrice, a day, then freshening it up with an astringent kind of after-wash, then using astringent-based "makeup" and on top of all that, *powder*—I'd have called them crazy. Or expected to be the Ms. Pruneface of the 1970s.

But twenty years ago was in my pre–Laszlo-education days, before I'd discovered that the answer to seemingly ageless skin lies in tightening that skin, tightening those pores, and never, never allowing one globule of excess oil to make my skin slide down!

And if you're going to follow my acid-balanced routine, which I expect you to do with no more cheating than you would with my diet strategies (it's you who gets cheated in the end), then you'll find that you must keep a close eye on that skin of yours if it's going to stay tight.

Want to know why? Because, as your skin becomes more acid balanced—meaning, more normal—your skin routine may have to be changed ever so slightly . . . just as the skin condition will change slowly, but surely, for the better. During my Laszlo life, my skin regimen has been changed three times. In the beginning, I used oil all over my face before I washed, and cream, which was washed off immediately by a milky, soothing sort of liquid brew.

As my new skin life progressed, so did my skin's normality. And I soon found that my skin was looking oilier than it should. But Dr. Laszlo indoctrinated me well. He hated nothing more than shiny, greasy skin, and I was taught and taught to keep my skin just a shade on the right side of dry; so soon my routine was changed from milky after-wash to astringent after-wash. And then oil under the eyes and on the throat *only*. For a while this was my summer routine, with oil all over the face in the winter. Now it's my year-round method. That should show you just how much one skin can change.

I have gone through bitter New York winters washing my face with soap and water and no oil at all, and using all the astringent-based products that go on afterwards, and still no sign of the dry skin I once vowed I had.

Forget about dry skin. The chances that you have it are as slim as the chances you have "glands" responsible for overweight. Just follow my acid-balance method and see what new skin turns up.

And one more word about creams. As I told you, being over twenty, over thirty, even over fifty, doesn't make creams a necessity. My own mother is a good example. She isn't old, by any means, but she's old enough to be my mother. And so, ordinarily, at her age, she'd be thinking "creams." Probably creams with a few useless, possibly dangerous, hormones thrown in for good advertising measure.

Now my mother lives far from me and I get to see her only about twice a year, so I am in a very good position to judge any change in her looks. On a recent visit, I noticed her skin looking oily, although she has the same thin-skin that I have. (Heredity will out.)

My sharp skin-eye caught that in a hurry and immediately upon my return to New York, I telephoned the Laszlo Institute where they (yes, this institute is still peopled by people—not computers) asked a few questions, confirmed my suspicions, and quickly put my mother on a much more stringent, and *astringent* skin regimen. Hers is more astringent than my own, in fact. And she is, in fact, still old enough to be my mother.

So you can see clearly that age isn't the factor in the condition of the skin—its oiliness or supposed dryness. And the idea that everyone needs cream as she grows older is pure malarkey. Just remember that, unless you have a very rare complexion-oriented dermatologist or a respected skin specialist in your neighborhood, your best bet is to train your eye to see your skin as taut, tight, and firm. And keep that "firm" picture firmly in mind.

The Cabinet of Dr. Laszlo

But let me tell you how I learned the debunk-the-myth facts in the first place. I may as well tell you the whole saga because it cost me a lot, in more ways than financially, as you will soon see. But there's one thing that I got and that's good skin—and I'm not asking for anything more, except that you profit from my skin experiences.

It all happened when Dr. Erno Laszlo's famous beauty remedies at last became available to the general public. Heretofore, they had been reserved for his patients alone, and to be a Laszlo patient wasn't easy, as I soon found out. First, you had to be able to afford the $75 per session fee. But, more important, you needed the cachet to get an appointment in the first place.

And that was the hard part. For, you see, an appointment with the great Dr. Laszlo was almost more difficult to get than an appointment with the president—of the United States, that is. One came armed with recommendations from patients-in-good-standing with the doctor and, even then, the lucky ones who entered those mahogany-paneled gates to beauty-heaven were a select group, indeed.

So, when the products (thanks to the insistence of one of the famous "faces" who felt the public had a right to beauty, too) became public property, I leapt at the chance. You see, I had decided to be a Beautiful Person, and I was determined. As you have learned, determination is an important factor in becoming one. (A B.P., that is.)

And so I collected the $65 I'd been told the products would cost me and rushed to the one New York store that sold the Laszlo wonders. There, I had questionnaires to fill out and later, when a collection of products was determined as "right" for me, more questionnaires, asking things that I thought had not much to do with my skin. (So what did I know then?) Questions such as, "Are you considered aggressive?" Or "timid?" "Do you blush easily?" (It might have asked "How's your sex life?" That was one of Dr. Laszlo's favorite questions. He realized its importance!)

I told the truth, I swear, and happily trotted home, sure that Garbo would have nothing on me by the morrow. (Oh, what a shock was in store!) Little did I imagine that my entire beauty life would change with that purchase.

And so I began, excitedly, my Laszlo life. The first shock came on the first morning when I bounded out of bed to splash cold water on my face—my usual wake-up morning routine. Then I realized—no more cold water for me! Now I am not a morning person. My eyes stay closed until almost noon. So without the splash of cold water, what? Hot water had never occurred to me, but if you want a real awakening, try it. It will get those "baby blues" open *fast*.

That problem was solved. But then the real (or imagined) ones began. I dutifully went through the beauty regimen that had been worked out especially for me. (In the beginning, it was pasted on the bathroom wall. All of this takes some learning, as I told you.)

First, there was my oil, applied with a piece of cotton the size of a quarter soaked with the stuff. Then a basin filled with the hottest water my hands could stand. Then *soap*. Yes, for the first time in many of my years, soap. The bar of soap rubbed onto my wet face and then lathered between my hands which deposited all this soapy stuff on me. Then thirty rinses with the same soapy water.

Fortunately, I have always been a rinser and, if you count, you'll see it takes about thirty lashes to get the soapiness gone. A friend of mine once laughed about how terrible it is when the phone rings somewhere about the count of nineteen. My advice: Let it ring. You'll be so beautiful, he'll call back.

O.K. I was clean. Then there was cream, dabbed (not rubbed) on with the fingers and removed with that milky brew. Then astringent-based (or so it felt to me) liquid makeup. And then powder! All on my (I then believed) dry skin!

Then I checked the mirror and realized for the very first time what was showing. It was *everything*. And at that point in my Laszlo life, everything was too much. For you see, I am a redhead—call it strawberry blonde, if you like —with a redhead's skin. That means parchment thin, unevenly colored (at least it was then), freckled, and, at that time, even peppered with a few little pimples and some broken veins to boot.

There it all was—not just for me to see, but for the world to see as well. And "let it all hang out" just didn't apply here, especially since I am a "fashion lady."

To make matters worse, I couldn't move my face and felt as if I couldn't even open my mouth (a boon for my co-workers, no doubt) and it was uncomfortable. Little did I realize that this was the tautening up process that was to save my skin from bad-cosmetics destruction. And so, as is

my custom, I screamed for help from the Laszlo Institute.
For the Institute was much like the Atkins office—manned
by a comforting staff to offer advice if things weren't looking better. Things, in my case, most decidedly looked
worse to me. My mentor at the Institute was Miss Gabrielle, Dr. Laszlo's right-hand beauty for twenty-odd
years, and a wonderfully patient woman with the humor to
humor me, and the knowledge to understand my problems.
She assured me that all was well, but that, if I really felt
naked, I should apply that liquid makeup twice.

Now, please bear in mind that all of my life I've been
anti-paint. I can't stand a face that looks as though it's
been covered with a layer of plaster of Paris, so I'd always
used the lightest makeup base I could find—just enough to
cover the things I didn't want to show—with a little bit of
moisturizer (oh, what an education was yet to come) worn
under that foundation. (Even then that "light" foundation
was in creases by the end of each day, and there were
creases in my face. That was seven years ago. And now
there are none. Well, maybe not "none" . . . I'm seven
years older, but a lot makeup-wiser.)

Still, skin-bare for all the world to see was too much. So
I applied the makeup twice, as directed. So what? The stuff
was still see-through and I had lots to hide, nothing to hide
behind, and was beginning to wish I'd never dreamed up
transparent makeup.

And then funny things began to happen. Odd red circles appeared under my eyes and across my nose. I looked
like a clown. One of my co-workers, who specialized in
beauty stories, asked me why I was painting those "funny
red circles" under my eyes. "New style," I flippantly re-
torted, thanking God that it was the sixties era of way-out
makeup. But secretly I had concluded that I was allergic to
the Laszlo products (allergies are another redhead's curse)
and I was giving up. Oh, woe! Never to be a Beautiful
Person. It couldn't, *wouldn't* happen to me!

And so it was back to the complaint department. I began
to pressure our beauty editor into trying to get me an
appointment to *show* this hideous mess to Dr. Laszlo himself. I even tried to sneak into the Institute through one of
the patients-in-good-standing, only to be told that she
wouldn't jeopardize her relationship with the doctor for

anyone—certainly not me. But I complained and tormented until finally I got that hoped-for call.

It seemed that my problems had been duly reported to Dr. Laszlo and he didn't believe me. In fact, he didn't believe me so fervently that he *insisted* on seeing me—and gratis, at that—for his own satisfaction and edification. Satisfaction is what he got, all right. The edification was mine.

An appointment was set—for some three weeks thence —and, I confess, I hid under my old makeup habits, and waited for the moment of skin truth to arrive. Three weeks can be an eternity if you're determined to be beautiful.

When that moment arrived, I sat nervously in that Oriental-carpeted, paneled waiting room in the place the Duchess of Windsor once called "The House of Silence." Everyone spoke in reverent, hushed voices. It was probably from fright.

Knowing that Dr. Laszlo always refused to see a patient who arrived even so much as an instant late (and the Duchess was not excused from this rule) I was, needless to say, well on time for mine. Enough on time to find the fabled doctor kissing the hand of a beautiful blonde with a Texas accent who, I was sure, had flown in via her private jet for her consultation with the man. I felt pretty intimidated.

Then there I was, settled into a deep wing chair opposite the stern mien and miss-nothing, piercing eyes of Dr. Erno Laszlo. It's a good thing that chair was deep, for by the end of that session, I had sunken into it as far as I could, doing my best to become invisible.

The inquisition began. I was told in no uncertain terms that the symptoms I had described were impossible, and that the red circles under my eyes simply were not there. Period. Miss Gabrielle sat in a chair nearby, taking notes on every word that was said—in Hungarian. The questions began. "When you were eight, did you have pimples on your cheeks?" I didn't remember any and so I said, "No." The questioning went on, with Dr. Laszlo's eyes never leaving mine and leading me through my skin life from age eight to the present.

And when we got to the present and my problems, Dr. Laszlo would coolly say, "I do not believe you. We will begin again. When you were eight . . ." I began to realize how suspects feel in a police question session. All that was missing was the light in my eyes (and that was soon to come). After reviewing my case from age eight enough times to have *me* questioning what my skin had been like, Dr. Laszlo looked straight at me and said bluntly, "What you are saying is not true. Miss Gabrielle, take her to the back!"

Not knowing whether "the back" meant internment or what, I meekly followed Miss Gabrielle to a blindingly white, blindingly lit, and smelling-of-something-beautiful laboratory peopled by bustling ruffle-capped assistants, all speaking in whispers. I was plopped into the examination chair and there was that bright light on my skin and Dr. Laszlo armed with a magnifying glass and having a good, long look at it. My desire to be Beautiful People almost faded right there.

The doctor pinched up the skin on the back of my hand and said, "Hmmmm. Too bad. The kind of skin that ages very early." Cheers. Then he informed me that yes, when I was eight, I had pimples on my cheeks and what is worse, "you squeezed them every one!"

It was pronounced like the death sentence. Later, I questioned my own mother about these supposed pimples and she can't remember any, either. But nothing missed Dr. Laszlo's eyes.

Right about then, I nervously declared—trying to get off that uncomfortable hook—that I was probably allergic to my new boyfriend. (Well, he did have oily skin.) Dr. Laszlo looked me straight in the eye and said, "Miss Gabrielle, write that down!" And so into my chart *that* went. Still in Hungarian. From that lame attempt at witticisms, Dr. Laszlo learned more about my character than I knew myself.

Back to his plush office we trooped—the doctor, Miss Gabrielle, and a by-now thoroughly cowed fashion reporter —and I was instructed to sit for sentencing. It was terrible, for the doctor told me, "If you believe you are allergic to my products, then I cannot give you any."

Visions of an Amanda Burden-me vanishing from my mind, I shrieked, "But I must have them! I want to be beautiful." And I begged and almost wept (really). I had been reduced, as was no doubt the doctor's intent, to a mass of jello, ready to follow any and all of his advice.

The doctor relented at last, when I swore that I would ever hereafter follow his instructions to the letter. Showing his fast analysis of my character—and the knowledge that people usually believe they can improve on a treatment by their own little personal touch—Dr. Laszlo instructed me, "In that case, you will kindly restrict your creative activities to your writing for *The New York Times* and leave your skin to me. You will never have a reaction again." And I never did. Which ought to tell you a lot about mind over skin.

From that day on, needless to say, I followed my skin regimen to the letter. If the instructions said thirty lashes of rinsing, it was thirty. No more, no less. Hot water was *hot*. Cream stayed on *exactly* the five minutes allotted it. And my skin bloomed.

The blotches disappeared. So did the broken veins (though I understand that no one is allowed to make this claim. All I can say is then you saw them, now you don't.) There were no more pimples, or blackheads, or makeup in creases at the end of the day. In fact, there were simply no more creases. My skin looked exactly the same with or without makeup. I had found beautiful-skin heaven—and I no longer had anything to hide.

One point I'd like to make "perfectly clear," before I'm accused of cosmetic-company favoritism. Dr. Laszlo's skin recipes, and his company, are now a part of that big boy, Cheseborough Ponds. I believe that the Laszlo name and products had been purchased by Ponds before I became a Laszlo patient, which is probably how they became available for public consumption in the first place. They were on the public market once before—about seventeen years ago—and I was a faithful, mail-order user at that time. But back then Dr. Laszlo discovered that he was unable to control the mail-order questionnaire bit to his perfectionist's satisfaction, so he withdrew the products immediately. Meaning that I only got about six months' good out of them before I was forced to return to the usual commercial misinformation via advertising, and therefore ended up needing Dr. Laszlo badly.

When I saw Dr. Laszlo, however, it was as my *doctor*—or perhaps I ought to say, skin specialist, for Dr. Laszlo never got his medical license to practice in this country, due, he always said, to his lack of facility with the English language (remember all that Hungarian notetaking?). I couldn't have cared less. What he did for my own skin was proof enough of his uncanny abilities.

Now Dr. Laszlo is gone. He died this year at an age, they tell me, of nearly eighty. I would have sworn to fifty-five. Miss Gabrielle has retired, and the Laszlo Institute has been removed from its mahogany-paneled "House of Silence" to sleek, new modernistic headquarters. I only recently met the Ponds people, and they are nice people, too. Only one of my old friends remains—she is Livia Inkey, who was with Dr. Laszlo for years. It is to her that I turn if problems strike (which they usually don't).

She hadn't heard my Dr. Laszlo stories until recently and, when I spoke with her last, she said that she checked out my checkered skin history on my chart. According to her, I must have a mind like a recorder. For the whole experience is now microfilm history. So if there are any skin-doubters among you, the whole thing is there—probably in Hungarian—for anyone to see.

Basic Beauty

The Laszlo life was the life for me, all right. It still is. But that doesn't mean that it's the only life. And I'm not suggesting for a moment that it *has* to be the way of skin life for you.

What I am suggesting—strongly—is that we consider together some of the basic beauty theories behind the successful Laszlo regimen (forty-some years' worth of success should count for some correct theories). I've been considering those theories for seven years now—time for me to come to a few logical, I believe, conclusions.

Obviously, Dr. Laszlo wasn't giving away his formulae —certainly not to me. And so I had to query and study and piece together what seem to be the basic points behind most successful beauty regimens. I am going to tell you all that I know. And I am again going to point out some of the unexpected slippery spots, where you may fall even though you're on the right road to good skin.

Here we go . . . on to the basics.

The pH Factor

The Erno Laszlo beauty-making technique is based on acid. That's right—on the natural acid balance of the skin.

And, while he never told me, this time he didn't need to, because all of the Laszlo products contain the letters "pH." And I was once a chemistry major, so I know that pH means a scale of acidity and alkalinity. I did not know at the time how important that acidity is to getting and maintaining perfect skin.

Did you realize that the natural state of the human body, both inside and out, is acid? (You'll see later about the state of your body inside, and I hope you'll learn something new.) Your skin, like your hair, your nails, and all of you, is protected by what is called the "acid mantle." That acid mantle is the only protection you have between your skin and all the bad bacteria that are out there in the air, just waiting to pounce on it, so you can see how important it is to make sure that nothing ever destroys the acid mantle of the skin.

Here's what California's progressive RedKen Laboratories has to say on the subject: "At birth, nature favored us with a slightly acidic mantle for the protection of our skin. This mantle, if kept in strict acid balance, will protect the inner structure of the skin from harmful bacteria. However, should this acid mantle be destroyed by the use of highly alkaline products and cosmetics, the destructive forces which cause wrinkles, infections, and other disorders of the skin, will take over and cause disastrous results."

Wrinkles, infections, and other disorders are things we are going to avoid. And the way we're going to avoid them is to test every single product that you're even thinking of putting onto your skin. I learned this little trick years ago, when I was working on a story on hair health. Now that I know that hair, skin, nails all have the same acid mantle, I merely take the same acid-precautions. There is a little packet of testing papers you can buy at your pharmacy. It is called Nitrazine, and it is similar to the litmus paper you worked with in Chemistry I. These little strips of testing paper are corn colored, and so they should remain. For that is the color of slightly acid—which is what your skin must be. The normal acidity of the skin is somewhere around 4.5—varying a bit with the oiliness of that skin. The Nitrazine paper at 4.5 will remain that yellowish color. If it turns blue, then watch out! Highly alkaline can mean highly dangerous.

If it turns purple, I think I'd leave it alone.

Cleanliness Is Next to Beauty

Whenever one goes for a treatment-visit to one of the great beauty-maker salons, the first thing one gets is a *thorough* cleansing. There is no other way to expect beautiful skin. All of the beauty-knowledgeables I have spoken with at least agree on that single fact: Clean is the beginning. And work is the continuation. But, as I told you, just get used to that sort of work. The beautiful results make it all worthwhile. And cleaning is the cornerstone for the gorgeous skin to come.

Cleaning means three little words:

Oil

Soap

Water

The oil is the tricky part. Because here is where you must learn to know your skin. You must put aside all of your preconceived notions about your skin—and stop saying it's dry when you don't really know that it is. I've already shown you that a great percentage of the so-called dry skins running about ruining themselves with unneeded creamery are not dry at all. Remember Myth No. 3 and try to look at your own skin objectively.

Some people, of course, do indeed have oily skin, and an oily skin is easy to spot. It is greasy, and that's not pretty. For, as Dr. Laszlo always said, there is a vast difference between greasy skin and dewy skin. Greasy skin can be spotted, usually, by largish pores, which run hand-in-hand with the condition. Greasy skin needs more cleaning than other skin. And it needs some of its natural oil removed, not added (we'll tell you about that later). But if oily skin is treated and cleaned properly, its overactive sebaceous glands will soon stop overacting and start behaving normally.

The sebaceous glands are, of course, those beneath your skin that produce its natural oils. Some work more, some less, some too much, and very few too little. But they almost always respond (or should do so) to a properly acid-balanced cleaning treatment. If they don't, which is unlikely, then there may be something else hidden-and-at-work. Some men, for example, have suffered for years believing they had acne, only to discover, too late, that it was ingrown beard all along. This is a good case for a dermatologist, and it's the sort of thing they're very good at spotting.

The point here is that you must begin to recognize that your skin should be kept, always, a touch on the dry side —or what you used to consider the dry side. If you ever see anything that even resembles a shine, then you will know that you must begin to dry it just a shade more. Soon you will know your own skin well, for it changes not only with the seasons, but with your moods, your health, any medications you may be taking, and you must adjust your beauty routine accordingly.

In just a moment I am going to give you a full run-down on the whys of keeping your skin on the dry side of oily. But first we will go to the next step in cleaning—soap. Did you realize that soap is the worst natural enemy of the acid mantle? It is a highly alkaline substance, although some soap is more harmful than others, some to be avoided completely.

So why are we telling you to use soap? Simple. Soap is the single best method of cleaning skin. And the point is that we aren't going to leave you at that. We're going to put the acid right back, the minute you dry your skin.

Now, many experts will tell you that your skin will revert to its natural acid state, no matter what you do to it. And so it will. But that process has been known to take as long as 3½ hours—the average is forty-five minutes— during which time your skin is left wide open to any bacteria that wish to enter. So the faster you get it back to acid, the better.

There are "soaps" being made these days that are already acid: I have not tried them on my face, for here is where I am going to let you down and not test *everything*. Laszlo saved my skin, and saved is the way I want it to remain. In spite of the fact that many of my best friends are in the cosmetics industry and are, therefore, endlessly offering me cosmetics goodies to test, I am never tempted. Once you've found perfection, why fool around?

That is what I suggest to you as well. When you get your routine going, keep it forever—changing only if your skin changes (which it will occasionally). By then, you'll know how to cope.

The cleansers that I am speaking of are high in protein, are properly acid, and, apparently, cleanse beautifully.

RedKen's Amino Pon bar is one, Jheri Redding's Milk 'n' Honee, another. There are more and more of these acid-balanced cleansing bars appearing each and every week, so check your health food store, or your local pharmacist, if he is health-oriented. Linda Clark claims that these bars work such wonders that her own mother "leaves it on all day as a skin tightener." So much for acid bars. They're here, to stay.

Last, there's water. And here's one indispensable beauty maker that comes for free. As Dr. Laszlo once said, the reason cosmetics companies are often so loath to prescribe washing is that they haven't thought of a way to make a profit out of water! Remember Laszlo's remark—the one that made him relatively unpopular with some people—about having to invent water had it not existed already. Well, he was certainly right about water's indispensability. You've got to have the water to clean with the soap, and, while we don't have to tell you where to buy it, we do have a few things to say about the kind of water-washing you must do. And so here we go beginning with oil, and taking you right through the cleaning-up routine to beautiful skin.

An Oily Trick

I've told you the oil is the tricky part. To use or not to use is definitely the question, and, since I can't see you from these pages, it will be up to you to follow my instructions on determining whether or not you need any supplemental oil before washing. Don't let anyone frighten you into making a wrong determination. I will give you plenty of expert opinion that shows that more oil is much worse for your skin than less oil. Never mind about the people who will tell you that their greasy skin will never age. It will, all right, and it will age just as ugly as it is now.

So be firm (your skin will be) and decide for yourself, following the rules of the game, whether or not you must use oil.

O.K.—you think you need it? Then I must tell you the sort to use. The acid sort, of course. I must admit that I was so cowed by my mentor, Dr. Laszlo, that I never questioned the makeup of any product. Why should I, as long as it was working beautifully? But, now that I must advise *you*, I needed to know more. And so I found out.

The Laszlo oil is, of course, made of top-secret ingredients. But the most important thing is that fatty acids are the most important ingredient. Apparently Dr. Laszlo tested plenty of oils before he came up with the one that satisfied him. And the reason it satisfied him was its high fatty-acid content.

Now, there are a great many cleansing oils on the market, probably many of which could be substituted for the Laszlo product in this routine, *as long as it checks out acid*. You could, for example, try wheat germ oil, with its extra added attraction of vitamin E. (And vitamin E, as far as I am concerned, is a beauty-maker supreme.) No medical opinion is going to back me up on vitamin E, because there is no real medical opinion, so far as I know. Doctors are doubtful, as most are about everything new unless it's drugs. There the medical profession often leaps before it looks. I have found vitamin E doing wonders for my skin, however, and wheat germ oil is one of its best sources.

Then there are the vitamin E oils—some containing, they claim, up to 28,000 units of the stuff. I am a bit leery of that, being unsure about their claims, unsure about what 28,000 units might do. You can try them if you like, but remember: at the first sign of any irritation, do as you would with anything else irritating. Forget it!

Avocado oil, cottonseed oil, corn oil, are all high in fatty acids, with olive oil being surprisingly low on the fatty acid list. But the vegetable oils are where you are going to find those fatty acids you need (*if* you do), so check out your health-food store where there's probably a cosmetics department set up with natural vegetable oils all ready for your cleansing use.

Once you've got your oil, you use it thus: Take a piece of cotton—not a cotton ball, as it's usually unnecessarily large—and soak it in the oil. Remove all of your eye makeup and lipstick with the cotton pad, and throw it away.

Take out another piece of cotton—about the size of a quarter is just right—and soak it to the dripping point. Then apply carefully to your face and neck. You should be plenty oily by now and ready to wash.

Now, with some of us, the only oil-needy spots are under the eyes and the throat. And so you simply apply the oil there and forget the rest. The soap takes care of that.

Hot Stuff

Here you are—either oiled by your own skin, or by the cotton-applied fatty-acid-filled oil, and ready to wash. Now, you know that I am hooked on what my own doctor taught me, so I will repeat it to you once more, for it seems to me to be the best possible way to wash.

You must start thinking hot (haven't you already?). Did you know—haven't I told you?—that the only way your skin can possibly receive the benefits of anything good you give it is when it is warm? For that is the moment when the pores are open to take it all in. That is the reason that the clients of most of the skin-beautifying experts I've spoken to suggest that you wash hot.

And by hot, I do *not* mean tepid. Nor do I mean that you should burn yourself. The best way to test the temperature of the water you are going to wash with is to make it just as hot as your hands can stand to be immersed in. Now your skin is delicate, all right, but believe me, if your hands can take it so can your face. It is going to feel surprisingly good, if you haven't tried it before.

The next part is the part that will, again, take some retraining of your thinking. For we are going to ask you to fill that basin with that hot water and leave it filled while you wash and rinse. This is, of course, the Laszlo method and the one I subscribe to so wholeheartedly. It seems to work, so let's use it with whatever product you've selected.

I feel a bit silly bringing it up, but you never know. I want you to make sure that your basin is clean. Meaning that if you have just done your nightly tooth-brushing, take the cleanser and give it a good scrub. We don't want any lurking household germs to get into those open pores. Sometimes getting the basin clean can be tricky—if you're someone's house guest, for example, or putting up in a hotel for the night. I will never forget having to ask my weekend hostess for a can of cleanser and waching her horrified expression when I told her it was part of my Laszlo routine. She was convinced it was to be used on my face! If you can't get hold of the cleanser, then forget filling the basin. Better to rinse with *running* hot water than to risk letting anything unpleasant get under your skin.

Now your basin is filled up with that free hot beautifier, water, and you're on your way to the next soapy step.

Lather Up

Soap—the worst enemy of the skin's natural acid mantle. And you're about to put it right onto your skin. That's right. You're going to do it because you want clean skin, for, without clean skin, you'll never have beautiful skin, and I assume that's what you hanker after.

The kind of soap, however, is, at this point, the question to answer. I've already told you I was brainwashed about my own routine, and so I never had tested any of the Laszlo products for their acidity.

You can imagine how horrified I was to dip my little strip of Nitrazine paper into my soap and find that it was turning brilliant blue. Alkaline! And very. I couldn't believe it.

Now don't believe for an instant that I stopped doing my beauty duty with that soap. Oh, no. For when I have the good results visible from all those years of using said soap, I'm not about to change a thing. Not at this stage of my skin life. But I did feel justified in asking why. And, of course, the Laszlo Institute had the answers. It seems that alkaline soaps still do the best possible job of cleaning, so Dr. Laszlo arranged to have his alkaline soap clean, and then his acid follow-up applied. Presto, acid-mantle!

There are, however, certain soaps that are to be avoided like the plague. They can literally take the hide off you. Detergents, for instance. Much too harsh for any skin that wants to stay beautiful. Deodorant soaps, *never*. These are dangerous not only to skin beauty but to you as well, for many may still contain the dangerous chemical, hexachlorophene—the same stuff that's been banned by the government as possibly deadly to newborn infants and therefore surely of some danger even to adults. A doctor warned me against deodorant soaps some twenty years ago, saying they were much too harsh for a thin skin like my own. I have, therefore, avoided them all these years. But I still see the advertisements, with new ones springing up each day, and so can only assume that somewhere out there, there are enough buyers to pay for the ads. I only hope that you're not one of them. If you are, I suggest you stop before it's too late to save your skin.

There's something else that can be irritating and that is, surprisingly, perfume. Some of the most expensive soaps on the market are highly perfumed (well, something has to justify their several-dollars-a-cake cost), and that same perfume that makes them expensive can wreak havoc with your skin—sometimes enough havoc to cause unsightly rashes and such. It happened to me, and it's a lesson I've never forgotten. So, when you're washing—your body, as well—get a soap that checks out as acid, or arrange a follow-up to acid-up all of you.

Back at the basin, you're going to wet that soap and rub it all over your face and neck, lather it between your hands and rub that lather into your skin. And then you're going to rinse. You're going to rinse a lot, right in that hot soapy water. My Laszlo routine says thirty times. Sounds like a lot, but you'll find you'll stay soapy with less. I often go more, if my face is still slippery at thirty. Here is one point where I am sure Dr. Laszlo couldn't have objected to improvisation. Less? Absolutely *never!*

There is a basic theory behind all of this. Apparently the hot, hot water stimulates your own oil glands to work so that you get the best possible moisturizer. Your own natural one. Lipids, they're called, these natural moisturizers, but do you really care as long as they show up as beautiful? And, while you're washing, you're combining the cleaning of your skin with the replacement of your skin's own natural fatty acids which, with the basin filled, are not allowed to run down and out the drain? Get the pretty picture?

By now you're clean and your skin will have a natural blush all its own. The good kind to have. The kind that makes the blood get moving, and start feeding your skin the good things you're putting into your body all the while.

And then it's back to acid, as fast as you can say "towel-dry."

Clean It Out

And while we're on the subject of a whistle-clean skin, let me pass on one recipe that I've been using for years. It won't interfere with your acid-balanced treatment (which you *must* be onto by now). What it *will* do is safely and naturally get rid of any and all awful things that might have hidden away in your pores. It's the invention of the G.O.M. of health (that's fashion-ese for "Grand Old Master"), Gayelord Hauser, and it's nothing more than an herbal laxative that is sold at practically any pharmacy. It's called "Swiss Kriss," and the ingredients are mainly dried leaves of senna, licorice root, fennel, anise, and caraway seed; dandelion, peppermint, papaya, strawberry and peach leaves, juniper berries, centaury, lemon verbena, cyani flowers, and parsley—quite a concoction, I'd say. Presumably you can whip up your own, but since this one works so well, and I'm usually so rushed, I once again lazily leave it to the lab, leaving my energies for where they're *really* needed!

Put a pot of water on the stove—about a two-quart boiler should do it—bring it to a boil and then put in a glob of Swiss Kriss. Mr. Hauser says three teaspoons, but I simply pour some in. Let the mixture brew on a low heat for about three minutes to make sure you've got essence of herb. Then remove from the flame, get yourself a towel, and cover your head with a shower cap if you have a hairdo you must save. (If you have a hairdo like mine, it won't make any difference. My no-set hair can't come un-set. Still, it might be a wise idea to try this treatment *before* your every-other-day shampoo!) Hold a towel over your head and your head over the pot and turn your face slowly from side to side for about five minutes. Make sure the towel is held so that the steam gets you right in the face!

Close your eyes, but of course. (They don't require this sort of cleaning!) Almost immediately you will find that you are, not perspiring, but *sweating*. Profusely. And that things are coming out. Just as they should be. According to Mr. Hauser, this herbalized steam is "made of the softest distilled water, soft as spring rain, and the glow in your cheeks is your own, brought there by your own red blood stream." Didn't we tell you that blood had to get to where you need it?

I will guarantee the relaxing effectiveness of this herbal sauna. I will also guarantee that plain old steam will *not* have the same effect. Don't worry. Having a natural reporter's kind of inquiring mind, I tested it. No dice. Just ordinary perspiration, not the kind of liquidating-all-evils sweat you get from this sauna.

Mr. Hauser recommends finishing it off with a splash of cold water. After learning my lesson on *that*, I finish mine off with my acid-balanced makeup regimen. *Hot* water and all. And I feel clean!

A Is for . . .

Guess what? You're all clean and ready to make very sure your skin is where it should be on the pH range. And so you're going to put on something acid.

Remember, we're obviously not talking about strong acid. We're talking about the kind of acid that comes with our old friend, cider vinegar, for example. Or lemon juice.

Now there are many new products on the beauty market, with a new one coming every day—just like a new you—and so you've fresheners and astringents galore to choose from. But first you're going to get out your trusty strip of Nitrazine and dip it into that product and make sure it never turns more than tan. That puts it safely into the protective acidity range of 4.5 to 5.5. No more, no less.

If you frequent the health-food store near you, and we hope you do, then you will no doubt find acid astringents there. If you *don't* want to buy a thing, then here's the easy answer. Let your lathery water go and wash that basin out again. (No more putting soap back onto your face.) Then fill 'er up again with fresh *hot* water, to which you add a small amount of cider vinegar. Or lemon juice, if you prefer. And then rinse all over again. And you're wearing your homemade acid mantle.

Bare Can Be Dangerous

Now that your skin is beautifully clean and blushing like a bride's (do they still?), you may think you're through with your work. You're not. For if you're one of those natural-look lovers who believes that you're giving your skin a treat by letting it go bare, forget it. Again, you're leaving it open to a lot of horrible things.

Your skin should never be left defenseless for even one red-hot (the condition your skin is in by now) moment. This means that some sort of protective skin covering is a necessity, and here's where I hit a snag. I am used to that thin-stuff makeup I once complained about so bitterly—the Laszlo treatment-foundation that is more the texture of watered-down calamine lotion than anything else I can think of.

You know I am not going to tell you that you must do it

my way. The trouble is that so many of the commercial foundation makeups available on the market today are greasy. It's Myth No. 3 at work again, and it's working harm on more skins than one imagines. Dr. Albert A. Kligman, professor of Dermatology at the University of Pennsylvania School of Medicine has submitted a paper on "Acne Cosmetica," in which he maintains that most cosmetics contain ingredients that can cause acne even on mature women. We certainly don't want to get on that hard-to-get-off-of road. As for many dermatologists' deep knowledge of skin, Dr. Kligman says: "They know damned little about it."

There are, I understand, a great many water-based foundations available. Revlon's "Natural Wonder" is one; Max Factor, I understand, makes another. Water-based sounds like a more sound foundation to build a skin on than oil, as far as I am concerned, for oil is one of the slippery spots I mentioned—one where your skin can fall and hurt itself.

It's very difficult for me to find the perfect makeup for your skin from this vantage point. Perhaps the one you are using now is perfect for you. But, before you decide it is, be sure you test it with your Nitrazine, for skin-safety's sake. My advice would be to look for the water-based, test with the Nitrazine, and avoid all makeup that smacks of oil. Grease is not the look we're after.

As for powder, which you ought to have, try to find the most lighter-than-air sort you can. And it should be practically colorless. In fact, that's a pretty sure way of making sure it's the light kind. What looks white in the box should look like no powder at all on the skin. Some theatrical makeup companies make "No-Color" face powder and many, many commercial cosmetics companies make what is called "transparent" face powder. That is the kind to head for. As for the way to apply it, I disagree with some of the makeup experts of my acquaintance. I have been told, by professional makeup artists, that the only way to apply face powder is with a brush. And I have tried the method and don't like it.

I prefer the way I was taught by Dr. Laszlo, which is to apply the face powder thickly (and here you *will* look like a clown—for exactly one minute) with a big wad of absorbent cotton. Leave the powder on for one minute and then take a *clean* piece of cotton and buff. That's right, buff. Polish your face until it shines, not with oil, but with cleanliness. It makes for a wonderfully natural, unpowdered look, but your face is further protected from the elements all the while. Only you are the wiser.

Hands Off!

During that first scary session with Dr. Erno Laszlo, I was caught red-handed in a gesture I hadn't even realized I was making. As the doctor was asking me for about the twentieth time, "When you were eight . . ." he suddenly looked at me sharply and said, just as sharply, "Stop it." Stop what? Then I realized that, as I mulled over my skin life at eight, I had been rubbing my forehead, deep in thought. It was a habit I didn't even know I had. But the doctor caught it, fast. I stopped it fast. He admonished me thus: "If you must touch something, then touch your arm where it can do no harm. But never, never touch your face again!" I have learned that lesson well, and it makes a lot of sense. For, after all, your hands are rarely as clean as your face should be—and the simple act of touching your face can deposit all sorts of harmful bacteria right where you don't need them.

So, *do* remember: *Never* touch your face for any reason at all—no matter how deep your thoughts.

And while we're talking tough, I'll remind you—although I can't imagine that you'd ever forget it—about the cardinal rule in good skin care. Should anything unpleasant ever show up on your skin—pimple, blackhead, whitehead—*do not squeeze*. If you do, you're opening your skin up to every hideous infection that's lurking out there. If you clean your skin by my methods, these things should never appear. If they do, I'm going to tell you how to stop them; but squeezing isn't the way. Hands always off!

More or Less Moisturizer

With Dr. Erno Laszlo gone, possibly the crown of skinstate belongs to his protégée and one-time pupil, Janet Sartin. Janet Sartin is a lovely lady of who-knows-whatage. (Certainly her looks don't tell you.) She began her career back in the nineteen-thirties, yet I would have guessed her age as early forties.

Ms. Sartin is the magnet that attracts the new generation of rich-and-beautiful to her quiet and competent salon. She has some devastating things to say about the world of commercial cosmetics and the horrible things women unwittingly do to their skins—such as moisturizing. "Why in the world are American women so brain-washed on moisturizers?" Ms. Sartin asked me. Don't ask *me*, for I don't understand it at all. Ever since Dr. Laszlo said to me, "So you think you have dry skin? You do not have dry skin," I just haven't had dry skin. But I rarely speak to a friend who isn't loading her skin with those moisturizers.

Janet Sartin swears that moisturizers smother the skin. And she goes wild at the idea of heavy creams. (Remember the tighten-up theory?) According to Ms. Sartin, skin is *never* dry, but its own *natural* oils may have been misused. A dry skin, says Ms. Sartin, means the outer layer is parched. (And that's what can happen when you overdo the sun. Sun is fine, in moderation, but during those hours when you want to be out there—between noon and 3 P.M. —better stay indoors. Or under a hat.) Having burned themselves to the peeling point, women invariably run for the moisturizers or the creams I mentioned before. Ms. Sartin says that the natural gravitational pull alone would be enough to make that skin sag, once its own elasticity is destroyed by weighty creams. Up up, and more up is the word for would-be-beautiful skin!

Now Ms. Sartin swears that, even with parched skin, nature's own oils are in there, trying to get out. A perfect acid balance of the skin, she maintains—achieved by the proper acid soaps and *water* (*that's* moisture)—is the answer to bringing the skin back to that condition in which it can lubricate *itself*. And, as for such severe, and unnatural, skin surgery as planing, for example—well, Ms. Sartin is horrified. According to her, *any* chemical or other kind of removal of the skin also removes the skin's vitality as well. That outer layer of skin is there, after all, for a purpose. And its purpose is protection.

So treat it carefully, balance it up, and *stay away from so-called moisturizers!* Have I made my point?

Suntanning

One more word about sun and your skin. You've probably heard all the pros and cons already. You surely know that sun is something to watch out for. Sure, it's great to tan—looks good, makes you feel good. But, if taken in improper doses, it can age you long before your time. It can give you distinctly unlovely sun spots, sometimes spots severe enough to require surgical removal. And sometimes those spots turn out to be skin cancer.

All of which should give you a pretty idea of how easy to take it when it comes to doses of Sol.

Besides all that, did you know that the very same sun that *gives* you vitamin D in the first place can work so your skin can't absorb that vitamin? For, the tanner you get, the less D your skin forms and, what is worse, the thicker your skin gets (which it most certainly does with overtanning—just think of the leathery skin you've seen at seaside resorts), the harder it is for *any* vitamin D—or any other good thing, for that matter—to be absorbed.

Even the experts have their own theories on sunbathing, for they understand the human predilection for the relaxing benefits of those lazy days by the sea. Erno Laszlo believed that sun is *not* harmful providing that you give your skin adequate protection and that you never, never take the sun between the hours of 12 noon and 3 P.M. Naturally, this is when everyone is out there, destroying all the benefits they might derive from a wiser sunbathing course of action. Janet Sartin, on the other hand, simply believes you should stay out of the sun. *I* believe that's pretty hard to do. But, on the other hand, I've seen too many erstwhile beautiful complexions wrecked by unwise sunbathing, so no matter how great it may feel for the moment, consider the consequences. And *whatever* you do, don't, repeat *don't*, think you should slather a sun-tanned skin with cream. It won't undo the damage over-tanning already will have wrought. It will just give you a leathery skin that sags down, down, down. Tan, perhaps, but ugly.

Let me also point out that a lot of exposure to the sun can eat up a lot of vitamin B. (After all, vitamin B makes the melanin—the pigment that makes you tan.) So, if you're out there, make sure you take plenty of B vitamins beforehand—so your skin is sun-planned.

Oiled from Inside

When he heard I was doing a health/beauty book, Dr. Carlton Fredericks, nutritionist and author, said, "I hope

you are going to tell those ladies that they *must eat fats*."
According to Dr. Fredericks, he receives literally hundreds
of letters from obviously unhappy non-beauties imploring
him for advice on what to do about dry hair or dry skin.
As Dr. Fredericks clearly points out, if you eliminate all
fats, how in the world do you expect to have glossy hair or
moist, young-looking skin? Instead, your hair is going to be
thatched-roof dry, and your skin more like a prune than a
ripe and luscious plum. And there is no reason to think, as
I have clearly pointed out in the Shape section, that fats
will necessarily fatten *you*. Necessary they are—both to
keeping your shape and keeping your glossy hair and
gleaming skin.

Not for a moment am I suggesting that you load up on
lard—even though the cholesterol scare has been questioned by some as being more scary than it need be. No—
what I want you to have are the good guys in fat land: the
polyunsaturates, or liquid fatty acids, that help your body
(and skin) to utilize its protein and then, as an added
attraction, beautify the rest of you. Some nutritionists even
suggest taking a tablespoonful of one of these beauty oils
each day (safflower oil is the one lowest in saturated fat.) I
personally am not mad for swallowing oil. But I do make
sure that I get a certain amount of fats every day of my
life, no matter which diet I spring for—the low carbohydrate or the low calorie. (Dieting of one sort or another
seems to be my way of life.)

And might I add that even skins with acne (which we
hope isn't yours, but even if it is, it won't be for long)
profit from the use of these unsaturated fats. Some say that
kelp, the same kelp that helps your shape, will help your
thyroid utilize and assimilate the liquid unsaturated fats.
But, of course, I believe in kelp every day anyway, for
everything, so that goes without saying.

Therefore, don't shy so much from the word "fat." It
has taken on an odious meaning it does *not* deserve. Fat is
one of the best beauty words in your beauty vocabulary!

If the Oil Is on the Outside

If you're one of those rare women who admits to having
oily skin, then the eat-fat, acid-balance routine is still for
you. For your skin has wonderfully intelligent ways of

repairing the damage you may have, unknowingly perhaps, done to it.

That hot, hot water, plus soap, plus those thirty (at least) rinses with the soapy water form an emulsion that works to balance up your skin's fatty acids and make it normal again.

Truly oily skins may need more stringent soap. Laszlo has one, Clinique has one, and the RedKen acid-balanced bar is just what it says—acid the correct way. The point here is, though, that in an acid-balanced regimen an oily skin may actually grow oilier for the first few days. Until that balance begins to get back to the 4.5 pH point.

Many of the cosmetics companies are now putting out treatment series—Laszlo may have been a pioneer, but many more have followed his leadership. Many of these treatment cosmetics are backed by a must-remain-anonymous "famous dermatologist" (each company to its own) who has worked out things to take skin types into consideration. Clinique and Etherea were two of the first commercial lines to appear with full, computer-analyzed skin treatments. Orlane has a recent computer addition in its Skin Scanner which takes imprints of your skin and blows them up for analysis. (Must be scary. Dr. Laszlo warned me against ever looking at my skin with a magnifier. I pass the information along to you—because it could set you back, and I won't have that.) Then Orlane-trained salespersons tell you what products you need. I think all of this shows that commerce is headed in the right skin direction.

I would still be wary. Wary enough to go right on testing every product with my Nitrazine paper. And I would still keep watch on my skin to make sure not an extra drop of oil appeared on its surface. Especially if your skin is already headed that way, watch it even more closely, and don't defend it with that "I'll never wrinkle" routine. If you keep up your oiling inside, your acid-balanced cleansing outside, and your hands off, your skin should shape up shortly.

Meanwhile, if—just *if*—something unpleasant pops out and you want to get rid of it in a hurry, telephone your druggist and ask for calamine lotion with phenol. Now be sure to get the ready-mixed variety, for phenol is carbolic acid, and that's too strong stuff for your face unless you plan to be Scarface. The kind the druggist has already mixed is perfectly safe and many a beauty swears by it for emergency measures. Which I hope you'll never need.

Here's Mud on Your Face

Not in your eye, where it won't help a thing. Mud, apparently, has some miraculous healing properties. A pretty good guess would be that those healing properties come from the mud-minerals. Primitive peoples have been healing their wounds with mud for centuries.

Mud baths have long been spa-favorite pamperers. Now mud is turning up more and more in the sometimes weird world of cosmetics, and it seems to do its best work on skin that goes toward oily.

An enterprising young lady named Lynn Beck became fascinated by the beauty secrets of Berber women while she was traveling in the Sahara. She was clever (or charming) enough to find out what those secrets were. One was something called "Rassoul"—a blend of earth found only in Morocco. Ms. Beck claims that it can be used not only as a facial mask which is supposedly deep-cleaning, slightly astringent, but as a shampoo as well.

Down-to-Earth is Arizona mud—discovered, quite by accident, by an ex-airline executive, George F. Denbow, Jr., who just happened to own eighty acres of that mud. Having nothing better to do with eighty acres of mud, Mr. Denbow decided to investigate the local ranchers' stories that the mud had healing properties, and that the Indian women of the region used it for cleaning their faces and hair. So Mr. Denbow experimented on his teen-aged children's problem skin—and the problems disappeared. Here again, the claims are that the minerals in the mud are the doers.

i Cosmetics, a health-oriented beauty product place in New York City, gives you English Clay—and it's called just that—which, i claims, does the same mud good. Mineral magic doing its beauty bit.

All of the mud products that are available commercially have been tested by the FDA and declared safe. They have also been filtered, cleansed, de-bacteria-ed, because I most certainly would not recommend that anyone put just plain dirt on her face. *Please!*

There is one more thing to watch about mud. It is highly —yes, very—alkaline. Which means that, should you choose to try it, you must remember to follow whatever directions the jar, or bottle, give you. But don't keep the mud in your basin. Wash it off and down the drain, and then follow with thirty hot slaps of your cider vinegar or lemon rinse.

As for not-so-oily skins—I think I'd steer clear of mud.

Skin Self-Destruction

There are plenty of ways we work at destroying our skins. Probably without even realizing it, for I can't imagine that anyone would *want* bad skin. The lives we lead, however, contribute a lot to the breakdown of a perfect skin performance.

Pills, for example, on which America spends $8,000,-000,000 per year. That's eight billion, you're right! And *the* Pill is apparently one of the very worst skin-offenders. The manager of the *i* Cosmetics shop in New York told me that she'd seen more really good skins ruined by the birth control pill than by any other single element. I wouldn't know, as I can't take the thing, and I don't want to. For I agree that the birth control pill is an unnatural disturbance of the body's hormonal system, and I don't like to fool around with anything quite that unnatural. If it's your thing, then it's your affair, of course. But I do believe you ought to be warned that less than beautiful skin may be the birth control pill's result. As for tranquilizers—they can cause real dryness and, what is more dangerous, an intolerance to the sun. Years ago, it happened to me and it was a pretty horrifying experience—real sun poisoning after only a few hours in a Florida sun. It's a relatively standard reaction if you mix sun and tranquilizers.

As a general rule, any of those $8,000,000,000 worth of pills—unless they're vitamins—are not going to do your skin any good and can do it a great deal of harm. Give it some thought, the next time you're about to pop an unnecessary aspirin.

Do You Still Believe It's Your Glands?

The last time I saw Dr. Laszlo as a patient was after I'd committed an unpardonable skin-sin. You see, I'd decided

I was too fat (which I was) and, thinking that I was dieting—since I didn't have the chart I'm going to give you—and still not losing any weight, I convinced both myself and my doctor that it must be my glands. (You see how easy it is to make excuses for one's own dieting ignorance?) And so I persuaded that doctor to give me thyroid medication.

I have already told you that my PBI (still stands for Protein Bound Iodine, in case you tuned in late) is at the lowest possible point on the normal scale. I used that as a convenient excuse for, I hoped, weight loss without work. And I most assuredly got what was coming to me. Acne is what I got. Or, if it wasn't acne, it was close to it, and this time it didn't require a magnifier and Dr. Laszlo to see the pimples on my cheeks. By now I was much older than eight—old enough for acne not to happen.

I was horrified when I saw it blossom, then terrified when it refused to go away. Naturally I rushed to the phone and tearfully (literally) described my hideous face to Miss Gabrielle who came up with some emergency measures for momentary help, and arranged for an appointment with the doctor. This time the appointment was going to be on me, but by then the $75 seemed minimal, in spite of my tiny bank account. For I was truly frightened of what had happened to my hitherto healthy complexion.

When I told the doctor about the thyroid medication, his attitude was one of total scorn. In his customary no-nonsense manner, he informed me that I was indeed too fat, and that I was too fat because I ate too much—not because of my glands. He followed that up with the statement that "I am sure you forced your doctor to give you those pills." He was right, of course. "Forced" is probably not quite the word, as my doctor is a strong-willed sort of man. "Wheedled" would be more accurate. The fact is I got them, by *my* will, and it should show you what can happen when you try to play doctor—even with your own doctor's possibly innocent cooperation.

Dr. Laszlo fixed me up fast. By taking me off the thyroid medication immediately, putting me back on the right road to good skin, and warning me once again about getting creative with medicine. He was right again. And when I tried to pay my bill, Dr. Laszlo gently removed me from his office by my elbow, and said to me in his best Transylvanian accent, "I do not need the money that badly. Besides, I will never see you again." And he didn't have to. My lesson in self-help was well learned. Don't ever try it!

Stimulation Your Skin Doesn't Need

When it's a matter of skin beauty, any *over*stimulation is bad. Except, perhaps, the sexual sort, for the sexual flush is real, medical fact, not phallic fantasy, and it works its wonders in getting the vitamin-filled blood up to the surface where it looks beautiful. We all know that blushing is good for the skin. So is the sexual flush. So is sex, and I'll say it often.

But other unnatural stimulants, such as too much coffee, too many cigarettes, and too much booze taken with too little sleep and too much tension, are wrinkle-making skin-wreckers that you neither need nor want. Your own vitamin-earned vitality should be stimulant enough for you.

The coffee can put your blood sugar down to sub-healthy, where it can wreak havoc with all of you. The cigarettes can eat up the vitamin C you must have for beautiful healthy skin. And the booze? Maybe it's because I gave it up entirely, but I'll keep hammering home the fact in every chapter of this book: Booze is bad. For your shape, for your hair, for your skin, for you. A beautiful boozer is still a dream (and a bad one at that). So if you want your skin to be oiled from the inside, manufacturing its own perfect moisturizers, then don't *you* get oiled. Alcohol is drying, both inside and outside of you. Unless you want to shrivel up your skin, stay off the juice.

Fresh Paint

If you want to know about makeup, you're probably asking the wrong person if you ask me. You see, I'm not particularly talented with my own. I am concerned with the state of skin, not what's brushed onto it. There are, thank goodness, scores and scores of experts who do know, and talented they are indeed. And there are scores of books on the subject, as well. There's a new one out on television makeup called—not surprisingly—*Film and Television Make-Up*. Whether you plan to make television your career—which is possible for some, but not probable for most—there are great tricks to learn with paint.

I myself have watched fashion models transform themselves before my very eyes with sticks and jars and sponges and colors of every hue. They can make eyes appear where they disappeared before, and noses or chins disappear when they were not as neat as they ought to have been. These models are so talented at their craft that I once stood at a store counter next to a model with whom I'd worked constantly and never even recognized her until she gave a salesgirl her passport for identification and the salesgirl read the name aloud. I was shocked and could only query, "Is it you?" For without her makeup, this girl, who was one of the reigning models of her day, had no face at all. I mean it was bland, characterless, and completely unnoticeable. But let her draw it on with paint, and in front of the lights, she came off superstar.

The important thing to remember is that you *must* protect your skin carefully before you start to paint. If your skin is wearing its protective, acid-balanced armor, then no amount of paint—assuming it is paint that is meant to be used on skin—can harm it.

One famous fashion model informed me that Dr. Laszlo (yes, the same) had saved her skin from the destruction it was getting from all the heavy makeup she was forced to use to look the way fashion models are supposed to on camera. Beautiful, elegant, bone-structured. (And for your information, plenty of a model's bone structure is the result of a clever paint job. In a photograph, it shows up real.) She was getting lines before her time, blemishes on a previously clear-as-crystal skin. Fortunately, models make money—lots of it—and this young lady was able to afford frequent private consultations with the doctor. After her skin was gotten into its perfect condition, and her protective preparations put on *first*, then the theatrical makeup could not work its legendary skin harm.

There are, however, a few things about makeup I've learned on my own. One important fact is that, the older you get, the less makeup you should wear. Sounds incredible, but it is quite the fact, for trying to pretend that we don't all get older *sometime* is absurd. But trying to hide it with a lot of paint is going to make you look like Methuselah's mother. I have discovered that I take it off as I go along. I have never seen a woman over forty who didn't do better with less, rather than more, makeup.

The only possible exception would be lipstick. It seems to my fashion reporter's eye that lipstick works the other way around. For a woman of, say, fifty, to try to get away with the teenage bare-mouth, big-eyed face would only look ridiculous. (It's going out of fashion anyway.) And by this, I don't mean she needs a bright red slash of a mouth or a forties kind of "camp" black lipstick. What I mean is she needs color. I guess what I really mean is that woman should look like woman, and a child can get away with whatever she wants.

As for the eyes having it . . . well, they're not getting as much these days, thank goodness. The Cleopatra look with the hard-edged black line drawn around the eye is definitely gone, although there are many more exciting ways to paint up the eyes. And it can be fun. So do as you like here but beware of one thing, for your eyes' sake: The moment a product burns your eyelids, take it off just as fast as you can. Remember, you have no protection there. The eyelid is one of the most sensitive areas of the body, and it is there for the protection of your eyes. Don't you forget that.

That is the reason you must be extremely careful about what goes on that eyelid. The eyelid can absorb things, right into your eyes, and occasionally those things can be dangerous. Beware of sunscreens, for example, that were meant for your nose, perhaps—your eyes, *never*. There are many substances that are good sunscreens, but contain substances that present a very real danger to the eyes—a danger that could result in blindness. So if the label says, "not to be used near the eyes," then don't think they're kidding.

One more warning about eye products. Be wary of the ones that you may buy abroad—or that a friend may have given you. I know of a fashion model who used fashionable French eyedrops to whiten her eyes. And all was well until the whites of her eyes turned blue and remained that color forever. This is a true story and is meant to frighten you. These drops have since been removed from the market, even in France. But that won't help this model's ruined career—or her ruined appearance. So beware of foreign products for the eyes, and, if in doubt, do the usual—check with your eye doctor. He will know.

The Dermatological Question

As for dermatologists—sorry, doctors, but I'm going to say what I think. You're great when it comes to skin diseases—there we couldn't make it without your medical expertise. But after skin-problem years of unnecessary, and possibly dangerous, X-ray treatments, and more years of being told such things as to wash my face with tar soap or live on antibiotics—well, quite frankly, I'd feel more comfortable if the dermatologists kept their hands off my face. And I've finally found a dermatologist who's good-doctor enough to agree with me. He is Dr. Albert M. Kligman, professor of dermatology at the University of Pennsylvania in Philadephia. I love him for not being uptight about the fact that dermatologists know a lot about everything except complexions.

Recently, Dr. Kligman gave a talk before the Fashion Group in New York in which he maintained that dermatologists actually are an insecure crowd when it comes to beauty maintenance. To them, it's a medical put-down, and, says Dr. Kligman, they are terrified someone might identify them with "cosmetologists." And, claims Dr. Kligman, the very worst thing to say to a dermatologist is "You're lucky . . . your patients never die." Apparently, it sends them into a flurry of defensive descriptions of their terminal disease patients.

But Dr. Kligman believes, as I do, that a good complexion is important to everyone, man or woman. For one thing, it has a pretty important effect on the state of your mental health. I know a tremendously successful business executive who is not only a dashing-looking man, but cuts an equally dashing swathe with the ladies. Yet this man still feels ugly, thanks to the emotional scars left behind by a teen-age case of acne. It's a common thing, and one important enough not to sweep under any dermatological rug.

Dr. Kligman claims that, if a patient comes to him complaining about a pimple, or a wrinkle, he listens and acts accordingly, feeling that this pimple or this wrinkle is important to his patient and, therefore, to him. And, as one skin-knowledgeable pointed out, "Whose ego can be 'up' with a pimple at the end of her nose?"

I have found, in my checkered medical career, that the dermatologist question is much like the G.P. versus the diet doctor. That is why I would choose either a cosmetically oriented dermatologist—and they are growing in number, I hear, although I have yet to meet one—or an exceptionally careful, medically oriented skin specialist. But I would be very careful in any case. There is a book called *The Skin Game* by Colette Dowling. Get it and read it if you want some frightening facts about who is out there doing what to skins. And sometimes killing patients in the process.

My advice would be to stay well away from any person, or doctor, who recommends anything that sounds like harsh treatment for the skin. The skin is delicate and should be treated like a blossom not to be broken—really. If X-rays or dermabrasion or hot-ice packs are recommended to you, then here's where I'd suggest you depart the premises to consider. Unethical doctors, unfortunately, do exist and they can put the onus on the good ones.

Now that I've doubtless infuriated the dermatologists to the extent that I'll never be able to see one again, let me say that dermatologists are the only people to see when something that looks tentatively dangerous turns up on your skin—pre-cancerous rough spots, for example. These must be removed by electric needles, occasionally by the knife, and for that you require nothing less than a licensed physician.

In this chapter my intention is not to "put down" dermatologists as a crowd. Far from it. I adore my own and he has removed a lot of that pre-cancerous sun damage I did to my own skin before I learned my lessons, but good.

It's just that dermatologists, like Dr. Kligman says, often don't find that one wrinkle any more important than your doctor found that one pound too many.

So when it's cosmetics beauty of the skin you want, turn to just the sort of person I'm recommending here. If it's a disease you think you have—psoriasis or anything of the sort—or any growth that looks suspicious, see your dermatologist at once. You will need him.

You're Protein

Now that we've gone through the basics on the outside, how about the basic things to put *inside*—inside your stomach—to help make that beautiful skin. The first basic to remember is that you *are* protein. Your skin is protein, your nails are protein, your hair is protein; and so protein is what you're all about.

Stands to reason, doesn't it, that protein is what you'd better get if you're going to have all parts of your beauty system "go." In the diet section, I've warned you against equating protein with meat. There is protein and there is protein, and there is as much protein in a cubic inch of cheese as in a normal serving of rib steak. You must learn to think of protein not only in terms of meat but in terms of eggs, cheese, milk, and many vegetables such as lima beans. Then there's fish—as full of protein as meat, and about half as fattening. I suggest again that you check out that paperback book by Frances Moore Lappé—the one called *Diet for a Small Planet*. It will tell you as much about protein as you could possibly digest.

The fact I want well-digested is that since you *are* protein you need protein, both in you and on you (as you will soon see). It would most likely be very difficult for you to get too much protein, although my doctor says that he has treated fanatical weight lifters who put themselves on such rigid all-protein diets, hoping to get those muscles bigger, that they end up with real health complications. Of course, my doc maintains they dose themselves with weird things along the way, as well.

Unless you're planning something silly like that, the chances are very slim that you'll ever be eating more protein than your body can utilize, and the chances are very fat that you're eating less. So eat all the protein you can—a minimum of fifty-six to eighty grams per day—depending on your size, your reference, and whether you're female and smaller, or hunky husband and bigger. Besides food protein, there are the protein supplements available today. Use them.

There are all sorts of good things in health food stores—and, to their credit, most supermarkets now have health food departments. There are protein powders to be mixed with your milk, protein from soybeans, from fish, from meat. Just remember your check-the-label training, though, and—if you're dieting to shape up your body as well as your skin—remember to add up those calories or carbohydrates. Otherwise, you have the go-ahead light on protein.

Don't believe for a moment, however, that egg on your face can be absorbed as the protein you need for your skin. The cosmetics folk are hard at work on it. So far, the best they've come up with are creams (watch it!) made of protein that do their beauty work by keeping your own natural moisture in your skin—in other words, making that natural moisturizer we talked about really work. But the protein molecules are not absorbed by the skin. Nobody claims *that*, that I know of. At least, they haven't said so to me.

There are the traditional egg-white masks that not-too-young actresses use for a performance-length face lift under their makeup. That's a temporary tightener and we've already worked on getting your skin permanently and naturally tightened. So forget the egg-on-the-face recipes and concentrate on putting that egg inside of you where it can do some real beauty good.

Lovely Liver

"Uggggh!" you say. Then, my would-be beauty, you'd better re-educate yourself. For liver, especially in its dried (what is called desiccated) form, is the easy-to-swallow route to the most beautiful, luminous, and translucent skin in the world. Not to say that real live liver isn't. You bet it is. But I wouldn't want it for breakfast, lunch, and dinner and I doubt that you would, either. And that's about how often you ought to be getting your desiccated liver into skin circulation. (By the way, if you're on the low-carbo-hydrate diet as well, where organ meats are not permitted, desiccated liver remains well below the allotted carbohydrate limit. No excuses there!) Desiccated liver is a gold mine of beautiful B vitamins; Linda Clark calls it a "wonder food." According to Mrs. Clark, liver probably contains more nutritional value than any other single food. It has a rich supply of vitamin B-12, which you may know well, since doctors often give it as quick-energy shots. (Remember what we said about doctors bearing shots! Even B-12 is better taken naturally as it appears with the other B vitamins; thus, the better nutrition of B-12 in liver.)

Desiccated liver is whole liver from which the connective tissue and fat have been removed and which has been dried at a low temperature, so that the vitamins are not destroyed.

Linda Clark tells of a woman with gorgeous skin and hair who told her, "I eat plenty of liver. It feeds and nourishes my skin and hair from the inside." She maintains that both were drab before she learned the beauty secret of liver. Now she downs thirty tablets of desiccated liver daily and apparently the radiance of both skin and hair are noticeable to all.

One of the most amusing liver tales I've heard was told by Adelle Davis in her book, *Let's Eat Right to Keep Fit*. It concerns a young man finishing his doctorate at the University of California who consulted Miss Davis because of extreme fatigue. Her suggestion was that he eat, temporarily, a half-pound of liver daily for breakfast. Through a misprint, the young man believed he was to eat *two* pounds of liver each morning. Miss Davis received the following doggerel:

My dear Adelle, it is plain hell to follow your directions
But I do try hard, avoid all lard and all the fine confections.

There is much to encourage and much to intrigue,
So much to be grateful for this lack of fatigue.

With devotion to you and in spite of my pride . . .
One thing that I can hardly abide

Is rising each morning at the clang of the clocks
    And facing the white vastness of the icebox
I withdraw with fright and begin to shiver
    On seeing that mountain of slippery liver.

But once it is down, my eyes open wider,
And I can drink deep of the milk from the tiger.

Shades of *Rosemary's Baby*, but I am sure that Miss Davis was quick to soothe this young man's queasy stomach with the *proper* dried liver prescription!

Well, I can promise you: Raw liver for breakfast is not on *my* prescription list. But the desiccated kind is, indeed. I take tons of it myself and, on a recent trip home, my very own *family* (and you know how *they* never notice) said, "Your skin looks *fantastic!*" That was beautiful.

The Never-Never Skin Foods

There are, of course, foods that are so anti-skin that they must be placed on your never-never list forever and ever. They are so basically bad, not only for skin but for your general well-being, that you may have already learned (possibly the hard way) to avoid them.

One bad teen-age experience with skin breakouts probably taught you that chocolate is a number one trouble-maker for skin. If anyone, including any dermatologist, tells you otherwise—shake him. For you will find hundreds of other equally expert dermatologists who will assure you that chocolate is indeed injurious to beautiful skin. If you're a chocolate addict, then I suggest you try carob powder as a chocolate-tasting substitute. Just to show you that commerce is getting health-conscious, or else health-conscious has become commercial, one can even buy ice creams these days, flavored with carob. I never thought I'd see the day.

White sugar, refined flour, and any and all overprocessed foods are horrifically drying to the skin. They won't do your health any good either. But I've lectured you on the horrors of that sort of eating in the Shape section. I just want to make sure you remember.

Olives are terrible for skin that tends to be oily—as most problem skin is—and so, naturally, are such greasy foods as French fries. By now you won't be eating those anyway, but I might as well mention this one more time. Greasy fried foods do not a pretty complexion make.

Then, oddly enough, you may add mustard, along with most hot-and-spicy condiments, as being too stimulating for a complexion that is less than perfect. Even if it is perfect, you should handle these with care.

And Drinks

Then there are the drinks. Cola beverages—yes, the diet kind as well—are just plain bad. And they're going to make your skin break out if you don't watch out. For your beauty regimen can't do it all—you still have to eat with the care you've learned to have by now. And you must work at eating well just as hard as you work at all the rest. Beauty never comes easy.

Too much of any sort of stimulant is definitely out. Coffee, tea, and (I'm afraid to say it again) alcohol are all detrimental and should always be avoided in excess. Avoid altogether if there's a skin problem already present.

Check the chart for the really good foods that contain the vitamins and minerals that are good for you. And then choose from that list when it's menu-making time. I've deliberately included the bad foods in my chart as well— just so you can see for yourself how worthless they really are.

Vitamin A, the Skin Vitamin

I have discovered, to my disbelief, that there are still people out there—would-be beauties—who are not taking vitamin A. I suppose that I live in a rarefied vitamin atmosphere, for I always thought that virtually everyone who aspired to beautiful skin knew the beautiful skin value of A. It's as basic as the B vitamins, something that no one should be without if that one wants to live up to her beauty potential.

A friend of mine put me onto the non-A-takers recently when she asked for advice on her skin. This friend is a young girl with beautiful bones and not-so-beautiful skin. I knew that she was well into the acid-balanced routine I'd suggested for her, so I couldn't imagine what could be missing. The reason I couldn't imagine is that I am still amazed to learn that the vitamin-uneducated are about in great numbers, usually complaining about their looks. (If that sounds like you read on.)

I asked this almost-perfect-beauty about her vitamins. She replied that she's a naturalist (so, who isn't?) and doesn't believe in them. Perhaps that's why a gentleman of our mutual acquaintance said to me recently, "What is it about her that keeps her just short of beautiful?" I couldn't reply.

For naturalists who scorn vitamins, let me say that I, too, prefer food vitamins. It would be wonderful if we could get *enough* of them—but we can't. Not by food alone. I'll grant you that the vitamin A that comes from cheese and carrots and all those good things you love to eat is probably much more potent than what comes in a capsule. But if you check my chart *carefully*, you'll see just how much food you'd have to eat to get the amount of units you'll need for beauty. I take 50,000 units a day. That's a lot of food A any way you look at it.

Now there has been a great deal of discussion, dissension, and investigation of late on the amount of vitamin A that we are going to be allowed, by government regulation, to take. And I am going to go along with them and say that too much vitamin A can be dangerous.

The reason is that vitamin A is an oil-soluble vitamin, meaning that it can have a build-up effect inside of your body. It is not thrown off by your body with its wastes, as are the water-soluble vitamins such as C (that's why C has to be replenished each and every day, or each and every cigarette, for example). Therefore, it is conceivable that there might be some danger if one were to try one's own improvised recipes with vitamin A. There *is* danger and I strongly advise you not to think about playing around with it.

But, for myself, 50,000 units seems the norm needed to keep my skin looking top shape. I wouldn't dream of reducing that dosage, for since I've been taking it for some fifteen years now, with no ill effects, I cannot imagine that it's harmful to me. But now I must get my vitamin A by prescription only. One can't buy 50,000 units of vitamin A in any other way. Thank goodness my own physician is a vitamin-believer. Otherwise I would simply take two of the 25,000 units, were I denied my fifties.

If you are just starting your vitamin habit, perhaps you should start with a lower A-count and work your way up until you see your skin improve. Just never, never dream of going above the top level I have given you. And don't even hit *that* without your prescription firmly in your hand.

While you're shopping for A, you might keep one other thing in mind. There are two kinds of A—the oil-miscible sort and the water-miscible sort. "Miscible" is a word that gets me when it comes to definition, and I will be slightly inaccurate by calling it "water-based," but I believe that's close enough for those of us who don't aspire to the scientific calling. The oil-based, fish-liver kind of vitamin A is fine for some people. (Remember cod liver oil?) But for others who may have skin that is already too oily, the water-miscible vitamin A is a wiser choice. After all, why add oil to an already overactive sebaceous sytem? Check your druggist. He'll know what to give you.

Vitamin D—The Other Skin Vitamin

And how could it be called anything *but* a skin vitamin? One of the few places you'll find vitamin D is *on your skin*. Because a combination of sunshine and skin actually makes vitamin D. So there! You see, your oil glands secrete a substance (ergosterol is its name) which is transformed right there on your skin into vitamin D—by the magical action of sunlight. And then, that good little D is health-fully reabsorbed into your skin, which is why you feel so good after a day at the beach. (Assuming, of course, that you've been wise enough *not* to overdo it. Better to take your D in pill form than to risk *irreversible* damage to your skin by the ultraviolet rays of the sun.)

The reabsorption of vitamin D is one reason why sea-soned sun-bathers say it's no good showering immediately after you sunbathe unless you want to wash away all the benefits of the beautiful skin-vitamin D. And if you must wash, make the water *cold*. (Never cold on your face. *Never*.) Where I come from—near the sunny, Southern beaches—the story goes that hot water makes the suntan go back in and not out there on your skin where you want it to show!

There are, of course, *some* foods that include vitamin D, but they are few. Check my chart—not much, right? That's exactly why it's always called the "sun vitamin." There is *some* vitamin D to be found in egg yolks, providing, as Adelle Davis picturesquely puts it, the hens sat in the sunshine (which they're never allowed to do these days, need I remind you) and preened their feathers well. If, Miss Davis says, you ate 50 to 200 eggs a day—well, you might get enough vitamin D by this method. Also, fish liver oils contain vitamin D (remember that cod liver oil again —the kind your mother used to force-feed you?). Still, be careful of this version if your skin tends to be oily. Caviar contains vitamin D, too, if you're on a rich kick. And some is found in the magic mushroom. Well, not *that* kind—it's only magic-seeming, since mushrooms are grown in the dark. So how did the sun vitamin get in them?

The best way to get vitamin D is still to get plenty of healthy sunshine. Healthy, we said. Don't overdo it! Alligator skin is not beautiful.

If you're going to get the dosage most nutritionists feel is minimal (some 20,000 units per week) then you'd better opt for the pill—the D pill—but get vitamin D somehow, for D is essential for helping you assimilate the calcium you need for virtually every good part of you. (That's why that good old sun is so relaxing. Calcium plus D—the natural tranquilizer.) There was once a television commercial about that that showed a terribly loving couple on a sunny beach while the voiceover soothingly said, "Warm climates make warm people." Calm ones, too, we might add.

Vitamin B

Vitamin B is so basic to beauty that I cannot conceive of any would-be beautiful person not taking plenty of it. In the final section of this book, you will find more and more about vitamins and how complex they can be—especially B, the most complex vitamin of all. There are so many parts to vitamin B, with more turning up every year, that it is difficult to break it down. Thank goodness, for I want you to learn to take it as complex as it comes, meaning take a B-complex capsule to keep on the safe side of the right proportions. In the final chapter, I will give you the experts' guidelines (you can always read ahead if you're curious) on the proportions to take to keep the B's working properly for your health and your beauty. When you've studied the situation further, you will also learn to study the labels on that vitamin B-complex and learn to choose the one that most closely matches the proportions suggested. I have seen enough empty B-complex capsules advertised (usually on "special sale") to know that many are practically worthless. Even on "sale," you're still paying for nothing.

But B is the Big-Beauty-B. It simply helps everything. It nourishes your skin, soothes away tension lines. It makes your thyroid make that luminous skin we talked about. So get hold of some B and take plenty, and then remember to leave off that bad B—booze—because alcohol thrives on B vitamins. It literally eats them alive, so that if you're thinking of drinking, you'd better load up on extra B. Better still—just lay off booze.

One more aspect of vitamin B that I didn't know until recently: When you're suntanning, you're losing your B vitamins all the while. I would suggest that you down an extra B-complex capsule before you head for the beach.

And never forget that basic B is beautiful.

Vitamin C

If you don't have enough vitamin C, your skin will know it. And show and tell. For a deficiency of vitamin C, the vitamin that can do a lot more than cure a common cold, will show up in ugly bruises that happen when an accident hasn't. In other words, your skin will be so delicate that a light touch can bruise it. (And some touches should remain your little secret.)

Not only that, a lack of C can give you a spotty suntan —ugly skin, indeed. Vitamin C is essential to the proper functioning of your thyroid, and your thyroid is one of the things that must be in good working order if you're going to have that porcelain skin you dream about. Remember my own experience with the improper thyroid medication and the distinctly un-beautiful acne that resulted. It would have been so much simpler for me and all of my doctors had I stuck to vitamins.

Now much has been written of late about megadoses of C as the cure for the common cold. Such scientific luminaries as Linus Pauling have recommended _enormous_ dosages of vitamin C—too enormous for me, I have to admit, unless I _do_ feel a common cold coming on, in which case I run for the ascorbic acid. For this synthetic form of vitamin C is the one that works on the common cold—the cold that works to give you an ugly red nose and, therefore, will be avoided. The natural vitamin C with bioflavanoids and rutin (found in the peel of citrus fruits, which is why you should always eat that part of the fruit; if you throw the peel away—or, at least, the pithy part close to the peel—you're putting the vitamins in the garbage) are the C-kind to take for beauty maintenance. They work best on the long runs.

I would say the best dosage for beauty would be anywhere from 1,500 to 2,000 units per day, but here again you must watch yourself carefully for any uncommon reactions. Vitamin C has been known to make rashes on some people—usually on the same people who have allergic reactions to citrus fruits. If you see anything peculiar happening, then, cut back the dose, but make sure you have your C, and daily. For C is one of those water-soluble vitamins that disappears and needs to be replenished every day of your life.

One thing you smokers ought to know: Every time you light that cigarette you are using up 25 milligrams of vitamin C. Perhaps that is why skin experts universally go against smoking as bad for the skin . . . drying, wrinkle-making, generally beauty-detrimental. That's 25 milligrams per smoke, 500 milligrams per pack. Therefore, if smoke you must, at least put back the vitamin C your smoking pleasure is destroying.

If I were you, I'd watch out for smoking. It's a real beauty-killer as well as a possible you-killer.

Vitamin E

Vitamin E has been called plenty of names—some good, some curious. It is, beyond doubt, the vitamin of the 1970s, and it will probably be in the 1970s that the true worth of vitamin E is determined.

As yet, we haven't learned everything about vitamin E by a long jump. (Do we ever learn *everything* about anything?) However, I have seen some of the beautiful skin action of vitamin E, and so can at least attest to my eyesight (which is good). One of the great beauties of this country, a woman with a baby's skin, regularly downs a dosage of 1,200 units of E per day. I happen to know her real age, which is closer to fifty than the twenty-odd she looks. Of course, I can't attribute all of her youth to E. For years I've been trying to pry her beauty secrets out of this friend, but women can be terribly evasive about such things, and so I only found out the E-dosage when she agreed to be interviewed (not by me—but there was a press leak there) for a beauty-and-health article; and I do know that vitamin E is noted for its supposed anti-aging merits.

Therefore, I'd wager a guess that it has a lot to do with this beauty's seemingly agelessness.

A lot of other skin claims have been made for vitamin E. Some E-fans claim that vitamin E can stop the formation of scar tissue. On a recent television interview program, Dr. Carlton Fredericks told who-knows-how-many viewers that vitamin E applied directly to some skin wounds had completely avoided the formation of such scar tissue. According to Dr. Fredericks, application of vitamin E topically (meaning directly onto the skin) may actually retard healing but does make for less hard scars when the healing finally comes.

I myself tried this treatment when I had some rather unappealing moles removed from my face. I never thought of them as so unappealing until the dermatologist I had gone to interview asked, "Well, do you believe they improve your looks?" He had me there, so I let him take them away. And there I was, with about ten plastic bandages dotting my face, looking like the victim of some sort of accident. And when the bandages come off, there were ugly red spots *in their* places.

This seemed the right time for me to do my own personal testing of E-power. I always keep the 400 I.U.'s of E handy, so I simply sliced one open with a razor blade and patted (don't rub!) the honey-colored, sticky liquid from the capsule onto each one of those scars, let it dry, and waited. This procedure was repeated every night at bedtime, and at the end of ten days there wasn't a scar in sight. For me, it worked.

Vitamin E also has other unpredictable qualities. It is, seemingly, a powerful bacteria-inhibitor. A large pharmaceutical company recently came up with a deodorant made primarily from vitamin E, and then almost as quickly removed it from the market because of complaints that it irritated the tender underarm area. However, with the sort of redhead skin I possess—the kind that's irritated by even the anti-allergy sort of cosmetics—I feel that if E were irritating to skin, mine would have been the first to notice.

Vitamin E, when let out of its captive capsule, is in a slight sticky liquid—somewhat comparable to honey in both color and texture—and it can do the same things honey has traditionally done, namely, tighten up. I tried it on those fine little lines that appear under your eyes if you've been overworked (which I always have been) or trying the candle-at-both-ends life. It worked for me. I still use the 400-unit capsule and I pat and never rub. As the liquid dries, it tightens as well and smooths away all those lines of fatigue.

Linda Clark gives an exciting and graphic description of the way vitamin E works to erase lines from the skin. She got together a group of men and women, herself included, and for approximately four weeks, the group experimented with the vitamin-E-on-the-skin treatment, used twice daily. The only difference between their experiment and my own was they used a 200-unit capsule, twice, rather than 400 once. At the end of four weeks, Mrs. Clark collected the reports and they were, she says, "enthusiastic." According to her, crepey skin was tightened and lines disappeared. In short, instant, unsurgical facelift—quite an experiment.

As usual, the medical profession seems reluctant to conduct such vitamin E experiments. And the FDA—those same friendly fellows who brought you filth in food and allowed excrement in your flour—apparently don't want E on your face. Not egg—vitamin E. Or, rather, if it goes into a product destined for your face, no claims can be made for it. Same thing as not allowing it, in my publicity book. Because, if you can't tell the public what something does, how likely are they to get the message?

Let us just admit freely that too many folk are leaping onto the E bandwagon these days, in my opinion—only because E is (they believe) the magic letter in beauty. Not much is known, therefore not much can be disproven. All I have to go on for my observations as to the skin benefits of E is just that—my own observations plus the observations of such sharp-eyed professionals as Adelle Davis and Linda Clark. (Much as I admire medical men, I find they often take more extreme care with something that smacks of what they consider "food-faddism"—meaning, in my book, plain old common sense—and less extreme care with delivering prescriptions for drugs that are far from tried and true.)

Whatever the FDA is thinking E-wards, it is permitting E to be used in creams, oils, lotions, soaps—you name it. It's usually called E. But I still believe that the simplest solution to E treatment is to try the direct application to scars, small lines—anything you'd like to clear up. On me, they disappear. I can't see how it could hurt you to try. If it hurts, wipe if off fast!

Iodine

And then there's kelp, our old pal. And kelp means iodine, and iodine works on your thyroid. You see, I haven't forgotten either the acne or the Laszlo-lashing I got when I tried thyroid medication as an easy means of weight-reduction. As you've learned, there simply is no easy means.

Which means it's healthier in every respect to get your iodine in a natural form like kelp. Have you ever checked the skin on those natural Irish beauties? The ones with the creamy complexions and violet eyes? If it makes you jealous, remember Irish seaweed, only one source of kelp. Kelp and more kelp is not only a giver of health, but of beautiful skin as well—and without any acne after-effects. It gives the skin a translucent quality that is hard to duplicate cosmetically.

Kelp is a little tablet that goes wherever I go. For it not only keeps my shape in shape, but my skin in shape, as well. And I don't know what more one can expect from seaweed. Needless to say, fish is another excellent source of the iodine that will work on both your body and your complexion. The more you get of it, the better. I just happen to be a lousy fish-cook, so when I eat out I usually eat fish, and when I eat at home I eat seaweed. Try it. You'll see.

Unbroken Veins

Now, broken veins are a delicate subject, I am told. For apparently no one is allowed to lay claim to making them disappear—except perhaps the dermatologists who are allowed to remove them with electric needles. The Laszlo people almost swooned when I mentioned, aloud, that my broken veins—the ones in my face, at least—had disappeared almost entirely, and they hurried to state that they were not allowed to make that claim for their products.

Well, I suppose that I am allowed to make the statement that my own became quite discernibly less visible. Who is going to know more about what's happening to my own skin than me? So, I believe, whether I am allowed to or not, that tiny broken veins can respond to the right kind of care.

Rutin and bioflavanoids are substances that are said to protect the blood vessels that are smaller than those strengthened by vitamin C; that is why I recommended the C with rutin and bioflavanoids for your day-to-day beauty maintenance. It is also why I suggest that while you're eating your C-filled citrus fruits, you always try to eat the white, pulpy part that's closest to the peel—the part you probably throw away as a matter of routine. Well, let's change that routine, for there is where you'll find most of the vitamins and the rutin and the bioflavanoids hiding. And you need those for the strength of your veins. Check the C chapter again!

One more thing about broken veins. They aren't called "gin blossoms" for nothing. I realize that you're going to hate me every single time you take a drink, but I'm willing to take the rap for the health-sake of your skin. Because alcohol is one of the prime villains when it comes to broken veins, especially on the nose. Consider W. C. Fields and decide whether or not you want to look like him. The choice is yours.

A Soft Touch

One thing about skin. You have to treat it to a tender touch or it will bite back with blemishes and those broken veins I just spoke about and wrinkles and other things you're learning how to avoid. What I am going to tell you now, you surely already know, but I will tell you again anyway—for your skin's sake.

When you apply cream (if any you need apply) under your eyes—or vitamin E, or foundation, or whatever you're putting there—do it with the lightest possible touch. And with the tips of your fingers *only*—and pat, *do not rub*. For rubbing can pull and stretch the skin below your eyes, which is exactly where you do not want it stretched. Stretching here leads to sags and bags and we will avoid those for as long as life lets us. Miss Gabrielle of the Laszlo Institute watched me apply a bit of cream under my eyes one day and she caught me, quite unintentionally, pulling rather than patting. Here again was a hand in motion without my realizing the destructive motion it was making. So watch it and make sure that you never *rub* a thing under your eyes. Just ever, ever so lightly touch it on.

As for washcloths, I think you can forget them forever for your face. Your hands are the only touch that's light enough for your delicate complexion. And everyone's complexion is delicate, in one way or another. Washcloths can't touch the touch of your hands, the same hands that have gotten *themselves* in shape with your wash-ups. The acid-balanced theory works on hands and nails just as it does on skin. Why wouldn't it? They're all made of the same thing.

Face Food

If your appetite for food on your face is still not satisfied, then I am going to pass on a beauty recipe that I consider relatively harmless. It's food, all right, but it also passes all the necessary tests for me to believe it won't hurt the good we've done your skin.

There is a model friend of mine, for instance, who swears by a yogurt-and-honey face mask. Now yogurt is protein, and probably cannot be absorbed but just may have the same cosmetic effect as protein creams—namely, it keeps your own moisturizer inside of your own skin. But more important than that, it is *acid* (test it with your paper; I did) and therefore not likely to do anything terrible. The honey in her recipe is a skin tightener that dates back to Cleopatra, and Cleo didn't do too badly with the boys. I personally would substitute vitamin E as a better tightener-upper. We don't know whether or not E is absorbed, but we do know that E cannot be washed off of the skin. So it's going to hang in there tightening things up. If it's face food you want, give this recipe a whirl.

Exfoliate or No?

A lot has been said, written, and advertised about "exfoliation," which, whether mild or strong, means peeling of the skin. I have already told you how I feel about skin. It's a delicate subject. It should be handled with care.

There are of course many famous dermatologists, with many famous and beautiful faces as patients, who believe in exfoliation as a route to beautiful skin. Your skin, however, exfoliates itself without any help from dermatologists. According to Dr. Earle Brauer, who is research director for Revlon, the skin rejuvenates itself via "shedding" about every two weeks. While Dr. Brauer points out that the shedding, or exfoliation, is almost imperceptible, he declares that much of the "morning dust" found on your sheets is *you*—or at least the skin you have shed during the night, for apparently most of your shedding takes place while you sleep. Thank goodness for that. Skin dandruff, we don't need.

Still, I think you can see that any severe chemical peeling or abrasion, except in cases where there is severe scar tissue, whether from burns, accident, or childhood acne, should be undertaken with great care. Even at that, it can be exceedingly dangerous, for with the skin left wide open after dermabrasion, for example, it is subject to extreme infection.

I personally do not believe in such violent assaults on your skin unless you have a psychologically damaging scar or birthmark. Or acne that has left hopelessly deep pits, thanks to maltreatment during its onset. If your skin is simply less than you want it to be, I'd stick to the less extreme approches and see if we can't get it together without taking off your hide.

What to Do If You're Spending the Night Out

Who am I to question your life? But I have been asked this question by the acid-balance brainwashed. "What do I do if I get caught out without my acid-balanced face things?" It took me a few moments to realize that the young lady questioning just might find herself spending a night out here and there quite unexpectedly—meaning she hadn't time to pack all that acid stuff.

Let me say that once you have your face in shape—meaning its acidity where it ought to be on the normal scale—you'd do better to leave your protective covering on overnight than to start fooling about with someone's (someone we haven't educated as yet) strong stuff—such as a deodorant soap, for example. Now I am not, *ever*, suggesting that you forget your nightly regimen in favor of going to bed with your makeup on . . . no matter how attractive your housemate may be. For if you have been on the proper regimen long enough, your skin will look good enough without makeup. But, whatever you do, don't go washing with deodorant soaps in the name of cleanliness, unless you want to undo all the good you've spent months building up. Better to wait until the next morning when you're home. Then take off your makeup with the proper things and start afresh. Your skin will be the fresher for waiting.

Laugh a Little—No, a Lot!

One final word on skin, and that is "humor." Have a little. Laugh a lot. For, as I told you, all of your thoughts are going to be perfectly visible right there on your face, and it would be better for us both if those thoughts were beautiful. And women who are afraid to laugh for fear of "laughlines" miss a lot of what a happy life is all about.

I am all for cosmetic surgery if you need it, because I believe that a woman (or man, for that matter) should do everything she can to make herself as attractive as possible. I am hoping that, if you follow the nutritional and other regimens we are giving you, you won't need surgery. And I am also hoping that you will not try to look twenty when you're eighty. But if you've fried your skin to a not-so-fine turn with unwise suntanning, for example, and you really do need surgical help, then you should have it for sure. As long as you check and check, to be sure you have a competent doctor who isn't going to make an unreal-looking mask out of your face.

I will never forget my own experience with a very famous plastic surgeon in New York. I went to check with him about having my nose straightened. For you see, I *wasn't* beautiful-bone-born, and I keep considering doing something about it. So far, I just haven't had the necessary nerve. But since I had been asked to pay $25 at the door, just to see this famous doctor, I decided to get my money's worth. And so I asked him what I could do about frown lines. And his reply was that he would simply inject me with silicone so that I couldn't frown. And *my* reply was, "Suppose I feel mean and *want* to frown?" At which point, he got reasonably huffy and made it clear I wasn't his idea of the ideal patient. Let me tell you, he most certainly wasn't my idea of the ideal famous plastic surgeon. I had already concluded that any doctor who would so blithely consider silicone injections wasn't the doctor for me.

So if a plastic surgeon, however famous, comes on like that, take lots of time to consider and discuss it with your general physician. I told my own this story and he almost had a fit! It took a bit of calming *him* down to assure him I had no intentions of siliconing it. Just remember: Humor, above all things, is going to light up your face and your life, in a way that no cosmetics can. If you're a frozen-faced, surgically sutured beauty, that's not natural. And, in my book, it's not beautiful.

Skin Foods

Here is a list of the foods that contain the good things I've just listed for you as "good for your skin." Use the list as a starting point, and then check my chart for the exact amount of the vitamin or mineral in question. That way you'll know for sure what you're eating and you'll be even more sure as to how much you ought to be "supplementing." Remember that food-vitamins are probably more potent than the synthetic sort, but the synthetic sort are essential to make up for the number of vitamin units you could not possibly obtain by food alone. With the list, and my chart, you should be well on your way to skin-beauty.

When you come to the foods that are high in the B vitamins, remember that those foods are good for your skin AND good for your hair, so we've mini-charted them only once—just to save you any extra chart reading. Just remember, and remember well: B vitamins are good for virtually *all of you!*

SKIN

VITAMIN A

Cheeses (except uncreamed cottage cheese)	Sour cream
	Baked custard
Cheese fondue	Eggs
Cheese soufflé	Whole milk (dry and fluid)
Light cream	Yogurt
Whipping cream	Butter

VITAMIN A

Margarine
Carp
Clams
Cod
Crab
Halibut
Mackerel
Oysters
Salmon
Swordfish
Tuna
Lake whitefish
Fruits—*except:*
  Apples
  Blueberries
  Crabapples
  Cranberries
  Dates
  Figs
  White grapefruit
  Grapes
  Lemon
  Limes
  Pears
  Pineapple
  White plantain
  Pomegranate
  Prickly pear
  Quinces
  Raisins
  Strawberries
Corn flour (yellow corn)
Hominy grits (yellow corn)
Johnnycake (Northern
  cornbread)
Spoonbread
Cornmeal
Egg noodles
Bran muffins
Corn muffins (made with
  cornmeal)

Dried beef
Chicken
Kidney
Liver (all types)
Liverwurst
Peas, mature, dry
Pecans
Pigeon peas, immature
  seeds
Soybeans, immature seeds
Black walnuts
Puddings
Green asparagus
White asparagus
Lima beans
Snap beans
Beet greens
Broad beans
Broccoli
Brussels sprouts
Common cabbage
Spoon cabbage (pakchoy)
Carrots
Celery
Chicory greens
Chives
Cole slaw
Collards
Yellow sweet corn
Cowpeas (including black-
  eyed peas), except ma-
  ture seeds
Garden cress
Dandelion greens
Endive and escarole
Fennel
Kale
Lettuce
Mustard greens
Green peas
Red chili peppers

VITAMIN A

Red sweet peppers	Tomatoes, green and red
Pimentos	Tomato juice
Pumpkin	Tomato paste
Rutabagas	Tomato purée
Spinach	Tomato purée
Squash	Turnip greens
Sweet potatoes	Vegetable juice cocktails
	Swiss chard

VITAMIN D

Milk (with vitamin D added), skimmed, whole, all forms	Tuna
	Mushrooms
	Eggs
Salmon	Cod
Sardines	Roe and caviar
Mackerel	

B's for SKIN AND HAIR*

FOLIC ACID

Buttermilk	Rolled wheat
Cottage cheese	Wheat flakes
Oysters	Shredded wheat
Avocados	Beef (all cuts)
Bananas	Liver (all types)
Blackberries	Desiccated liver
Cantaloupe	Brewer's yeast
Sweet cherries	Almonds
Dates	Coconut meat
Nectarines	Mature dry peas
Strawberries	Pecans
Bran, plain	Soybeans
Degermed cornmeal	Soybean flour
Oatmeal or rolled oats	Walnuts
Rice (white and brown)	Green asparagus
Rye flour	Common beans
Whole wheat flour	Lima beans
Wheat germ	Mung beans

* NOTE: Also see table on pp. 196–197 for other hair vitamins.

FOLIC ACID

Snap beans	Endive
Beet greens	Kale
Broccoli	Lentils
Brussels sprouts	Mustard greens
Cabbage	Parsnips
Cauliflower	Green peas
Chicory greens	Pumpkin
Collards	Spinach
Sweet corn	Squash
Cowpeas (including black-eyed peas)	Sweet potatoes
	Turnip greens
Eggplant	Swiss chard

PABA

Whole milk	Whole wheat flour
Bananas	Brewer's yeast
Oatmeal or rolled oats	Spinach
Whole grain wheat	

PANTOTHENIC ACID

Skim milk	Brewer's yeast
Lobster	Cashew nuts
Dried apricots	Pecans
Avocados	Soybeans
Cantaloupe	Soybean flour
Dates	Walnuts
Light pearl barley	Lima beans, mature seeds
Plain bran	Broccoli
Brown rice	Cauliflower
White rice	Mature, dry cowpeas (including black-eyed peas)
Whole-grain wheat	
Whole-wheat flour	Kale
Beef, short-loin cuts	Lentils
Beef, round cuts	Mushrooms
Heart	Mature peas, dry
Liver, all types	Pumpkin
Desiccated liver	Sweet potatoes

B$_{12}$

Eggs	Scallops
Canned crab	Canned tuna
Haddock	Beef (all cuts, dry cooked)
Herring	Heart
Oysters	Liver, all types
Sardines	Desiccated liver

NIACIN

Dry whole milk	Potato flour
Dry skim milk	Brown rice
Fish	Enriched, common white
Shellfish	rice
Seafood	Rice cereals
Dried apricots	Whole-grain rye
Avocados	Medium rye flour
Banana flakes	Dark rye flour
Cantaloupe	Enriched spaghetti
Casaba melon	Whole-grain wheat
Dates	Wheat flours (all types,
Guavas	especially enriched)
Mangos	Wheat cereals
Orange juice, fresh only	Wild rice
Peaches	Canadian bacon
Raspberries	Beef (all cuts)
Strawberries	Brains
Bagels	Chicken
Light pearl barley	Duck
Plain bran	Goose
Bran flakes	Heart
Breadstuffing	Kidneys
Whole-grain buckwheat	Lamb
Dark buckwheat flour	Liver
Canned bulgur	Pork
Corn flour	Rabbit
Whole-ground cornmeal	Knockwurst
Cottonseed flour	Sweetbreads
Cracker meal	Turkey
Enriched macaroni	Veal
Whole-grain millet	Desiccated liver
Enriched egg noodles	Yeast, all types

NIACIN

Almonds
Almond meal
Cashew nuts
Peanuts
Peanut butter
Peanut flour
Mature peas
Pigeon peas
Safflower seed meal
Soybean flour
Sunflower seed flour
Asparagus
Common beans, raw (all types)
Fresh lima beans
Raw, dry, mature mung beans
Broadbeans
Chick-peas
Collards
Sweet corn
Fresh cowpeas
Lentils
Mushrooms
Green peas
Mature peas
Potatoes
Tomato juice
Tomato paste
Tomato purée

RIBOFLAVIN (B₂)

Buttermilk
Cheese soufflé
Dried cream substitute
Whole milk, all forms
Skim milk, all forms
Yogurt
Fish flour
Canned herring
Pompano
Pink and red salmon
Avocado
Cottonseed flour
Whole-grain millet
Wild rice
Heart
Kidneys
Liver
Brewer's yeast
Almonds
Almond meal
Safflower seed meal
Defatted soybean flour
Sunflower seed flour, partially defatted
Mature, dry peas
Turnip greens

THIAMIN (B₁)

Condensed milk
Dry whole milk
Dry skim milk
Grouper
Atlantic mackerel
Mussels
Pike
Pompano
Lake whitefish
Avocados
Fresh orange juice
Canned pineapple
Light pearl barley
Breadstuffing

THIAMIN (B₁)

Whole-grain buckwheat
Dark buckwheat flour
Corn flour
Whole ground cornmeal
Cottonseed flour
Enriched macaroni
Whole-grain millet
Enriched egg noodles
Oat cereals
Potato flour
Enriched white rice
Enriched rice cereals
Whole-grain rye
Medium rye flour
Dark rye flour
Enriched spaghetti
Whole-grain wheat
Whole wheat flour
Enriched flours
Crude wheat bran
Wheat germ
Wheat flakes
Wild rice
Canadian bacon
Heart
Kidneys
Pork (all cuts)

Brewer's yeast
Shelled, dried almonds
Broadbeans
Cashew nuts
Boiled peanuts
Peanuts
Defatted peanut flour
Pecans
Pigeon peas
Safflower seed meal
Soybeans
Soybean flour
Sunflower seed flour
Walnuts
Bamboo shoots
Fresh lima beans
Chick-peas
Collards
Immature cowpeas, including black-eyed peas
Frozen black-eyed peas
Lentils
Green peas
Mature peas
Tomato paste
Tomato purée

3. Hair

Here's to Healthy Hair

I've been writing about hair health for so long that I'm beginning to feel like one hair-head. I practically am, for that matter, for my hair has become so healthy that it grows like those weeds you always hear about and, what is better, it remains thick and very together all the while it's growing.

My hair is healthy because I've always been practically paranoid about it. A friend once said to me, quite accusingly, that if I had all the riches the world could offer, and one hair was not quite right, I'd be unhappy. He was right there. For what good is a real crown if your crowning glory isn't up to it?

Probably that hair paranoia of mine is the very reason why now my hair is the one thing about myself that satisfies me completely. For one thing, I have found (finally) the man who can cut it perfectly into a style that means no "hairdressing" and, therefore, no trouble to me. And I have found hair health.

Once you've gotten perfectly healthy hair, cut into a perfect shape that is perfectly simple for *you* to handle, then you're well on your way to hair heaven.

But first, it's hair health, here we come.

Experience Counts as Hair

If you want to profit by my hair experiences, you'll doubtless be dizzy. For I've been through virtually everything the hair-heads could dream up, from short and geometric to Orphan Annie curls and from boy-short to long and straight, which is where I am right now, but yearning for a change. We fashion folk never like to let well enough alone . . . we like changes, swift and often. And those changes are sometimes disastrous, but there's one thing about hair. It will grow. If it's healthy, it will grow fast, so if you get a haircut you could cry about, don't bother. Just do what I tell you, and you'll get your hair where you want it again before you have a chance to feel less than beautiful.

You will see just what foods got my hair out of a disastrous skin-head haircut and into long. You will also discover, once again, how many myths about hair exist. It seems to be the one truth about beauty. Practically nothing you've heard all of your life is true. So once again, you must prepare to re-educate yourself to a new way of thinking about hair, and possibly a new way of eating, as well. You must realize, first and foremost, that your skin, your nails, your hair, and your body are all basically the same thing, and that thing is protein.

Protein ... Pro-Hair

We've already told you—you *are* protein. So learn to think protein before you think anything else for hair health as well as for all the other beautiful parts of beautiful you. And if you want to thicken up your hair and nothing else, then aren't you lucky? For protein, the very thing that can make you thin (if you've chosen the low-carbohydrate route to weight loss) is also the very thing that will make your hair thick, lustrous, long, vital, and vibrantly alive.

Your hair is ninety-seven percent protein (the rest is ash, so we'll forget it for here), and it contains nineteen of the twenty-two amino acids in protein. That should give you a pretty good indication of just how important it is to get protein into you. And protein is one more ingredient that *cannot* be stored by the body. It's like those vitamins that run away with body wastes and must be replenished each and every day. You simply must get your daily protein and lots of it besides. The experts recommend dosages of fifty-six to eighty grams per day. (They don't all agree, as usual.) Here, once again, I suggest you check your own doctor, for this is a spot where it is impossible for me to judge. Your needs, naturally, depend upon your height, weight, and body build. But with protein, more is better than less, and, as I have pointed out in the chapter on skin, the chances of your getting an overdose of protein are scant indeed.

You will find all of the protein grams contained in every conceivable food listed in my complete chart. I suggest that you count them carefully every single day to make sure you are getting the amount of protein your body needs to manufacture beauty. You might even consider keeping a protein notebook, much like the calories notebook I suggested, and adding it all up at the end of the day. Protein is so essential for both you and your family that I'd hate to see anyone get cheated on that, whether it's beauty you're after or just sound good health. As for hair—without protein, it won't be hair. It just won't be there.

Where to Find It All

Protein, as you all know, I am sure, is most prevalent in meat, fish, fowl, milk, cheese, and eggs. And we will have more on the egg in a moment.

But, lest you still consider protein as meat and meat alone, keep remembering the other proteins—the kind found in raw grains, nuts, seeds and beans, all of which are chock full of that valuable protein but also contain iron, silicon and sulfur which are some of the very best minerals for healthy hair growth. Plant sources contribute seventy percent of the world's protein supply. And check those soybeans. They're the best possible source (they're the commercial source, in fact) of our old friend, lecithin—the same lecithin you're using (I hope) to lithen up. But what you don't know—yet—is that lecithin contains two of the B vitamins that are most vital to beautiful hair. So you're getting, with those beans, both the protein you need and the lecithin into the bargain. Pretty good for a bean.

As for eggs, let's consider them for a moment. For eggs are perfect in more ways than shape. They're considered the most perfect protein of all. Protein gram for protein gram, the egg is said to have the most ability to support life itself, and eggs contain larger proportions of the amino acids that work on hair than any other protein, complete or otherwise. (Complete protein simply means that all twenty-two amino acids are there. It's complex, but, if you eat enough different kinds of protein, you'll get them all.)

Now when we talk egg and hair, we're not talking egg shampoo. That's something else, and it's just about as valuable as egg on your face—meaning it's not valuable at all. What we are concerned with is getting that egg into your body where it can do your hair some real good.

Many people are, of course, needlessly frightened by the

egg. It's that old cholesterol bogeyman again. I personally am more frightened by the idea of no hair, especially now that the validity of the cholesterol theory is being seriously questioned by medical men and scientists. Still, I'd be the last one to insist that you eat eggs if your own doctor says no. Yet I hear many people (with rotten hair, I may add) say they wouldn't dream of touching one. And I'll bet they haven't even bothered to have that cholesterol checked. It's an easy test and one your physician can do in a flash. Before you give up eggs, and possibly do a great deal of harm to your health and your hair, why not have that cholesterol checked? You may be in for a nice surprise, and find your cholesterol level beautifully low. If so, then you're free to discover the egg and its wonderful effect on hair.

The Egg—It Goes Inside

I learned about eggs, and what they can do for hair—and what can happen to that same hair without them—in a sadder-but-wiser-making experience I had when I was in college. I lived in a dormitory, of course, and the food was horrible. Horrible is really too nice a word for it. It was practically inedible. The breakfasts particularly, when the eggs arrived looking slightly green, making me slightly green as well.

Now, as a well-fed Southern girl, I'd been brought up on a life of big breakfasts—some kind of a holdover from the English way of life, I suppose, for Southerners have always gone heavy on the breakfast bit. And that's as it should be. Nutritionists will quickly tell you that breakfast is the most important meal of any day, doing exactly what its name implies: breaking the fast you've been on for the past eight hours—or however many hours you've chosen to spend in bed the night before. If you're ever going to skip a meal, which is something I never recommend, then for your health's sake don't ever skip breakfast.

In any case, back at the dorm, I was faced with a difficult choice—a sick stomach from green eggs—or a sticky-looking sweet roll and coffee. I opted for the sweet roll, which was my first hair-mistake. And my hair certainly showed my error.

Soon it was thin and sickly-looking where it once had

been plentiful. If I went swimming, I appeared almost bald, and my friends took notice enough to question what was happening. This is one time it wasn't my active imagination at work.

But I was lucky, as I always have been. For back in Alabama, I had a super-knowledgeable, way ahead of his time, hairdresser. He was Mexican (don't ask me how he got to Alabama), and you know the kind of hair the Mexicans have—thick, black and shiny. I've heard it comes from the corn that is the staple of the Mexican diet. It's possible. Corn is not only relatively high in protein, but is extremely high in phosphorus. Phosphorus is a mineral that is not only found in every one of your body cells but a mineral that helps create lecithin, and lecithin is what helps create hair. It looks like the Mexican connection from here.

In any case, on a weekend trip to my Alabama home, this hairdresser took one look at my scraggly locks and was duly appalled. His first question was, "What are you *not* eating?" You can see right there that he was, indeed, ahead of his time, for while I won't tell you the year, I will tell you it was long before the consciousness-raising toward food for beauty. When I replied, "Eggs," he delivered a tirade I've never forgotten, warning me that if I wanted to keep my hair, I'd better forget about forgetting eggs. He instructed me to get at least one egg per day, no matter how. I did (not at the dorm, however) and my hair miraculously, it seemed to me, grew back to its former healthy state. It was many years before I had another hair health problem, and I will tell you about that one, too. Both were due to my own diet stupidity, and now that I know the food facts, I don't expect it to happen again, ever. Because now my hair gets its daily health foods, and one of those foods is eggs.

Some people say that the best way to take egg—the best for the best benefits, that is—is raw. I can't take that. But I can give you a recipe for a raw egg milkshake—one that supposedly does wonders toward restoring a thick, lush head of hair, if that isn't what you already have.

Dale Alexander, who had his own hair problems with baldness, swears that he re-grew his hair with what he calls the Alexander Hair Cocktail. It is one way of getting that raw egg into you, and here is Mr. Alexander's recipe as given in his book, *How I Stopped Growing Bald and Started Growing Hair:*

1. Take three-quarters of a glass of whole milk. This should preferably be raw certified milk. (Most health food stores have it.) However, if that is not available, regular homogenized cow's milk will do. Pour the milk into the blender.

2. Add one raw egg to the milk in the blender. This should preferably be a fertile egg (again, try your health food supermarket. Even some supermarkets, now that the public is catching onto health). But if fertile eggs cannot be secured, use regularly available fresh eggs.

3. Add one tablespoonful of raw wheat germ oil.

4. Add two tablespoonsful of raw wheat germ. Do not use the toasted variety.

5. To improve the flavor of the blended ingredients, you may add a piece of fruit in season. This can be a section of pineapple, orange, banana, papaya, or apple; or you can add one or two tablespoonsful of sunflower seeds or sunflower seed meal. The sunflower seeds, available in health food stores, will give the cocktail a fine, nutty tang.

6. Blend at low speed from thirty to sixty seconds.

7. Drink this blended mixture promptly.

8. This drink should serve as your complete breakfast.

9. Do not eat or drink anything else for two hours after drinking this mixture.

10. The wheat germ oil, milk, and eggs used in this drink should be kept under refrigeration at all times. The raw wheat germ should be kept in a sealed container, preferably under refrigeration.

    Do not supplement the wheat germ oil you take in this drink with wheat germ oil capsules during the day. Once you notice changes in your hair, you may cut down on the daily intake of the hair cocktail and take it only twice a week. Of course, since it is a healthful drink, you may prefer to continue taking it daily indefinitely.

So there's Mr. Alexander's hair recipe. Of course, I can't imagine cutting down one's intake of either eggs or wheat germ (I'll get to that shortly) to twice a week. I believe in getting it inside of you at least once a day, even if I am chicken and take my eggs cooked!

One raw egg believer I know suggests combining that egg with skimmed milk, a high-protein supplement and, if you insist, a sweetener. If you must sweeten, then I suggest carob powder, which is a wonderful, naturally chocolate-flavored substance that comes from St. John's bread (breadfruit). It can't do your skin and hair all the harm that chocolate can and it will satisfy your sweet tooth all the way. If your diet allows sweeteners of any kind—you've by now checked on your blood sugar—then you could use a touch (and that's all it will take) of blackstrap molasses, that wonderful wonder food that's filled with iron and B vitamins. Of all the sweeteners, blackstrap is probably the most good-things laden of the lot. As for sugar—I've already told you the harm it can do to your looks. That goes ditto for your hair.

Throw this concoction into your electric blender and you've got your own brand of instant breakfast. If you don't have to worry about weight (lucky you), you can have it *with* your breakfast. Or double the dose if gaining weight is what you're after. Your whole body is bound to benefit.

Protein On

Your next question will be, I am sure, "What about protein conditioners and protein shampoos? Do they really work, or are they simply a put-on?" You're right to question, but put them on and find out. What you'll find out is that they do work!

I questioned their validity myself until, as usual, I had a problem. And this was my first hair-health problem since my re-discovery of the wonders of the egg. Do you remember what happened to me when I'd been too long at the carbohydrate counter? When my body needed the protein it was busily converting into the carbohydrates I'd been withholding from it?

If you'll check back, you'll find that it was through my hair, and a sharp-eyed scalp specialist, that I discovered how my body had by-passed the low-carbohydrate regimen in the first place. When your body needs that protein for its own health use, it really doesn't care how your locks look. And, if you'll recall, it was right about then that I wanted a fashionable permanent, and my hairdresser asked me to sign a release—just in case my hair all fell out. Well, that ought to give you a pretty clear picture of how my hair looked back then. Limp, lame, unlovely, and certainly not the picture of anything *you'd* want.

Once I had put the "not-enough-protein" diagnoses together—the ones from my trichologist (scalp specialist) and my dermatologist and my general physician—and come up with that realization that my diet had to be reversed and fast, I got on with the rebuilding of my once-healthy hair. By the way, one of the very first places to spot protein deprivation is in the hair, so look to that first, and then to your diet.

So, on with the cure and the protein. I marched myself back over to Nicholas at Vidal Sassoon—Nicholas, the man who'd refused my perm in the first place—and I said, "Okay, baby. You said I had lousy hair; now you fix it." And he did.

Now if anyone had told me before that there really were products that really did produce seemingly miraculous results on damaged hair, I would probably have called him a liar. For there's not a claim to be made that I haven't already heard in my almost-eight years of reporting on beauty products. Most of those claims are taken with more than a grain of doubt. For here's where our old friend, advertising, gets into the beauty act, and makes it hard to separate truth from moneymaking fiction. And if it will make money, they will push it and as long as it does no harm . . . well, I have to admit, the "truth in advertising" routine is paying off somewhat, although it seems to zero in on such things as little cigars more than hair healers. Still, possibly that "truth" is yet to come. I promise to do my bit, in any case, to the best of the knowledge I can root out.

At any rate, I placed myself in the competent hands of Nicholas and prepared to keep an open mind on the whole treatment. And the whole treatment is what I got. Now bear in mind that Nicholas was the resident trichologist at Sassoon. And also bear in mind that swinging London, back in the 1960s, had discovered swinging hair, while the U.S.A. was still into the teased phase of hairdressing. And to wear that swinging Sassoon-styled hair, you needed *good* hair. Therefore, London was filled with trichologists and their hair-knowledge long before Vidal Sassoon opened his salons here and started a new wave (via the non-wave) of hair ecology. Thank goodness it all happened. It just may have saved a lot of hairs.

Now Nicholas, like most of my other beauty-gurus, turned out to be a brusque sort. I don't know whether I attract that kind or whether, because I can be a tough customer myself, it takes that sort of strength to make me believe. Perhaps the whole formula for being a successful diet doctor, skin specialist, or trichologist is the "fear" approach—to frighten the patient into following instructions. For it is true, indeed, that if you don't follow any given regimen to the letter, you certainly aren't going to get the results. If *you* don't work, *it* won't work . . . and there goes that "work ethic" again.

The first thing Nicholas did was jerk (yes, he did) a strand of hair from my head and insert it under his microscope . . . a contraption that was originally designed to measure the muscle structure of animals but was now set to work to analyze my hair's protein content (rotten) and its elasticity (lousy). In short, my hair needed a lot of help.

And so my treatment began, and it was to continue for eight weeks at the rate of one treatment per week with Nicholas, plus my own hair homework. Some rapid-fire instructions were issued to an assistant who took me off for a protein shampoo, slathered me with protein conditioner, heated to shorten the soak-in time. Then still another protein shampoo and a dry-by-blower non-"set" by the man who's responsible for the shape of my hair—Roger Thompson, whose formidable title was International Artistic Director at Sassoon, but who is, more important, an old friend from London who has the cool to cope with that hair paranoia of mine. By the end of that session, I looked fantastic! Or at least my hair certainly did. It was swinging beautifully and shining like a jewel. And two days later it was bedraggled again.

On my next weeks's visit, you can bet that I complained. Or at the very least demanded some explanations as to why the jewel-look wasn't lasting longer than two days. For it seemed to me that my hair had looked better on its old

regime of creme shampoos and creme rinses and I was
questioning whether or not it was better to have pretty,
shining but unhealthy hair, or bedraggled getting-healthy
hair.

And so Nicholas gave me a little lecture and I learned a
bit more about healthy beauty. First, I was told that my
hair hadn't gotten into such bad shape overnight, so there
was no reason for me to expect it to get gorgeous overnight. There it was again—that old truth that you cannot
hurry beauty. Whether it's hair, shape, skin, or whatever,
miracles do not happen overnight. They happen, all right,
but they sneak up on you. Now I never expect to see real,
lasting results from anything in less than six months. And
then suddenly one morning you look in the mirror and see
something beautiful. You. ·

I was lectured on the fact that all those things that had
formerly shined up my hair—namely, the creme shampoos
and creme rinses—were not only just cosmetics, designed
to cover up any damage, but they were most probably the
very things that had caused the damage in the first place.
For they were probably highly alkaline and (does it surprise you now?) hair—just like skin—is and must remain
acid. The acidity of hair came as a surprise to me, for I
was uneducated then, but we'll get into that in a moment.
For now, let's keep that protein on.

Each week I kept complaining, for each week my hair
looked as sad as ever except for the few days right after my
treatment-session. I was given the same protein shampoo
used in the salon, to continue my hair work homeside.
Work at it I did. I washed every other day, for, as Nicholas
pointed out, dirt is the very worst enemy of beautiful hair.
(*I* will point out, dirty hair is the worst enemy of beautiful
skin, wherever the two happen to meet.) And in New York
City, dirty is a common word.

Each week I was tempted to slide back into my creme-
rinsed beautiful-but-sick hair routine, but I hung on dog-
gedly, determined to see whether this protein-on stuff really
worked. It did, but certainly not in the eight weeks I
worked on it with Nicholas. Just as I have said, it takes, in
my own experience, close to six months before the real end
result turns up on you. Suddenly one day I looked and had
hair. Lots of it. About twice as much as before, it seemed,
and so many people commented on the thickness of it all

that I find it hard to believe it was my overactive imagination again. This job was done by protein.

Now the whole protein-shampoo-conditioner theory is pretty technical stuff, for a protein molecule is much too big to be absorbed by the hair. That's the very reason an egg on your hair isn't likely to do any more good than that egg on your face. Before a protein molecule is in any condition to do your hair condition any good, it must first be cut down to size. I would prefer to let the experts do the technical explanations and so I will quote from a letter written by Dr. Ron di Salvo of RedKen Laboratories in Van Nuys, California, to a dermatologist who stated that protein shampoos were no better than ordinary shampoos. Here is Dr. di Salvo's reply:

> Protein technology is no simple matter. . . . Proteins first of all have to be hydrolyzed (broken down) to the correct molecular weight and size to become substantive (become fixed) to the hair. You see, it isn't enough for a manufacturer to simply decide to put protein in a product to be used on the hair (or skin, for that matter) because protein molecules are simply too large to be absorbed into the hair's complex microstructure. In order to be absorbed when topically applied, proteins must be broken down (hydrolyzed) to smaller molecular components. This process must be carefully governed. If broken down into too small a molecular size and weight, amino acids (the building blocks of proteins) will be absorbed, but cannot find a site of chemical attachment, so serve little purpose. The secret, then, is to strive, through chemical hydrolyzation of protein, to achieve numbers of amino acids chemically bonded together (called polypeptides) of the correct molecular weight and size to be small enough to be readily absorbed, yet large enough to find sites for chemical attachment.

I can assure you that all of that is too technical for my own mind, which is why I don't think there's one chance in a million you'll be whipping up an effective protein shampoo in your own kitchen. It would be far better to use that kitchen for getting that protein into your stomach and leave the hydrolyzing to the laboratories. There are plenty out there doing the job with more onto the process every day—so many, in fact, that I can't keep up with them. There's Fermodyl, originally Swiss; Jheri Redding, who was one of the original founders of RedKen; and Wella, to name only a very few. For protein seems to be as magic a word as vitamin E. Suddenly it sells anything. But "protein" is a word that is popping up on practically any old product, so once again I'll advise you to try any one of them carefully. RedKen works for me, and yet others loathe it. Some of my friends love the Jheri Redding formula, while I don't. Here again, you as a person are unique and so is your hair, your skin, your shape. You must be the ultimate judge of just which product is the one for you. But before you judge the protein-on routine, I think you *must* give it time. I would have given it up at once had not Nicholas been there insisting that I stick with it. Yet the results I got at the end of six months made it all worthwhile. You couldn't get me back into hair cosmetics for the world. My hair is jewel-shining all by itself!

Label Caution

Beware of the word "protein" on the label, because of late it's being bandied about all over the place, from every ten-cent store to every health food shop cosmetics counter. And, frankly, I am suspicious. I have learned to be a cynic during my cosmetics life and I don't trust advertising and the fact that advertisers will say almost anything for salability's sake. For example, the other day I picked up a mascara wand of the sort I've been using for twenty years. And suddenly the label says, "with protein." I have no doubt that there's protein in there all right, but where is it getting to me?

I am sure that all the protein shampoos that are making great use of that salable word probably contain protein. But it may be simply one more egg-on-your-face routine. In other words, has that protein been properly hydrolyzed so that it doesn't just lie there doing nothing, but gets inside your hair shaft where it can help? My suspicious nature tells me that the extremely inexpensive "protein" products probably have just had any old protein plopped in—so they can use the word on that label. Hydrolyzing is an expensive procedure, and, while I have no proof, of course, that all these cheap imitations are not hydrolyzed protein, I am allowed to doubt. If I were you, I would stick to reputable companies; I would question my beauty-supply house (yes, they are helpful whether you're a beautician or not), and I would ask for any and all literature on that particular product. As for my protein mascara—I returned it for my old non-protein kind. And you can be sure it's not because I don't believe in protein-on power. In that case, I simply don't believe it's there to work. Just to sell.

Acid, Acid Everywhere—Hair, Too

With my hair education came the acceptance that acid is all over the place, as it ought to be, when it comes to both the health and the beauty of your skin and your hair. For your hair is not so different from your skin, though they may look different, indeed. That hair is protein, as we've shown you, and that's what your skin is. And it's got to have the same acid mantle to protect it.

The acidity of your hair is normally, so Nicholas tells me, set at 4.5 to 5.5. The big problem with hair is how to keep it there, for there are certain cases where hair will have to go alkaline—deliberately. If you color your hair, for example, or perm it, you will have to make it alkaline in order for the color or the curl to "take." The ideal thing is, of course, to take it as little to the alkaline side as possible, and then get it back to acid as fast as you can. That is one reason why jobs like tinting or perming are best left to the experts who know the best products for the job. And the best products for these jobs are the ones that will do the least damage to your hair, because this is the way bleaching and perming work on your hair (I wouldn't want to try a do-it-myself job here):

Your hair, you see, has a cuticle just like your nails and a strong (we hope) center shaft called the medulla. When all goes well and the hair is properly nourished and acid balanced, this cuticle is smooth and tight and hanging in there protecting that medulla, which is the strong point of your hair.

Now, with bleaching or perming, that cuticle must be deliberately opened out—a little like peeling a banana—so that the tinting or permanent wave solution can penetrate. Now you can see how such a process leaves your hair wide open for some pretty severe damage. As these solutions are, by necessity, alkaline, you can see just *how* severe the damage could be. Most of the hair-products manufacturers are busily educating salon people, these days, as to just how important it is to re-condition the hair with both protein and acid after such a deliberate alkalinization of the hair. Otherwise, you just could end up with the hair equivalent of a hangnail, i.e., your hair cuticle hanging out, instead of holding in close to that medulla. If it does, your hair will look scraggly and hang-hair, not sleek and shining the way we want it to be.

Therefore, please leave any alkaline doings to the salon experts. And when it comes to doing it yourself, do it up acid. Here, once again, your Nitrazine papers become the indispensable little beauty-testers you must always have handy. I am sure that, if you try them on some of the products you're using on your hair right now, you'll probably be surprised if one of those strips turns bright blue. If it does, drop that product immediately. With hair, blue won't do!

Blue Shampoo, You're Through!

There's one more point where hair differs from skin, even though they're made of the same thing—and that's from the cleansing angle. For here's one place where, even though alkaline may be cleaner-making—it had better not touch your hair.

I think I have told you my own experiences with alkaline creme shampoos and other such coverups. While I was covering up, I was ruining my hair in the process. Now I think I've learned that lesson well, for, while my face can get back to acid, there's a lot more to my hair and I'm not about to let anything alkaline or harsh have a go at it. Not now that it's thick and lustrous all on its own.

Soap is a definite no-no for hair. It simply won't do. The protein-filled, acid-balanced beauty bars that are everywhere these days will do beautifully, however. In fact, if I'm traveling, I find it much easier to take along one of these bars, which is, in actuality, solidified shampoo, than to lug a leaky shampoo bottle. It works just fine.

But as for ordinary soap—the kind we've been told cleans the best—well, skip it. That's not the sort of deep cleaning your hair wants. Your protein shampoo should have your hair-cuticle tight in there where it belongs and we don't want anything alkaline making it loose. Detergent shampoos are particularly to be avoided at all hair costs. They can actually make you *lose* your hair, I've been told, and here's one more time where I refuse to experiment for my readers' sakes. I'll take the researchers' word for it and assume that you will, too. It's safer for us all that way. One way to spot detergent shampoo is through its rapid-lathering quality. The *best* way to spot it is by poking your ever-ready strip of Nitrazine into the bottle. Just once more: If it's blue, then blue won't do.

Cider Vinegar ... My Old Pal

Now that I think about it, what did I do before I discovered cider vinegar? Looked a mess, no doubt. Because everywhere I look now I see cider vinegar ready to do a perfectly natural beauty job on practically everything. You can see, I am sure, that cider vinegar is a natural for rinsing your hair with acid. Our grandmothers knew more than we gave them credit for, it seems. Vinegar rinses are as old-news as the hills. But I wonder whether anyone ever questioned why. Well, now that you've learned about your hair's acid mantle, it's easily understood. Cider vinegar on your face, cider vinegar on your hair, cider vinegar inside of you. It all adds up to the acid that protects you all over.

So if you want to give your hair a double dose of acid for extra protection, mix about a half-cup of cider vinegar in a basin of water for that last rinse. We've always known vinegar left hair shining. Now we know why.

Thickeners—Do They?

I see that there are reams of so-called hair-thickeners on the market these days, and, while I cannot imagine using one, I will attempt to explain what they do. The reason I cannot imagine using one is, first, that I tend to distrust the cosmetics industry which seems to feel that selling comes first, health later. And the FDA seems to be ignoring hair cosmetics for the moment, while they concentrate on the facial ones. Second, my own hair has become so very much thicker, thanks to my new-found knowledge on what makes it so, that I don't need one anyway.

Apparently the thickeners that contain protein actually wrap themselves about the hair shaft and adhere to it, thereby giving the appearance of thicker hair. They take up more room. And that's all there is to that. To me, the answer is to get your hair thicker by the proper care and the proper diet. Remember to eat your wheat germ daily and make sure you get all the B vitamins you need and avoid all of the things we've suggested you forsake for the sake of your hair. I don't believe for a moment you're going to need a false thickener. But don't forget to give your own hair six months to a year before you make that judgment. Should you decide, after that time, to try one of these products, test it first with your Nitrazine; if it's blue, then don't use it. Less thick hair is better than no hair. So you might as well concentrate on getting that protein into your body instead of wrapping it around your hairs.

It Won't Come Out in the Wash!

Remember all those old stories about how too much washing could ruin your hair? Forget them, just the same way you've forgotten all the other myths I've exploded as nonsensical. For clean hair is the only kind of hair that can possibly be healthy. And if you're using the proper kind of shampoo—protein filled and acid balanced—then you're actually giving your hair a beauty treatment each and every time you wash. You're putting protein back into your hair, which is where you want it. I still see people who tell me that they have bad hair and are therefore afraid to wash it too often. It's hard to say to someone that the reason their hair is so bad is probably just that. They don't wash it often enough.

Of late, I've been listening to a commercial which advertises a shampoo that can be used every night. That shows that even the world of commerce is getting the natural beauty message. For every night, or every morning, is just about how often your hair should get its protein bath. Just make sure that the shampoo *is* protein and *is* acid. That way you're bound to be helping and most certainly are not hurting. No way.

Healthy Glands, Healthy Hair

I have had several disastrous bouts in my life with un-necessary thyroid medication. In most cases, it was a case of my searching for any easy way out of fat and blaming my glands instead of my gluttony. In all cases—save one, which I blame on the doctor—I wheedled my way into thyroid medication with hideously nonbeautiful results. You have seen what happened when my skin blossomed with ugly, festering pimples until Laszlo gave me the last word: "Stay away from thyroid medication!"

But I have not yet mentioned that years ago, back in Alabama, I played around once again with my metabolism and got just what I deserved. For, once again, I blamed my thyroid for my fat, instead of blaming myself; and I per-suaded my doctor to at least try the little pills. Thank goodness I have learned, after a lifetime of nonsense, that you simply can't mess with a good gland, especially when it's doing all you should ask of it and it's *you* who aren't doing your part. My part, in my case.

The result I got this time was not acne but dull, dry, and listless hair. Now don't ask me why the thyroid medication would make me come up once oily, and the next time dry. My Protein Bound Iodine index was right where it had always been. So my only guess is that the *kind*, or brand, of thyroid medication was different—plus the fact that the hair bit happened twenty years ago and a body can change a lot in that time.

I, of course, was too uneducated at that time to even connect my suddenly dried-out hair (it never had been) with the thyroid pills. It took that same aware Mexican hairdresser to guess that I'd been doing something wrong. And, of course, he was right again. Don't, *please*, play around with thyroid pills. They're not candy drops.

Fat Again—For Shining Hair

Don't believe for one single moment that you can have that thick, shining, swinging, luxuriant length of hair you ob-viously want unless you eat fats. For your hair, as we keep pointing out (hope you aren't bored, but just let it bore into your brain) is exactly like your skin. It craves fats and

without them, your hair will be dry, dull, listless, and limp
—but not beautiful. I'd be willing to swear to that.

Again we'll say that most people consider fat a dirty
word. But fat doesn't mean *you're* fat. Heavens, no! That's
what we're fighting against. If you've read the chapter on
Shape, and read it carefully, then you know that fats are as
important to keeping your shape in shape as they are to
sleeking up the rest of you—meaning your hair, your skin,
and your nails.

In fact, if you try leaving out fats, you can get into
plenty of trouble, most of it ugly. Like real dandruff, or
other unbeautiful things. Some nutritionists feel that fat is
so important to all of you that they recommend that no
less than a quarter of your diet be made up of fat. And, as
we know, the unsaturated fats are the kind to recommend,
not only because they're the best for shaping you up, but
because they're full of vitamin E—the E that's so essential
for the beauty of your hair.

While we're on the subject of unsaturated fats, let me
just remind you that they're the vegetable oil fats, the ones
that needn't worry your cholesterol, the kind that remain
liquid at room temperature for easy recognition on your
part. There is only one vegetable oil, however, that is saturated and that is coconut oil. I bring it up because recently
I discovered something curious on my weekly Saturday
supermarket trek. I was trying to track down safflower oil
margarine because I find that it is the kind that gets any
unnecessary fat off of me the fastest. (That's me. I don't
know about you, but safflower is still the least saturated of
the oils.) And safflower oil margarine is practically impos-
ible to find, thanks, I suppose, to the public's disenchant-
ment with the whole idea when Dr. Herman Taller and his
safflower remedy fell from grace. Too bad, for he was
right, as many other doctors have shown. Calories don't
always count. And so I have to search far and wide in
obscure and very out-of-my-busy-way health food shops
for that sort of margarine.

What do you think I found in my supermarket then? A
margarine made of coconut oil. So if you automatically
think that eating margarine means eating unsaturated fat,
think again, and learn to read those labels carefully, even if
it means reading the very fine print. You can bet they print
it as fine as possible.

Always remember that no matter how well you follow all the rest of the hair regimen, without fats you will never have shiny, beautiful hair. Fat is definitely the best shiner-upper for hair.

What Are Those Flakes on Your Shoulders?

If you've got dandruff, then here's one place where I'll recommend, without qualification and without hesitation, that you see a dermatologist, and fast. But the problem is that perhaps it isn't dandruff at all. Possibly you've mistreated your scalp for so long and so much that you've literally made it fall off of your head.

I thought I had dandruff once and I was duly horrified. It turned out to be a simple case of dried-up scalp which was scaling off and falling onto my "little black dress" where it looked like dandruff to me. For you must always remember that your scalp is your skin—no more, no less—and it must be treated as carefully and as gently as you would treat the skin on your face.

That is where your acid-balanced hair regimen helps your scalp just the way it helps your complexion. That is why I am leery of so-called dandruff shampoos and other dandruff remedies. Unless they test up, via your Nitrazine, as acid, then I would avoid them. Most dandruff remedies are pretty strong stuff and have about the same effect on your scalp as detergent or deodorant soaps have on your complexion. Let's just say that probably won't keep it as healthy as we want it.

Before you try the dandruff treatment, why not try the acid regimen first? Shampoo, conditioner, the works. If, after, say, six weeks of the proper sort of shampoo plus conditioning treatment of protein and acid, your hair still shows up as flakes on your shoulders, then get yourself to a doctor and have him check it out. For dandruff (real, not look-alike dandruff) is a disorder that only a physician can cure and, I am sorry to say, here again they often fail.

But at least try our gentle method before you break for the dandruff remedies that television commercials take such delight in trying to sell you. You will probably find you don't need them.

Wheat Germ—At the Root of Healthy Hair

One balmy spring day, a few years ago, I wandered into my (then) hairdresser for my regular trim-up. That session went like this. "Hey, man (they talked that way in those days—really), it's spring! Let's cut your hair." Me: "You're right. It is. Why not?" Several hours later I could clearly see why not. For my hair had been clipped to within ⅛″ of my scalp and I looked like one of those World War II collaborators—the kind that had been sheared before they were tarred and feathered.

To make matters worse, I was giving a dinner party that evening for my good friend Pablo Manzoni, creative director (and great-beauty maker) of Elizabeth Arden. What a day to get caught with my scalp showing through the no-hair! To show you just how awful I looked—for I know I exaggerate occasionally—when I opened the door to greet my guests, Pablo screamed. So you have a pretty fair idea of just how I looked.

Actually, I had to laugh. What else could I do? For these things happen occasionally, in a so-called fashion lady's career, and laughter is about the only thing to see you through. I got through my dinner party with a lot of way-out makeup and a great deal of swagger that I didn't feel at all inside. The next day, however, I wasn't laughing. I was crying. But when your hair's gone, "Man, it's gone," as my hairdresser might have said. When this kind of disaster happens, as it's bound to sometime in everyone's beauty life, there's only one thing to remember. As long as your hair is alive, *it will grow*. If it's lively and healthy enough, it will grow fast.

But my hair, at that time (though I didn't realize it), was not lively enough to cover me up as fast as I needed. For then I was on my strict low-carbohydrate diet, under the watchful supervision of Dr. Atkins, and I wasn't straying one iota. And my hair wasn't growing one iota either. But that was long before I learned that protein deprivation shows up first on your head, in a lack of hair, so I was stuck with that skinhead cut and feeling miserably ugly.

And then, quite by chance, I found myself pleading with Dr. Atkins one day to allow me to return to my favorite breakfast of wheat germ and cream. I vowed that I could no longer face even one more egg in the morning. (For me, P.M. is the best M. for egg.) Dr. Atkins relented, even though wheat germ contains carbohydrates, but he allowed me only three level tablespoons of wheat germ per day. If you'll have a look at that amount, you'll see it's quite enough—even for a lover of the stuff, as I am. Three tablespoons make for nine carbohydrate grams, so I was still well within the safe limit to keep my weight going down.

Delighted, I went on my merry wheat germ way and I got a very unexpected reward. The hair that had lain ugly and dormant for all those months began to grow in spurts. It grew fast. Now I know that every hair expert in the world says that hair can't possibly grow more than six inches per year. If that's true, then mine grew six inches between that spring day and September, because by that month it was touching my shoulders in back, and those crew cut bangs in front were by then hiding my brows.

Now, this isn't *True Confessions*, but it is a pretty good illustration of what wheat germ can do for hair growth. For bear in mind that I was under the very strict supervision of Dr. Atkins and his diet during this whole hair-growing time and the only single element of my diet that changed was the addition of the wheat germ to the low-carbohydrate regimen.

It wasn't until much, much later that I discovered much, much more about wheat germ. First, according to Carlton Fredericks, wheat germ has a protein value of high quality and of percentage exceeding that of meat. Check it out on my chart if you're a doubter; just remember to keep the weights equal. So wheat germ is valuable protein and therefore good for your hair health.

But wheat germ is also chock full of vitamin E, and vitamin E, as you will soon find out, is a must-have for beautiful hair. The little germ doesn't stop there: It's also a powerhouse of B vitamins—the Beautiful B-complex crowd —and the only part of the wheat grain to contain vitamin A. This germ is one germ you'll want your hair to encounter; and, besides all those vital-for-hair vitamins, wheat germ contains the fatty acids that are essential to keeping your hair glowing and glossy.

Personally, I am a wheat germ freak, so it's easy for me to take. I love it, especially as a morning meal cereal with cream poured over it. To me, it makes commercial cereals taste like so much wet cardboard. I'll grant you that, when I started my wheat germ love affair, I eased in on the honey-covered kind. (That was long before I discovered I could never have sweets again.) I went on to toasted, plain wheat germ, and now I have graduated to the raw, for, although toasted wheat germ is still wheat germ and therefore still great for you and your hair, the heat required to toast it removes some of the vitamin content—particularly the vitamin E. Since E is Essential to lovely hair, I don't want to lose a bit.

At first, the raw wheat germ tasted just like it sounds. Raw. But I am of the unshakable opinion that you can get used to anything if it's making you beautiful. And so I not only learned to love raw wheat germ—I'm firmly hooked on it.

Not only do I eat it daily—*never* failing—but I top it off with that tablespoon of lecithin I also have each day, taking care of many of my beauty must-haves with one meal. For lecithin, while it's keeping your fat moving off of you, is also thickening up and shining up your hair via those two hair vitamins, choline and inositol. They're part of the B-complex, but the part that is sometimes omitted from the usual B-complex capsule. They act directly on the hair—hair-vitamins, they might be called. And, since you're eating your lecithin anyway, why not have it this way?

It's an easy way to take beauty-care of two parts of you with two of what Linda Clark calls "wonder foods." Try it. Your hair will show it likes it.

The Beautiful B Vitamins—Best for Your Hair

The B vitamins work their big, beautiful best to keep your hair strong, healthy, and looking it. B vitamins are so important to every part of a healthy you that I simply cannot imagine anyone's not getting enough of them. Not being *sure* they're getting enough, I should say. Check the chapter on Vitamin Vitality in the last section of this book to see just how much of the B's ought to be going into you every day.

The B vitamins are so vital to hair that Leonard of London, the hairdresser who lopped off model Twiggy's locks and thereby made her into a superstar—prescribes B vitamins for all of his clients. It's part of his beautiful-hair program. And Vidal Sassoon, in his London salon, kept a

registered nurse on hand to administer shots of B vitamins
as instant salvation for hair that looked on the way out. It's
pretty sturdy proof of B-power when these gentlemen, who
are well acquainted with hair, consider the B vitamins the
basic beginnings of beautiful hair.

At the risk of being repetitive, I will say once again that
I never like to dissect the B vitamins. But if you can get
hold of those two elusive B's—choline and inositol—
you've got hold of two of the greatest hair-helpers extant.
Brewer's yeast is possibly the best, natural (as opposed to
capsule) way to get all the vitamin B-complex in one food.
Brewer's yeast makes for beautiful B-full hair, so get it
inside of you if you can. I have to confess that I cannot.
For, after all my lectures on learning to love things that do
beautiful things for you (or me), brewer's yeast is one
food I just cannot swallow. And so I take my extra super-
duper B-complex capsules, instead, following all the pro-
portion instructions found under Vitamin Vitality.

And, while we're onto B, always bear in mind that too
much sun or too much alcohol both have a way of taking
all of the vitality out of the B vitamins. (By the same
token, extra B vitamins can cure a hangover pronto. I'd
still prefer you didn't have one.) If you're contemplating
lots of either—sun or drink—then be sure to double dose
on vitamin B, and save that hair beauty.

And if you save those Bs, you're in for a lovely surprise.
For B vitamins, it is claimed by both hair experts and
nutritionists alike, are the ones that can change your hair
from white to color again. Sounds phenomenal, all right,
and it is. So phenomenal that we're going to give it a
chapter all its own, next.

Gray, Gray, Go Away!

I *believe* you can recolor your hair naturally. I've seen it
happen and more than once. And the beautiful B vitamins
—the very ones you're already getting loads of if you've
taken my advice at all—are the boys who can do it.

Consider these personal encounters of mine:

When I was quite small, a great-aunt of mine became
critically ill. So ill she could not, or would not, eat. Eventually, she had to be hospitalized and fed intravenously. I
did not see her at that time, but my parents did and,

apparently, the change in her appearance horrified them both. For my always-rambunctiously-alive aunt was, by then, shriveled up to eighty pounds of weight and that beautiful, blue-black Irish hair of hers had turned a deadly snow white. Both of my parents are willing to swear to that. She remained in the hospital for some months, during which time she was given shots—megadoses, in fact—of B vitamins by a truly farsighted, for that era, physician.

When my aunt left the hospital, she came to spend a few days with my family, so I do know what *I* saw. And what I saw was hair that was far from white. It was black again, with just enough gray scattered throughout so that you knew it was her own. Anyway, I don't believe hospitals have much time for tinting jobs. My aunt's hair remained dark until she died in her eighties.

An experience I have watched from start—well, not to "finish," for I am still watching—concerned a man—a friend of mine who, when I met him, had the *most* hair you ever saw (this was long before the Beatles made the long-hair breakthrough for men), but it was white. This man was young, indeed; he was twenty-six. (At least that's what he told me. I've since discovered that men lie about their ages more than women.) An explorer, he had just hit New York after a lengthy sojourn in the jungles of New Guinea. And he was undernourished, weighing in at 126 for a height of 5'10". So you can see the Spartan sort of life he'd been living. Obviously, survival was on his mind more than nutrition.

As he was an attractive young man, I took a less-than-maternal interest in fattening him up. In the fattening-up process, I watched his hair turn from white back to its natural black-brown. We have been friends for many years now and in those years I have watched his hair color change continually from black to white to black again. Much of that change contiguous with our friendship—meaning who was doing the cooking for him and whether or not she watched his vitamins. This man is married now, to a gourmet cook, but gourmet or no, she apparently doesn't give him all the vitamins he needs. For his hair is white and his paunch is apparent, and he's still only forty-five. Unless he's lying again.

Now there's plenty of hair-moral to these two stories. To me, they prove beyond doubt that hair color can indeed change, and that proper diet has plenty to do with it. Nutritionists and coloring laboratories alike are taking more and more interest in the work that vitamins can do to recolor gray hair. Here is what Adelle Davis, as quoted in Linda Clark's book, *Secrets of Health and Beauty*, has to say on the subject:

> Adequate amounts of iron, copper, and the following B vitamins are essential in maintaining the natural color of the hair: pantothenic acid (calcium pantothenate), PABA, folic acid and inositol. Gray hair at any age, particularly prematurely gray hair, probably indicates a deficiency of one or more of these nutrients.
>
> The natural color of gray hair has sometimes been restored by an adequate intake of all the anti-gray-hair vitamins. The most marked results in restoration of color of gray hair have come from a liberal use of natural foods supplying B vitamins: brewer's yeast, blackstrap molasses, wheat germ, rice polishings, liver and yogurt.
>
> When liberal amounts of yogurt are taken daily, the yogurt bacteria growing in the intestinal tract apparently synthesize or produce the B vitamin inositol, and other anti-gray-hair vitamins. The richest sources of inositol are whole wheat breads, brewer's yeast, blackstrap molasses, and wheat germ.

And I would like to add, lecithin, which you're already taking and which is already filled with that inositol.

Most of the elements mentioned by Miss Davis are the B vitamin foods, and B vitamins seem to be the ones that are there to keep our hair colorful as well as healthful. Take pantothenic acid, for one more personal-experience example from me. I know a gentleman who is in his nineties (he won't let me tell his exact age—told you about men!) and who is still outlasting and outdancing everyone—including his twenty-year-old grandson—at his birthday parties. (He likes his toddies, too, but at over ninety I feel he has that right.) This man has been loading up on calcium pantothenate, or pantothenic acid, for years, in addition to his regular daily B-complex capsule. According to his wife (a beauty in her seventies who looks fifty, thanks to the same vitamin regimen), this man's hair had, at one point, turned white. It has now returned to steely gray. Not bad for over ninety. And not bad for pantothenic acid.

I don't agree with his method of separating the B vitamins. But, on the other hand, it is just possible that his B-complex didn't contain enough pantothenic acid to start with. Until you reach the chapter on Vitamin Vitality (unless you wish to look at it right now), you won't be sure about the B-complex you're taking. Perhaps you should check that chapter this very minute.

PABA, which is short for para-aminobenzoic acid, another B vitamin, is apparently one of the very best of the B's for natural hair recoloring. I imagine you have read of the experiments being done in Europe with procaine, which is a first cousin of novocaine. Reports credit procaine with remarkable abilities to bring color back into graying hair. If it is true, which I do not know for sure, then I think it can safely be attributed to the fact that procaine is filled with PABA, our old colorful friend . . . or so Carlton Fredericks informed an astonished me.

The third anti-gray factor among the B vitamins would appear to be folic acid, which Dr. Fredericks tells me contains PABA, as well. Folic acid is another B vitamin that's hard to get—or at least hard to get enough of, thanks to the FDA, which fears toxicity problems. I cannot imagine such problems with the B vitamins, but I am not going to step beyond the limits of the FDA and say they don't exist. I just simply go right on taking the number of micrograms of folic acid that make up the amount I need to keep all my B's in proper line.

With all the B vitamins working on color, there's still protein, and that's what your hair is still all about. A group of scientists (nutrition scientists, they were) at the University of California at Berkeley have shown that *protein deficiency* can cause loss of hair color. Didn't I tell you that your hair was the very first place to show such deprivation? The Berkeley experiment involved eight healthy male volunteers who were kept in a research ward for three months and fed a liquid formula diet three times a day. One group got seventy-five grams of protein daily while the other received none at all. I'll give you just one guess as to which group turned white in three months. The no-protein crowd, of course. And even more horrifying than white, their hair roots were atrophied. It's enough to make you even more pro-protein, right?

The Natural Way to Color

Herbalists have been touting the beauty-powers of the camomile flower for centuries. According to them, camomile flowers—or rather the extract from them—make a very good semi-permanent lightening rinse for fair hair. And, they add, dark hair can be brightened by it as well, although not bleached in any way. Until I read this, I had completely forgotten that it was a matter of childhood routine for my mother to rinse my hair in camomile. Or was it camomile shampoo? It has been a while—since I was around three—so my memory is a bit foggy there. And so the other night, when I had brewed myself a cup of camomile tea (for camomile is good for other things, too; for one thing, it's a soporific—puts you right off to sound sleep), I decided to make more than sleep use of that cup of tea and I dipped that strip of Nitrazine paper into it, and guess what I found? Acid, which means that no wonder camomile is a perfectly safe and natural way for you to make fair hair more fair. In fact, now that camomile tea can be gotten in tea bags, it seems a pretty simple way to mix up a camomile rinse for yourself. Just remember to brew the rinse in boiling water, but be sure to let it cool down before pouring it over you. No cooked heads of hair, please.

Henna is, of course, another much-recommended form of coloring hair and one that has been around just as long as camomile, if not longer. English nutritionist Charles Perry believes in henna as a "perfectly harmless and beneficial dyestuff." He does, however, go on to say that only Egyptian or Indian henna is to be used, since Tunisian henna is not henna at all but a toxic metallic compound. He also warns against "henna" found ready-mixed in bottles as being non-henna henna, and probably suspect. Some hair salons tout henna, but I had heard some stories that make me wonder, and therefore, before you consider henna, insist upon testing it first. What do you care if the whole salon thinks you're crazy? Better be paranoid than bald, I always say. And if you're thinking henna, think red.

That's the color your hair is going to be, if the henna you're going to use is the kind you'd want.

If You Still Want Unnatural Color

If you really insist on tinting your hair, then at least try to do it in the least harmful way possible. There are, thanks to modern-day research powers, products on the market now that are also acid-balanced. No, they cannot color your hair and keep it acid. I have already explained to you how your hair cuticle must be literally peeled away from its medulla, or center, in order for any color to penetrate. Frankly, the idea of that alone is enough to make me allow my own hair color to go in any direction it chooses, as long as it remains my own natural color.

But the point is, if I can't talk you out of coloring, then at least I can warn you to use products that will get your hair back to acid just as fast as possible. Talk it over with your hairdresser. I am sure he, or she, is very up on what's happening right now in the busy world of hair cosmetics; and I am very happy to say that what is happening is happening for the good of your hair.

Hunza Hair

Returning to the subject of wheat and the one germ you want, let's consider the Hunzukuts, because these people are a wonderful example of what the right sort of eating can do for the hair on your head. And for you.

Hunza is a tiny state in the Himalayas. So who goes there? Well, people who want to find out how the Hunzukuts manage to remain sexually potent to age ninety, and maintain enviable health until they die—which is usually somewhere around the age of 120. According to our hair expert, now non-balding Dale Alexander, the Hunzukuts keep their hair at full head-value until the 120 years makes them give up living altogether. Mr. Alexander is only one of many who have studied the diet of the Hunzukuts, and most are convinced that it is their diet of naturally grown foods that include lots of whole grains such as millet and barely, wheat and buckwheat. Plus plenty of *fresh* vegetables such as turnips, peas, beans, carrots, tomatoes, corn (remember the Mexicans), cheese, butter, and milk.

It's a health-maintenance sort of diet, all right, and, according to Mr. Alexander, there are only two men in all of Hunza who are partially bald. And those two spent part of their lives in England where, no doubt, they caught on to the "refined" way of eating.

The Hunzukuts have long been examples for health food fanciers. But to me it is more fascinating to find an entire nation of healthy hair-growers and to know how they did it.

Vitamin E—The Sexy Hair Shaper-Upper

As you may have guessed by now, I believe that vitamin E is good for every part of you. But that's my belief, for since E is the seventies' baby, there's lots and lots of research still going on to determine any and everything about vitamin E. One thing I do know. I know that wheat germ got me out of that Indian-scalp cut that was *that* hairdresser's undoing. And do you know why? Because wheat germ is filled with the very best kind of vitamin E—the natural kind.

And since vitamin E has been called, among other names, the sex vitamin, let me point out that sexy hair is, in my beauty book, hair that is alive, vibrant, vital, and swing-free. Vitamin E can help you have it.

I have discovered a little secret about vitamin E. It works as well from the outside as from the inside. I assume that by now everyone's taking her daily dose of E—whether from wheat germ-and-lecithin, or in capsule form. But have you ever thought of adding vitamin E to your shampoo?

I hadn't either until one day, back before my hair hit its beauty stride with the protein, acid-balanced treatment, I complained to my hairdresser about the lack of shine—something a straight-hair like myself needs, since we have little else in the way of interesting shape. This hairdresser (haircutter, for it was my friend, Roger Thompson) suggested that I try a few drops of wheat germ oil in my shampoo.

Now, you know by now my fondness for improvisation, and also that I prefer the fastest result whenever possible. Therefore, I decided to go right to the vitamin E capsule rather than take the wheat germ oil way around. As we have discovered, vitamin E is the one vitamin that can't easily be washed from the skin. Doesn't it stand to reason the same would apply to hair? And so I slashed open my vitamin E capsule, and poured it into the bottle of acid-balanced protein shampoo. And guess what happened? I had hair that was gloriously shiny and, furthermore, looked about twice as thick as it had before. Now vitamin E, as we have said, is a bit on the honey-textured side. And it clings to hair. So here, then, is your "natural" hair thickener. I was so fascinated by those results that I wouldn't dream of giving up this magic shampoo mixture.

I use two of my 400-unit vitamin E capsules, slashed with a razor blade, and squeezed into an applicator-sized bottle; that means the size your hairdresser uses to apply shampoo. This is 800 units to the bottle and on me it works. I expect you'll not only be surprised with the results but delighted as well.

Now vitamin E, once put into a shampoo bottle and let out of its protective capsule coating, doesn't retain its vitality, so you are going to have to replace that 800 units every three or four days if you really want the results to show up on your hair. I realize that vitamin E is not the least expensive of vitamins (here again, everyone's in there selling the hottest item at the highest possible prices), and thus it turns out to be relatively expensive shampooing. But, as far as I'm concerned, you can't put a price on natural beauty like that.

I wash my hair with this concoction every two days, which means that I'm not only putting protein on and maintaining that protective acid hair-mantle, but putting E onto it as well. Believe me, it keeps my hair looking very together.

One thing I really must bring to your attention, and that is refrigeration. You wouldn't leave your meat out at room temperature, would you? So why should you expect to do the same with your protein shampoo? Or anything with those volatile vitamins in it? This means that any and all organic beauty products really ought to be refrigerated, for longer beauty-life, if you expect the freshest beauty from them. Occasionally, I get lazy and don't do it. But I make up for that laziness by mixing a fresh batch of shampoo every time I wash.

Just remember—organic is non-preserved and therefore, for safety and beauty's sake, should be kept on ice.

E and A—Inseparable

A word of caution here, now that I've told you how good vitamin E can be for your hair. It *is*, and don't suspect that I am going to tell you now that there's a danger. It's not that. It's just that vitamins A and E are two that work together. Now I've already touted A as the skin vitamin and I assume that you're taking it every single day. But just in case you consider yourself skin-perfect and aren't downing that vitamin A, let me warn you here that vitamin E tends to act against vitamin A—which means nothing more than the fact that you must take them both, especially if you are taking the amounts of E that are recommended to produce beautiful results. You should never have one without the other!

I don't want you losing your skin-beauty in favor of hair shine and therefore want you never, never to forget that, as long as you are taking vitamin E, you must take vitamin A as well. They're both beautiful, so why not? And, as of this red-hot moment, there is now available a water-miscible vitamin E—just in case you're not into adding any more oil than necessary. Maybe you're one of those rare creatures who manufactures quite enough of her own natural oils, with no help needed. So now you have no excuse. For vitamin E is one more oil-soluble vitamin, just like vitamins A and D, and, although there has been no research on vitamin E as there has with the other two when taken in large doses—you might want to play it safe, and head for the water-miscible version. Just thought I'd let you know there's an oil-free kind.

Diet vs. Doctors

Here's where I hope my way—the diet way—will win. For, unbelievably, many doctors still inevitably refuse to admit that proper diet has anything to do with the health of the hair—or any other beauty part of you. One famous New York dermatologist, who has said that I may quote him, came flat out with the statement that, "Diet has nothing whatsoever to do with hair." I choose *not* to name him, for

I see no reason to destroy an otherwise good reputation . . . especially since this is the general reaction of the medical profession when the question of diet's effect on beauty is put to them. To me, this sort of statement is blithely irresponsible and just the sort that makes the medical profession look less than beautiful when it comes to prescribing for less-than-serious ills. On the other hand, what is less serious today may be quite serious tomorrow. For a woman who loses her hair could have some pretty damaging psychological scars—perhaps even some suicidally damaging scars. Only then would the medical profession consider the desire to look one's best and preserve one's natural good looks as serious business. Therefore I am not going to name the doctor that made that statement, but you can bet he isn't going to be my doctor, either. For again, when it comes to hair, lead me to a trained trichologist or a hairdresser who is up on his product-research and is going to know what's really happening—and that's quite a lot, as you've seen—in the world of hair care.

As for saying diet doesn't matter when it comes to hair —just try telling that one to an animal breeder. You can be sure the high-gloss coats in champion animals aren't there by accident. Surely you deserve the same sort of diet-for-beauty care.

To Cut to Grow? Is That the Question?

Do you want to know whether it's truth or myth that cutting your hair regularly makes it grow faster? The truth is—it's one more beauty myth. Some hair researchers say that there may be a sudden *spurt* in growth immediately after a cutting—sort of a making up for lost hair-time, so to speak—but, in the long run, it all averages out to about six inches growth per year, no matter who you are.

This is assuming, of course, that your hair is healthy. If it isn't, it may grow barely at all. Remember my experience with the low-carbohydrate diet, when my hair was sheared to the scalp and then refused to cover it up by growing as it should? Until, of course, I added wonderful wheat germ and unknowingly, at that time, added the B vitamins and the vitamin E that were destined to get my hair growing within a matter of weeks.

O.K. I'm assuming you've got the healthy-hair matter

well under control by now. At least, if you've been reading this carefully, you should have. But there *are* some things to know about cutting besides the fact that regular trims won't—repeat, *won't*—give you more than six inches of hair per year, no matter how well they're done.

Dr. Norman Orentreich, a New York dermatologist whose specialty is hair as well as skin (he pioneered hair transplants—something you should never need if you are as careful as I hope you'll be), scoffs at the cut-and-grow theory, but does compare hair with an old sweater that has been washed and washed and washed until it's frazzled. That's about what becomes of the ends of your hair— which, after all, are the oldest part—if you don't cut them off regularly. According to Dr. Orentreich, it's not so much a question of hair health as of hair beauty. Frazzled ends? Forget them!

Split ends are something else again, and they have to go—and not just for beauty's sake. For, when the end of a hair starts to split—meaning that if you look closely, you'll see a little inverted "V" shape at the end of each hair— then, chances are, that split will soon travel straight up the shaft of your hair, thereby destroying it. That we do not want, and so I will recommend that you get rid of any and all split ends by virtue of a proper haircut just as soon as you spot one. Even one.

What's a Proper Haircut? It's Your Hair's Choice!

A proper haircut is the one that suits you. It's the haircut of your hair's choice. I am very anti the idea of trying to force your hair into a style that it just won't wear. I still don't understand why, in this age of do-your-own-thing living, people usually are unhappy with whatever kind of hair they happen to have.

I have never, for example, met a curly-haired person who liked his/her hair. Yet curly hair can be one of the very easiest kinds to deal with if properly cut by someone who understands it. It can be the wash-and-shake out kind of thing that every woman ought to be yearning for (more on that in a moment) no matter what her age. And yet the curly-hairs go on complaining, and occasionally resorting to the damaging habit of straightening those curls. I think it's not only damaging, but absurd as well, to try to force your hair into any image but its own.

And the straight-hairs—that's me—do just the opposite. They perm and set and tease and do all the things that are so injurious to the health of those straight hairs that *can* be the shiniest things in town. For straight hair, if left alone, can light up a room with its highlights—something the curly-hairs have to make up for with other advantages. But if you torment it into some unnatural shape, you're going to have no highlights, and possibly very little long straight hair. I will soon show you the dangerous chic of some straight hairdos—namely, the ponytail and chignon. But perming, straightening, teasing, spraying, setting, and all the rest of the unnatural routines that used to be so routine to us all, are so injurious to your hair that I would find a way to avoid them. In fact, I have.

My Way

I have my hair cut twice a year. That's because I have one of the best haircutters around for me and my hair. He is Roger Thompson, who was the International Artistic Director of Vidal Sassoon. The title is impressive, but Roger is friendly—in fact, we've been friends since about 1965 when he cut my hair in London. You see, Vidal Sassoon and his crew have been my men since back in 1964 when I muscled my way in for one of the original swinging-hair Sassoon cuts by the Original Sassoon himself. (At that time, I was in retailing, and I can only surmise that Vidal Sassoon assumed I was a retail heiress, or some such thing. Anyone who would come to *London* for a haircut!) That is when my hair became fem-liberated and I was never again to turn, or return, to the sit-under-the-dryer routine for hair. Not for my looks and most certainly not for my hair health.

At any rate, my hair is straight, as I've told you. Very. And it's cut that way—straight around. It only has to be cut twice a year because it never loses its shape, it never gets split ends. It is, some say, a phenomenon. Roger says it's my hair. I say it's Roger's haircut. It's probably the cut combined with the fact that, thanks to Nicholas's re-educating me on the subject of care and feeding of hair, my hair is now in better condition than ever before.

My hair used to grow in scraggly, and it was, in fact, one of the sore points of my looks-life. I have spent more unnecessary time having hair-hysterics than on any other part of me. But now it just grows longer and nothing else happens. I suppose it could grow straight to my waist without losing its Roger-given shape, except that I feel I'm a bit old for that look—which is pretty much gone-with-the-fashion wind in any case. Strong and straight forever—that's my way.

Wash-and-Wear Hair

Fem-liberated hair is almost here for everyone—thank goodness. For that will be the day when heads can get to be their very healthiest and hair ecology, rather than hair*do*, will be the order of the beauty day. I only wish it had all happened when I was young, before I put my own hair through such tortures to keep it in style. Nowadays, the style is good hair, period.

I have already said that "hairdo" ought to be an obsolete word. For I feel that every woman in the world, once she has been liberated from the weekly "set," will be liberated forever. I have Sassoon to thank for setting me free from all that rigamarole. On the other hand, I am well aware that there isn't a Vidal Sassoon, or a Roger Thompson, in every town in America. (I am not limiting my list of A-one remarkable haircutters to these, but fact is fact. The Sassoon sort of cutting was what started hair swinging again—swinging away from "set.")

I realize that age and hair type and bone structure and all of those things enter into a woman's choice of hair style. I wouldn't be in the fashion business if I didn't know *that*. But I still maintain that the proper cut, on any kind of healthy hair, should be the cut that *you* can maintain all by yourself, with no worries about damp weather, rainstorms, wind, hail, or even a swim in the dark of night. A really good haircut ought to come up looking just as good after any and all of those things.

I will never forget taking a friend of mine to my beach house for a weekend, only to find her spending half of a beach-ideal Saturday afternoon with her hair in curlers, in preparation for the usual weekend bash. My only emotion was pity. No woman should have to worry about her hair at the beach. Or in an open car. Or making love. Or wherever. Not if she's gotten the right kind of haircut by someone who understands the kind of hair she has and the kind of cut that will look best on her.

Sooner or later, wash-and-wear hair will be an accepted part of woman's liberation—just like the disappearance of the girdle. (I can't say "bra." I wear one.) Everyone's hair is going to be a lot healthier for it. It's the "wave" of the future!

Strip Tease

That's exactly what teasing is going to do. Strip your hair of all its own natural good looks. First of all, teasing simply isn't the look to have these days. But what is more important, teasing, or back-combing—one more unnatural way to thicken up limp hair—is highly injurious in that it can break your hair and break it badly. I feel that most hairdressers today who are worth their titles avoid teasing like the plague. They know exactly what it can do. And I am relieved that both the cosmetics industry and the hair-dressing profession have turned their thoughts to ways of keeping you looking your own *natural* best rather than dreaming up unnatural looks that will rob you of nature's own handiwork. No—they all seem to be thinking right on that subject these days. A few years ago, during the bee-hive boom, it would have been hard to convince even a teenager that swinging-free hair was the kind to have. Ecology has gone a lot farther than saving energy; it's helping save our looks as well.

But if a hairdresser ever attempts to tease your hair, or if you should ever let your own thoughts drift in that direction, start thinking about what you will do when your hair is broken off to the scalp. It won't be a pretty hair-picture.

Dangerous Chic

On the subject of hair styles, I feel I'd be treating you unfairly if I didn't give passing (that's all *this* style deserves) mention to one that is literally *dangerous!* That is the ponytail, or, for that matter, any sleeked-and-secured back hairdo you can think of. Sure it looks chic, but how chic will you feel when you realize you're going bald? This kind of hair-wearing is one of the primary causes of female baldness (and there's more of *that* than you dream of; and we don't want it to happen to you). I have heard that one of the world's most famous ballerinas has a part in her hair that's almost one inch wide—from all that sleeking down. Now ballerinas have to keep their hair out of the dance, but you don't. So *don't pull.*

A co-worker of mine wears her beautiful, thick, long hair hanging down her back in a heavy braid. I have watched, helplessly, as her hairline receded to bald at one point. I have warned her. So have her other friends. But she's either oblivious to all warnings—including her mirror's—or she finds her hair style easy. It won't be so easy when she finds herself in a hairpiece.

Should you ever, even for one evening (and not for any longer) try the sleeked-back look, for heaven's sake, don't use a rubber band. It's a sure way to break off your hair. We won't worry about rubber bands.

Cold Weather Shrinkage

If on a cold winter's day you should find your hair lying down and looking limp—don't worry! That's natural. Nothing can flatten out a head of gorgeous hair faster than a cold snap and a little static electricity. Your hair is just like the rest of you: It shrinks (yes, it does!) in cold weather. Just like your hands and your feet. (And that same cold is not noted for making your skin look its best either. That's the reason for protection, protection, and more protection.)

Not only does that hair look flatter and lanker in supercold, the truth is that you have less. For people, unlike animals, who obviously know a lot that we humans don't, tend to have *less* hair in the winter than in the spring.

Dr. Norman Orentreich, the New York dermatologist, has done research and more research on the growth habits of hair. He has found that May is the month when you'll have the most hairs on your head (about 140,000 if you're blonde; 108,000 if brunette; and redheads get about 90,000). All during the summer, you'll have Godiva locks, for summer heat and humidity make the hair swell, so that you not only have more hair on your head, but it will look double that.

One answer to the cold shrinkage subject is to keep a humidifier in your bedroom. At least that's the answer I got from one shiny-haired beauty who managed to look like May on the coldest day in January. She swears that without it her hair looks like a rag mop. Not a look we hope for here!

No Hot Stuff Here!

This is one spot where hair makes a rapid departure from skin—same protein-makeup or not. For here is where I want to warn you about the danger of heat on hair. I recently read an article in *Vogue* magazine on "Hair Fall-out" and the phenomenal rate at which it is happening to women. And one of the very things *Vogue* blames are the heated hair-beauty aids. Or supposed beauty aids.

I learned long ago, from an enlightened hairdresser who had burned off his own, that even blow-dryers are very likely to dry the hair right to a crisp, crinkled turn if they are held too close to the hair itself. If you use one of these nozzle-like dryers, as I do, and if you have ever had an opportunity to watch an experienced hand holding one, as I have, then you will notice that the experienced hairdresser will work the dryer quickly back and forth across the lock of hair he is holding out from the head with his plastic-bristled brush. The plastic bristles let the hot air through, the back-and-forth motion eliminates the possibility of frying your hair. You will also notice that he never holds the blow-dryer directly *on* the hair, but rather at an angle, ever-moving. You will learn to do it this way, too, if you want to have any hair to dry.

Heat—lots of it—is injurious as all get-out to hair. I am reasonably sure there isn't a woman out there who hasn't managed to curl her eyelashes by peering inside a too-hot oven. True? I know I've done it many times—though I'm learning. This, then, is the kind of frazzle you'll get from too much heat. Heated curlers—which I was astonished to realize have been around for ten years now—are one of the worst hair-hurters. My former hairdresser used them on me until even he decided they were harmful. Your hair simply won't take too much heat, even from the dryer in a beauty salon. That is why I am so hopeful that one day soon, the great cut will completely eliminate the good "set," and thereby eliminate that heavy heat that setting requires . . . the kind that does so much (especially when used in combination with metal pins) to destroy the health-and-shine of your own *natural* hair.

Creme Rinse—Do You Need It?

Here we are again, asking the same question we asked about skin, except that this time I don't think you're asking for trouble nearly as much by using a creme rinse on your hair as by the indiscriminate use of facial creams on your complexion. There's one qualification only: that creme rinse just must be acid. Acid is in there for hair and hair is one place we aren't going to forget it for even a second.

The purpose of creme rinses is to add highlights, and to make your hair easier to comb, if it tangles after a shampoo. I personally use an acid-balanced creme rinse, but I have to admit that it is more for non-tangling purposes than anything else, though it helps luster-up things when I'm feeling less than lustrous myself. Still, with hair, you can't hide your feelings, and if you're not feeling up to par, it will show up fast on your hair. (That's why I want you so healthy.) Tangles, of course, can cause breakage and therefore are to be avoided, and here is where a creme rinse can come in handy. In its miraculous way, it gets rid of them before you comb, making breakage unlikely.

Beware, however, of a creme rinse that tends to make your hair lie limp—especially if you have fine hair to start with. With hair, as with skin, softening is not what we want. On the contrary, strength is the sought-after quality. Tensile strength, combined with elasticity but most certainly not softness. For softness does to your hair what it does to your skin—i.e., makes it droop. Droopy hair is not the prettiest sort to have, whereas springy is lively and that's where we're headed.

A friend of mine has true "problem" hair. Baby fine, soft, difficult to deal with. She tries to force it into a style it didn't grow into and she tints it to boot. And, one assumes, to offset that damaging routine, she douses it with creme rinse after every wash. And then she wonders why it's so soft and flyaway. This is not the kind of hair for which I would ever recommend any sort of creme rinse—even the acid-balanced sort. But this young woman is deaf to any suggestions that possibly creme is not her need. So I simply let her fly away—her own way.

However, if you want strong-looking hair, consider your own hair as carefully as you do your own skin before deciding if it needs any extra, artificial lights. If you think it does, then make sure you test it first for no-blue. That will do fine.

Circulation from Stimulation

There are two kinds of massage, of course. The soothing, relaxing sort and the zingy, vigorously administered kind that's meant to set your blood tingling, so that it will get up and do its beauty work. And your scalp is one spot that can use plenty of stimulation, if it's the proper sort and done with care.

Don Lee, a scalp specialist in New York, who has given lion's mane locks to such luminaries as model Veruschka, counts as a large part of his scalp treatment a vigorous massage, administered by a crew of Mr. America-sized men with Mr. America kind of muscles. Believe me, when you get a massage from Don Lee, your scalp gets the message!

George Michaels, a New York hairdresser who only half-jokingly calls his salon "The House of Long Hair," has turned out more real longhairs than you can possibly imagine, with clients in almost every musical show on Broadway. You know, those long-maned dancers with the gorgeous swinging tresses. Mr. Michaels has his own ideas about the kind of massage that makes hair grow long. And he must know, for his assistant has hair that is long enough to sit on! It would be a bit in the way in my own fast-paced business, but to each her own hair-length!

Mr. Michaels' recommended massage is done in the shampoo shower and consists of a gentle back-to-front motion, all done with the head hanging down. The reason for the shower massage? Mr. Michaels doesn't believe in massaging dirt into the hair. Sound hair-thinking, I'd say.

And then, of course, there's massage with a hairbrush. Mr. Michaels thinks it ought to be done first thing in the morning—even before you put the coffee on to brew. Once again, this kind of massaging should be done by bending forward from the waist, and brushing from back to front. And he believes in the two hundred beauty stokes, all right. He also believes that the only way to brush at all is with a natural-bristled hairbrush. Here, he and I part theories. For *I* believe in, and use, the plastic-bristled rubber-based hairbrush so often used by the no-set, Sassoon sort of hairdressers. The advantage to this brush is that there is no way the hair can get tangled up in those wide-apart plastic prongs. And since the plastic "bristles" are based in a rubber pad, the static electricity, which could conceivably cause hair breakage, is calmed down. In any case, I have a lot of hair to show for this kind of brush. While we're onto brushing, let me warn you about one possible danger. Never, *never* brush wet hair. For when your hair is wet, it's at its most elastic—meaning it might stretch just one shade more than it can, and break off. Save the brushing for almost-dry and use a comb to get out any wash tangles.

New York hairdresser Ian of Davian Inc. reminds me that an awful lot of people don't know how to comb wet hair. I must admit I hadn't given it that much thought myself. But, as he puts it, comb it slowly from the *bottom* —starting to work out the tangles from there. If you start from the top, you'll have a whole length of hair to untangle and it will be a lot harder on your head and your hair. Remember: bit by bit, from the bottom upward.

Keep Calm—Stress Is a Sure-Fire Hair-Killer

Every single one of the hair experts I've met, and interviewed, has stressed the importance of avoiding stress. It's "cool" you need if you want your hair to keep on growing —and you most certainly do—for stress is not only a beauty-killer, but a hair-killer as well. It is such an adept hair-killer, in fact, that if you can't keep calm you may find that your scalp has actually constricted to the point where your hair *can't* grow. That, I certainly do not want for you.

Your hair and your psyche are so intertwined that an experienced hairdresser—or one who's aware—can actually guess your state of mind from the state of your hair. If your hair's just lying there looking sorry for itself, chances are you're feeling that way, too.

Psychiatrists have told me that one of the first places to spot real depression is in the hair. If it doesn't look lively, the patient isn't, either. So it's relatively easy to get that message, for you want to be alive and lively and showing it. Therefore, I have to stress stress, so that you may avoid it all the way.

One hairdresser could always spot my mood the moment he took hold of my hair (and would often say, "Not feeling well today, huh?"). He had, as part of his without-charge client-regimen, a lovely massage with a protein conditioner, all administered gently by the best scalp-masseur I've every known. This hairdresser believed strongly in the protein routine (and he was one of the first to pick up on it—I'll give him that—even though he was the one who gave me my crew cut). And he believed in it so strongly that he insisted on it for everyone who entered his doors—man, woman, or child. So we all not only got that protein into our hair, but we got that wonderfully relaxing massage into the bargain, which helped it work all the better.

Don't overlook calcium as the best natural tranquilizer around. Adelle Davis swears she keeps a bottle of calcium lactate tablets by her night table and downs a handful whenever sleeplessness hits. Certainly calcium is the only sort of tranquilizer you should consider unless it's the B-vitamin complex—another tranquilizer of the best natural sort. Unnatural tranquilizers are just as bad for your hair as they are for your skin, and their unlimited use will show up as limited hair. They simply aren't good for you, and whatever is not good for you will never make you beautiful. Stick to calcium for beauty's sake.

Happily, the things that relax you are often the very things that get circulation going to your hair as well. Massage is only one way, but it's one way that's used by most of the hair experts around. A beauty editor of my acquaintance swears that the yoga-style neckstand has made her hair grow by inches. Not only does it pinch off the tension but, according to this lady, it pinches the thyroid gland in a manner that actually stimulates it, and hair growth goes hand in hand with healthy thyroid—just like skin growth. I haven't tried this method—my neckstand isn't too expert—but if you're careful and don't do it too vigorously, it shouldn't hurt and just may hair-help a lot.

Nutritionist Linda Clark recommends daily headstands as a way of getting blood to the scalp, relaxing it (and you), and getting that scalp in good shape to grow hair, because the good things you eat are no good to your hair if they never get up to your scalp where they belong. Miss Clark also suggests that one more way to getting things into scalp circulation while you relax is by lying on a slant board, feet up and head down, of course, for about fifteen to twenty minutes every day. If you don't feel up to a headstand.

The point here is relax, relax, *relax*. It's not an easy order, I realize, in this era of hectic living. But, for good looks and good health, you'd better try it.

Here is the quick-reference route to hair-growth eating. For these are the foods that contain the things I've told you to eat for the health of that hair. Don't forget all the beautiful B vitamins, which I have just given you after the "Skin" section. That's where you'll find those (why tell you twice) and then you'll get the whole vitamin picture in my big, beautiful chart.

HAIR

VITAMIN E

Eggs	Barley
Margarine	Oatmeal
Corn oil	Whole-grain rye
Cottonseed oil	Whole wheat flour
Olive oil	Wheat germ
Palm oil	Peanuts
Peanut oil	Brussels sprouts
Safflower oil	Cabbage
Soybean oil	Leeks
Sunflower oil	Kale
Wheat germ oil	Mustard greens
All cooking and salad oils	Spinach
Lecithin	

Buttermilk
Cottage cheese (small and large curd)
Cheese soufflé
Swiss cheese
American cheese
Whipping cream (light and heavy)
Eggs (prepared any way)
Milk
Skimmed milk, all forms
Yogurt
Fish
Shellfish
Plain prepared bran
Buckwheat, whole grain
Buckwheat flour
Corn flour
Cottonseed flour
Oat cereals (cooked)
Rye, whole grain
Rye flour
Wheat flour
Wheat germ
Cooked wheat cereals
Wheat flakes
Wild rice
Bacon
Beef
Chicken
Capon
Duck
Goose
Heart
Kidney
Lamb
Pork
Blood sausage or blood pudding

Liverwurst
Frankfurters
Headcheese
Knockwurst
Salami
Thuringer
Squab
Sweetbreads
Tongue
Turkey
Veal
Desiccated liver
Granola
Almonds
Almond meal
Cashew nuts
Coconut milk
Peanuts
Peanut butter
Peanut flour
Peas, mature seeds
Pecans
Pigeon peas, mature
Safflower seed meal
Soybeans
Soybean curd
Soybean flour
Sunflower seed flour
Walnuts
Common beans, all types
Lima beans
Mung beans, mature seeds, dry
Broadbeans
Broccoli
Chickpeas
Cowpeas (including black-eyed peas)
Lentils

4. Nails

The Nails Nobody Knows

Nobody knows the troubles I've seen trying to find somebody—just *anybody*—who knows anything about nails. Because fingernails (and one assumes toenails, too) seem to be the stepchildren of the beauty world. Which is sad, since they are the best indication of one's general state of health. And the general state of health is what is going to determine your beauty.

I have problem nails of my own, which is one reason I've been on a nail crusade for so long, only to find out that the medical profession, once again, seems to know little more than I do about what makes them healthy and strong, or unhealthy and brittle. I've checked out companies that manufacture nail products, dermatologists, skin specialists, and general physicians and the answer almost always comes up, "We just don't know."

One reason there seems to be so little concern about nail health (a dangerous lack of concern, if you ask me) is that people worry, according to one researcher, if their hair looks frazzled or if their skin breaks out. But if their nails break off, they chalk it up to bad luck and let it go at that, little knowing the health implications. For if your nails are O.K., you're O.K.—and the reverse applies as well.

Therefore, we have very little information to work with when it comes to nails. We *do* know that they're made of—I'll give you less than one guess—protein. Just like everything else. And, therefore, protein can go at the very top of your list of things that make nails hard. For the nail is actually a horny extension of the skin (sounds hideous; if properly cared for, looks beautiful) and should be treated in exactly the same way you would treat your face —namely, with care.

Nails—Treat Them Like Your Skin. They Are!

All of the things you've learned about skin—the acid mantle, the protein importance—apply equally to the nails. And the things you put on them should be tested just as rigorously as you would test your facial cosmetics. For alkaline—with detergents coming most rapidly to mind—is just as harmful to nails as to the skin on your face, and that's awfully harmful.

So let's simply consider that your nails are an extension of that beautiful skin you probably (or ought to) have by now and treat them accordingly. Never let anything touch them that you wouldn't let touch your face. That should keep them safe until the medical profession and/or research can tell us more nail secrets.

I mean, would you *really* go around washing your face in detergents? After all I've told you about that acid mantle your skin had for its own protection and the importance of *keeping* it there? No, I know you wouldn't! Just remember that detergents are the harshest of the alkaline sort of cleaners that can come along to destroy your skin. And that's your nails. According to the editors of *Prevention* magazine, with the onslaught of "miracle" cleaners, hands are not only dishpan-variety, but even real skin disease has been traced to the grease-cutting strength of detergents. Can you imagine how constant immersion in that kind of water can destroy even the best and hardest of fingernails?

That's another point. Constant immersion in *any* kind of water is going to make your fingernails soft. And while they're in that shape, watch out! That's the time they peel off. I know it's an old axe to grind, but rubber gloves, if you have to handle water *all* the time, are the *only* solution for helping save those nails. Or at least for keeping them as hard as you'd like them.

Nail Myths to Disbelieve

Well, those old wives have been at it again, tongues wagging with tales about what's good for your nails that all turn out to be every bit as false as the myths surrounding the rest of you.

One perfect example is the gelatin myth. You know, the

one that tells you that a packet (of gelatin) a day will keep the breaking nails away. The simple fact is that gelatin has absolutely no effect on the growth of your nails. I have had gelatin recommended to me by general physicians and dermatologists alike as a nail problem cure-all. That should tell you what they know on the subject.

It is quite true that some years ago—in the twenties, I believe—a radio-isotope study was done to determine whether gelatin turned up in the nails. Sure, it turned up all right, as would almost any food you might put into your body and thereby into your blood stream. But does that mean it does those nails any good? Emphatically no.

Recently the Federal Trade Commission barred one gelatin product from making false nutritional claims about gelatin drinks. The F.T.C. claimed that, in ads, the manufacturer falsely claimed that the protein in gelatin is high-quality protein that provides nutritional benefit. To the contrary, the complaint alleged, gelatin protein is a low-quality protein of very little nutritional benefit. Does that sound to you like the sort of protein that is going to benefit those protein-hungry nails of yours? Not to me it doesn't, and since I find the stuff not only unpalatable, but downright un-swallowable, I prefer to get my protein in more edible ways. By eating practically any other sort . . . fish, cheese, yogurt, milk (you know how I feel about beef, so we won't go into that), and fowl. As for gelatin capsules, forget them entirely. I even got a dermatologist to admit that it would take approximately fifty capsules to equal the contents of one packet of gelatin. So why bother, if it's low-quality protein in any case? Leave the gelatin to making congealed salads containing all the good fresh vegetables and fruits you need for good health, and take your nails on to valuable proteins . . . the kinds that harden them up.

The second myth we come to is the calcium one. Back in the days of my protein-deprivation—thanks to that low-carbohydrate-for-too-long nonsense—I had calcium recommended to me by all sorts of doctors. For, by then, I was losing my nails (as well as my hair) at a rapid clip—and I was losing them down to the quick, which not only hurt, but got infected as well. Now that I have studied the subject more carefully, I am astonished that many of the physicians I respect mightily were among those recommending calcium for nails. Now calcium is important, all right, and you should never forget nor ignore it. *But your nails are not made of calcium.* Your teeth and bones are, but your nails are pure protein and that's what's required to keep them strong and healthy. Remember my protein recommendations from previous chapters and continually check the chart to make sure you are getting enough. For protein is what is going to salvage those nails for you, and, as your health improves, so do your nails.

Dr. Norman Orentreich has done as much research on nails as on hair, it seems, so let him say it for me. "Fragile nails that break and split are a problem to many. Such nail problems are apparently *not due to calcium deficiency;* there is little calcium in the nail; furthermore, people with calcium deficiencies do not necessarily have fragile or split-ting nails." Convinced?

Shape Up Your Nails

Dr. Earle Brauer, Research Director of Revlon (you know them—the nail people) warns that, if you have let your nails get into less than lovely shape, *be patient.* Once you start to care for them *properly,* it is still going to take six months before you have a *wholly new* beautiful fingernail.

Didn't I tell you? Six months seems to be the limit for re-doing *you.* It's the same with hair or with skin. (But hope-fully not with shape. There, we can speed things up with our four little fat-removing friends—lecithin, B-6, cider vinegar, and kelp.)

Just *don't* expect overnight results or you're bound to be disappointed and perhaps tempted to give up. *Don't!* It's stick-to-it-iveness that gets the beautiful results. And those results are always worth the waiting. As for caring for the nails you've grown, our nail friend Dr. Orentreich cautions about manicuring. Not too much and certainly not the wrong sort. The wrong sort, for one thing, means excess cutting of the cuticle. That cuticle is there for a purpose. It protects (like the cuticle of your hair) the nail fold from infections and should *never* be cut unless it is torn or ragged. A painful hangnail should most definitely be trimmed. But the best thing is not to get a painful hang-nail!

Instead, pre-manicure, try soaking your nails in warm water, to which you've added some acid-balanced soap—

suds. Or some wheat germ oil. Or even some vitamin E—squeezed from the capsule, of course. Then those cuticles should be pushed back *ever so gently* with the fingertip—not the fingernail—of the opposite hand. Better still, do it with a soft towel.

Finish everything off with an E-oil massage if you want to keep the cuticle soft and invisible.

Everybody should know by now that there's only one way to file nails and that's one way. In one direction, that is. Watch any competent manicurist and you will see that that's how it's done. It seems that to saw back and forth with a file (and I hope you're using an emery board) is injurious to the nail itself. So think one-sided and you'll have stronger, better-shaped nails. And keep the emery board at a 45-degree angle.

As for nail polish—well, Dr. Orentreich thinks it's O.K. I personally hate it. I hate the way it feels. I much prefer polishing my nails with a paste polish and a chamois buffer. Buffing stirs up that blood and spurs the nails' growth, and anything that does that is fine with me. But do it gently. Buffing too hard can actually *burn* the nail! I've had that unhappy experience. A mixture of honey, wheat germ oil, and egg yolks, mixed into a paste and seasoned with sea salt, will nourish the nails when rubbed into and around them.

Polish does, however, protect the nails when they're getting some rough use. It can serve as a shield against the world of hard knocks. But when you're removing that nail polish, be sure you add a little wheat germ oil to soften up that strong action of the (of necessity) acetone-based polish remover. After all, you don't want to remove your nails in the process.

As for nail-hardeners—watch out. Dr. Joseph Jerome, Secretary of the Committee on Cutaneous Health and Cosmetics of the A.M.A. says, "In recent years, products to prevent the nails from chipping, fragmenting, and peeling have become popular. Most, if not all, of these products contain formaldehyde. Several physicians have reported severe reactions to nail hardeners containing or releasing formaldehyde. Reactions have included discoloration, bleeding under the nail, pain, dryness, and loosening or even loss of nails." You wouldn't want that to happen to you, would you? Read on.

Harden Your Heart to Hardeners

Apparently some cosmetics intended to beautify the nails end up doing a lot more harm than beautifying. Hardeners are just one such so-called cosmetic. There is even a case history of one woman who applied fingernail hardener to her nails, only to discover that, a few hours later, they had turned blue! They don't tell us whatever happened to the blue-nailed woman. But I'd be willing to bet she stayed away from hardeners for the rest of her life. Although some experts recommend polishes (Norman Orentreich is one), others say that polishes contain resins—and that *those* can cause trouble.

So, instead of hardening up your nails with fake hardeners, or plastic nails (Ouch! These can *really* be a danger and I've heard horror stories of nails being lost through too constant wearing of plastic—the kind you brush on— nails) or resin-filled polishes, why not just protein-up your diet and exercise your nails with buff, buff, and buff?

Nail Tidbits to Chew On

So where does that leave your nails? Back at good health. And good nutrition. Same thing. For as nail-knowledgeable Dr. Norman Orentreich said to me, "There are no specific foods for the nails. Just good nutrition." I would disagree with the doctor on only one thing. *Never let up on protein!*

But a few more Orentreich-finds about fingernails: Bosses take heart! It seems that the best nails grow on the *workers*—the ones who really get in there and pitch. That's right. The harder the work, the stronger the nail grows—a sort of built-in *non*-self-destruct device for protecting those nails. And when the work lets up, the nail grows thinner again. How's that for keeping every worker at it!

Remember that bit, ladies, if you're complaining too much about work (as long as that work doesn't involve keeping your hands in detergent). For—here we go again —alkaline detergent is your old destructive enemy. And while nails are practically indestructible, enough alkaline soaks can do the dirty, destruction work.

The most fascinating nail-bit of all is that nail-biters' nails grow 20 percent faster than anyone else's! But since the nail biter never lets them get long enough for anyone to have a look at, we don't recommend *this* sort of stimulation.

Stimulation, however, is what it takes—just as with the hair—to get proteins and all those good vitamins into circulation and out on you in the form of good, strong-and-long nails. That's why buffing (but no biting, please) gives the nail that little push out—to long.

And nails, like hair, grow faster in warm weather. Some believe it's because cold can make them brittle. (Cold makes me brrrrittle.) Others say that vitamin D is essential for healthy nails. This might be the reason that good old Sol brings the nails out of you.

Dr. Norman Orentreich also tells us that the rate of nail growth varies in each and every one of us (here's the one spot where nails break away from hair; hair grows at six inches per year and that's that!). And, of course, according to our various, and very personal, metabolic systems. It must be the truth. I haven't forgotten my own very personal and very nail-disastrous experiments with taking thyroid pills. Rotten health, naturally, can affect your nail growth. (That's why I want you in great shape all over!) But—get this—piano-playing, pregnancy, and *typing* (whew!) can *increase* the growth of your nails. And apparently growth decreases with age—diminishing almost fifty percent between the ages of twenty-five and ninety-five. Tell you what. If I'm still kicking at ninety-five, I promise not to worry Dr. Orentreich with my nails!

And, if you care, there's this little tidbit. The middle fingernail on *everybody's* hand grows fastest and the nails on the right hand grow faster than those on the left. (Presumably this applies to right-handed people—lefties, you're opposite.)

Nail Nutrition

As for good-nail-nutrition, well, I've got a secret of my own—one that none of the experts seems to understand, admit, or even believe. So I guess you'll just have to try for yourselves, find out for yourselves, and for heaven's sake, if it works for *you*, let the world know. That little secret is bread. That's right. Good old bread, plain and simple.

Plain and simple may be the answer, because naturally I'm
referring to *natural* bread, preferably homemade and baked
with unbleached flour, perhaps a bit of wheat germ, or
sprouts. *Natural.*

I learned about bread when I was going through my
withdrawal symptoms from the low-carbohydrate deprivation diet I'd been on, after that clever little body of mine
(it *was* little) turned on me and began to turn my protein
into carbohydrates and put *fat* on me! My nails began to
break, as I've told you. Viciously. And painfully. And to
the quick. And, what is worse, there were infections and all
sorts of horrors more real than simple vanity. Then along
came Christmas and my annual journey to my beloved
Southland—biscuits, grits, and all. (Remember?) It was at
this point that I bid a temporary good-bye to my friend (he
is, and I am his fan) Dr. Atkins and decided, "The hell
with it. I'm going home and eat. Everything my mother
sets before me!" (It isn't too often one gets a mother's
home-cooked meal, and, while I'd firmly resisted in visits
past, *this* time I'd had enough of the experiments and the
greater and greater stringency imposed on me in order to
stop the tide of fat that had inexplicably begun to show up,
no matter what I or my doctor did.)

So eat I did. (Not *over*eat, you understand.) But I ate a
modicum of everything that everyone else ate. Most especially biscuits. Now the South is where biscuits taste like
no place else in the world. And I am, and always have
been, a bread freak. Sweets you can have (I suppose I'm
lucky there; I can take 'em or leave 'em and mostly would
rather leave). But bread loaded with butter? *That's* my idea
of a real Christmas present. Believe it or not, after only
one week's vacation from dieting, my nails began to grow,
visibly so and back to where they had been. (In my line of
work, long nails are not so practical, and, while typing may
stimulate growth, it's pretty hard to hit the keys with
talons.)

I was as puzzled as all the experts I've consulted since.
Some of them even refused to believe it. But there were
those nails staring back at them, strong, healthy, and apparently there to stay. I concluded that the bread I was
eating—the good stuff—was loaded with B vitamins, and
while I can't find a soul who will admit that B vitamins

work directly on the nails, I don't see why they shouldn't.

Your nails are practically the same composition as your hair. And we know how important the Beautiful B's are to *that*. So why not admit they work wonders toward making strong nails as well? Face it. It's a delicious sort of treatment.

Home-Baked Nail Food

When I say that I arranged to get *bread* in my body each and every day (after seeing the miracle it performed on my fingernails, I *never* again intend to eliminate bread from my diet; it is not called "the staff of life" for naught), I am *not* referring to that snow-white, marshmallow glue that is sold as bread and still eaten, to my horror and disbelief, in so many, many homes in this country—served up by supposedly intelligent mothers and housewives to their unsuspecting (probably) families. Most bread, unless it is of the health food variety, is little more than, as Jean Mayer of Harvard University School of Nutrition described it, "an edible napkin"—something to eat *off* of rather than something to eat!

No. What I am referring to when I refer to bread is *real* bread—made of unbleached natural flour, with no possibly-cancer-causing chemical preservatives. Many commercial bakeries—among them Arnold and Pepperidge Farm—are jumping on the health bandwagon, much to the benefit of us all. Pepperidge Farm's Sprouted Wheat bread is a delight, as is Arnold's Seven Grains loaf. Both of these companies have been pioneers in producing breads from natural flour. And I understand that Pillsbury, that paragon producer of flours, has been the first of the big companies with unbleached flours on any grocer's shelves.

Raymond A. Sokolov, when he was food editor of *The New York Times*, found to his surprise that American food tastes may be changing—for the better. He stated that in 1972 the most-asked-for recipes were for desserts. In 1973, there was a sudden switch to home-baked bread. It certainly gives one hope that there's a food-revolution going on. Mr. Sokolov gave one recipe for Cornell bread, that famous nature loaf that is totally nutritious bread.

And here is the recipe:

> 3 cups lukewarm water
> 2 packages dry active yeast
> 2 tablespoons honey
> 6 cups (approximately) unbleached enriched bread flour
> ½ cup full-fat soy flour
> ¾ cup nonfat dry milk solids
> 3 tablespoons wheat germ
> 4 teaspoons salt
> 2 tablespoons oil

Melted butter, optional

1. Place the water, yeast, and honey in a large bowl. Stir to mix and let stand in a warm place five minutes.
2. Sift together the flour, soy flour, and dry milk solids. Stir in the wheat germ.
3. Add the salt to the yeast mixture and about one-half to three-quarters of the flour mixture so that the batter has a consistency that can be beaten. Beat for two minutes in an electric mixer, or 75 strokes by hand.
4. Add the oil and work in the remainder of the flour mixture, adding extra flour if needed to form a dough. Turn the dough onto a floured board and knead 10 minutes or until the dough is smooth and elastic.
5. Place in a greased bowl, grease the top of the dough lightly, cover, and let rise in a warm place until almost doubled in bulk, about 45 minutes.
6. Punch the dough down, fold over the edges and turn upside down in the bowl. Cover and let rise 20 minutes longer.
7. Turn onto a board, divide into three parts. Form into balls, cover and let stand 10 minutes.
8. Roll out one ball into a rectangle twice as big as an 8½-by-4½-by-2½-inch loaf pan. Fold the long sides into the center. Pinch to seal layers and fit into a greased loaf pan. Repeat with the other two balls.
9. Cover pans and let rise in a warm place until doubled in bulk, about 45 minutes.

10. Preheat oven to 350 degrees. Bake loaves 50 to 60 minutes. Cover with foil if tops begin to overbrown. Bread is done when it sounds hollow when tapped on the bottom. Brush tops with melted butter for a soft crust. Cool on a rack.

Yield: Three loaves.

5. Eyes

Bright Eyes

I am going to have very little to say on the subject of eyes, except to say that, if you've followed your regimen to the letter—the regimen for healthy living, that is—your baby blues should be bright and sparkling. For, once again, health shows up all over, and a sprightly sparkle to the eyes usually means a person's feeling sprightly. A dull and listless look means just that—less than perfect health.

But the main reason I'm going to have very little to say about eyes is that here is one part of you I believe belongs strictly in the hands of the trained medical doctor. Your eye doctor, to be precise. Your vision is nothing to fool around with and, in the chapter on cosmetics, I've already told you a few things to watch for when it comes to such things as eyedrops that could possibly be injurious to your eyes. Eyesight is precious, and, if you've lost it, there's no regaining it, no matter how well you eat. And so I would prefer to hand over any and all eye health problems to your eye doctor. I do not mean one of those people who will give you discount eyeglasses. I am suspicious of those, though they may in some cases be perfectly legitimate. I am talking about medical doctors, specializing in eye problems. Those are the people to see when such problems arise.

There are, however, a few little hints I might give you. Watch out for sun, which is, as we already know, one of the worst enemies of beautiful skin. It is also possibly injurious to your eyesight while you're suntanning, unless you take great care to protect your eyelids. That's the problem—how to protect them. For your eyelids are thin-skinned and they have a tendency to absorb things right into the eye itself, causing possible blindness if you don't watch out.

I have queried a great many cosmetics people on the best possible sun protection to use on eyelids when one is tanning. Mainly because, in my later (read that as older) years, my eyelids have suddenly begun to burn and swell to frog-eyed non-beauty, while the rest of me goes on to a fine-turned tan. The cosmetics flock don't have many answers other than to say that any sunscreen that does not—repeat, does *not*—say "avoid contact with the eyes" is probably safe for use on the lids. I am not thoroughly convinced. I would prefer to have a product that is made especially *for* the eyelid, rather than take my chances with its safety probability. One cosmetics researcher told me, by the way, that zinc oxide ointment was one of the best things to use. But by the same token, I have read, of late, that zinc oxide can be toxic and therefore dangerous. So how does one find the truth?

There is, of course, the possibility of wearing sunglasses, if you don't object to white-ringed eyes, which I do. Or you can do as the South-of-France crowd does and wet small pieces of cotton to be placed over the eyes while you're flat-out. But if you have skin as delicate as mine you'll still end up with white circles. It's a problem, and one I'm still searching for the answer to. One answer I know already. If the label on any sunscreen tells you to steer clear of the eyes, you'd better do it. I'd rather have circles than no sight, and I'm sure you would, too.

Eye Lines

I've given you my feelings about eye makeup along with other makeups in the section on "Fresh Paint." I will again stress that you should take care and more care when it comes to eye makeup. Beware of those foreign-produced eyedrops, for example. Beware of any eyedrops unless they are okayed by your eye doctor. Just generally beware of anything you are going to put close to those precious eyes of yours.

Generally, cosmetics in this country are rather rigidly tested for safety's sake. Unless you have an allergy all your own, you are pretty safe with them. But be careful of picking up goodies in other countries. Kohl, for example—one of the oldest eyeliners around and still in use in India and other far-Eastern countries—is made from a deadly poison. Leave it to the Indians to worry about their eyesight. You just take care of your own.

As for your lashes: in case you decided to use an eyelash curler, remember one thing. *Always* use it *before* you use mascara. Otherwise you stand a pretty good chance of pulling out those lashes when the mascara glues itself to the curler.

As for false eyelashes, watch that glue. I once had some applied for an elegant dinner dance by one of our most famous beauty experts. A drop of that eyelash glue fell into my eye, and, while it burned like anything, that too passed, and I gave it no more thought. Until later, when I looked in a mirror and saw a crater-like depression in my eyeball. I rushed to an eye clinic (it was Friday afternoon, wouldn't you know? with no New York doctor to be found) only to be told that I had a serious condition of the retina. Needless to say, I was frightened to death. Later (on Monday) my own eye doctor assured me that it was nothing more than irritation from the glue. Still, if glue can do all that, I'd be careful. I don't like false eyelashes anyway. Oil your own with wheat germ. That should help them grow long and lustrous on their own. Natural is always more beautiful.

As for eyebrows, you can do anything with them you like. But if you pluck them all out over an extended period of time, don't expect them to grow back. Many a twenties flapper found that out, to her distress. Eyebrows don't do much for eye health (I've checked) but are mostly there, as are eyelashes, to help protect the eye. As for how you want to paint them up—make it red, yellow, green. I don't care, as long as you're happy.

Smoke Shows in Your Eyes

It's a delicate subject to broach, but then I've never been one to worry about being delicate—especially when health is at stake. So I might as well come right out and say it: Don't let your eyes go to pot. Literally.

Some time ago I was afflicted with an ugly and painful, albeit relatively common and minor, eye inflammation brought about by doing what I've been preaching against— too much work with too little rest. Its name is episcleritis and it simply makes the eye that's got it bright red. Sort of a one-eyed Dracula effect. I rushed off to my eye doctor, as I always do when such things strike and, as this doctor examined my eye and confirmed my already-guessed diagnosis, he said, rather tentatively, "Dear, may I ask you a personal question?" Wondering what on earth anything *that* personal might have to do with my eyes, I quickly answered in the affirmative. The question was "Do you smoke pot?" I couldn't help laughing with relief. The answer is I don't. Not because I so whole-heartedly disapprove of the idea. (I just disapprove of the unsureness of the whole bit at this point. I mean, does anyone really know—or can anyone really prove—what it might do to you later?) But I don't even smoke at all.

My doctor, who couldn't be a more dignified man, hastened to explain that his practice had changed with the times—to such an extent that it was imperative he ask this question. It seems that marijuana is a sure way to make your eyes bloodshot—and for as long as you're smoking. Something about the way it dries up the mucous membranes. Now I'm not here to moralize, believe me. But if it's sparkling eyes you're after, better forget this sort of smoking. Better forget any sort, if it's true beauty you want.

P.S.

I have not mentioned vitamin A because *everybody* knows how vitally important it is to good eyesight and happy, healthy eyes. *Take it!*

6. The Beautiful Body Machine

Sex and Sleep—The Greatest Youthmakers of All

Let's take first things first. Which means sex, of course. A friend asked me recently, "Are you *really* one of those people who believes that one's sex life shows in every pore?" You can bet your beauty I do! Remember the old "radiant bride" routine? Well, I don't know if they make *those* any more (blushing brides, I mean), but I do know that a solid satisfying sex life is good for your skin, good for your figure, good for your nerves. In fact, I can't think of a single thing it isn't good for. And it's fun besides. I think you might say I'm a sexual activist.

I can almost tell just by looking at a woman whether or not there's a good (for her) man in her life. There's always a dewy look to the skin, a bounce to the walk, a swing of the hair, and an air of cool relaxation. One of the greatest skin specialists in the world has been known to counsel his patients to "keep up the good sex life." Seems the two— great skin, great sex—go hand in glove. Perhaps it's due in part to the sexual flush, which is real and very well medically proven. You know—all that blood that rushes to the face, making for a pretty terrifically natural skin treatment.

Not only that, you'll *never* see tense little lines in the face of a sexually well-cared-for woman. The relaxation practically seethes from every pore. There we go again, full circle: It does show up in every pore. And before I could answer her question, my friend, whose lovely skin tells *all* about *her* love life mused, "Yes, I suppose it does!"

In the dazzling discotheque days of the mid-sixties (remember then?), my favorite dancing partner, a young man at least ten years my junior, used to pick me up at, say, 11:30 P.M. for a round on the town. He'd exclaim, "You look great!" and then add in a somewhat accusatory tone, "You took a nap, didn't you?" Natch. First of all, you really can't burn the candle at both ends and look like anything but a burnt-out candle. Sleep is, always has been, and always will be better than any cosmetic, manufactured or natural, for an unlined skin, a radiant vitality, and a relaxed view of the world, no matter how harrying that world may become. But sleep, in this harried world, seems to be increasingly elusive. Millions of Americans resort to sleeping aids of one sort or another, from pills to booze to an often fatal combination of the two. And it has been said that a drugged sleep is simply a paralyzed body rather than a healthfully rested one.

The answer to sleeplessness is so simple as to be practically unbelievable. It lies deep in the roots of folk medicine. Remember that warm-milk-at-bedtime story? Right! For *calcium* is the great *natural* tranquilizer, and, though it's doubtful that our forebears understood the workings of the warm milk remedy, they most certainly had the right answers. Adelle Davis believes in calcium as a sleeping aid so firmly that she suggests that you keep those calcium tablets right on your bedside table, with a glass of milk beside them, and that you swallow several each and every time you awaken during the night.

I can personally attest to the put-out power of calcium. I *am* a light sleeper, and in the hubbub of New York City, where apartments have practically paper walls, that's bad. Besides, sleeping pills can put me away for days and leave me with a hangover that wasn't even fun to get! So I tried Miss Davis' remedy . . . I took *six* giant-looking calcium lactate tablets before bedtime (calcium lactate seems to be the form most recommended for sleep-help) and pow! Instant knock-out. I felt as though I had been hit with a hammer, slept soundly, and awoke feeling like a kitten.

The herbalists have long recognized the value of camomile tea as a soothing sleep-giver. Fortunately for lazy herb-users like myself, such teas are on the market in tea bag form (purist herbalists may recoil in horror, but the sleep-effect is the same). Camomile tea is made, of course, from the camomile flower—the same camomile flower that works so well on your hair. Its taste is enchanting and I guarantee that this is one tea that will, even when drunk in the middle of the night, *never* keep you awake.

If you don't have a comfortable mattress *plus* a comfortable pillow, then get one! And this means comfortable for *you* and never mind what the alarmists tell you about brick-hard mattresses being the only kind to have. That may be true if you like brick-hard mattresses. I don't. After all, at 103 pounds, I'm not going to make a dent in a super-duper-ortho-firm affair, whereas a 300-pound man might truly need just that. Of course, trying to find a *medium* mattress these days is a bit of a problem. I have even gotten mattress manufacturers to admit that they don't make 'em like they used to any more—the reason being the great backache scare. Apparently those tales about backs and hard mattresses have frightened people into buying bricks, and, according to one salesman I spoke with, those same people often come around complaining that they can't sleep. So I say go with what's comfortable for *you*. And forget what you read about backaches. If you happen to like hard, then fine. But do be sure that, whatever degree of firmness you choose, your springs are good and non-sagging.

As for that pillow . . . well, remember, that if you're given to puffy eyes, never, but *never* sleep without a pillow. You're sure to awaken looking like the frog-princess, and when the swelling subsides you'll have not-so-neat little stretch-wrinkles to show for it. *Always* sleep with your head elevated. It's O.K. to put your feet up now and again, and to practice those ever-so-relaxing headstands we spoke about. But not for an entire night!

If you live in the big city, as I do, where the clangor and clamor simply never stops and the sirens scream about the streets all night, and electronic alarms go off for hours with nobody, but nobody, caring—except for poor little you, trying to get your beauty rest—then consider buying one of those marvelous little machines that just sits there and hums like an air conditioner. Really! That's *all* it does. No breeze, no heat, no nothing except a heaven-sent drowning out of street noises, neighbor noises, radios, and TV sets. (Apartment living is definitely not for the light sleeper's life-style—but what is one to do?) These are relatively cheap, but if you are feeling flush you may even want to go for one that makes sounds like waves. Or rain on the roof. I bought mine to drown out the snoring of a certain gentleman who was sharing my pad at that moment. (He swears it kept him *awake!* I don't know how, since he continued to snore.) Since that time, I've used it to drown out the basketball player upstairs who dribbled that ball across a bare floor at 4:00 A.M. And the little old lady downstairs who forgets to turn off the tub water and has not only a flood on the floor, but one rushing through the pipes that makes Niagara a piker. Let's just say the investment in rest is well worth the $29.95 spent. P.S.—If you're a newly-transported-to-the-country girl, it drowns out crickets, barking dogs, and early rising birds, as well.

And, since we've linked them together once, let's do it again. Remember *sex is the greatest of all soporifics*. As Dr. Abraham Friedman put it, if, after a good go at sex, you head for the refrigerator, you're doing something wrong. What you should feel like heading for is bed! And if you're not sleepy yet—well, you're already *in bed*, now, aren't you?

Vitally Beautiful Vitamins

I *believe* in vitamins. I mean I believe in megadoses of vitamins. Not just for common colds and other cures. But for *beauty*. We all know that healthy food is beautiful, that vitamins found in food are beautiful. But we *have* seen, and you can check the chart again, if you don't believe, that food alone won't do that much beauty work. It can't. You just couldn't hold that much food. And, while the vitamins you get from your food may be more potent than the ones that come in a capsule, you couldn't prove it by me.

Now I'm not telling you to give up good, natural, healthy food for a pill. I'm saying you ought to *supplement* that same good, natural, healthy food with plenty of vitality-giving vitamins. Beauty-making vitamins. Youth-making vitamins.

But watch that bottle! Vitamin labels need to be checked just like any others (and I hope that by now you've learned to do that without a second thought). You ought to know what you're popping into your mouth, whether it's food or a pill. I know a few bargain-minded people who will travel all over the city to find vitamins a few cents cheaper. Of course, they haven't checked to see whether there's anything *in* that bottle. They only check the price.

Believe me, some of those so-called bargains in vitamins are bargains only to the manufacturers who foist them off on an unsuspecting health-minded public. Learn to know how much you need of each vitamin and then make sure it's in that bottle! (Don't worry, I'll tell you soon.)

Why Should Physicians Fear Them?

It took doctors to discover their healing powers. Why are those very same doctors now so reluctant to admit that vitamins—their very own life-saving discoveries—may just have the power to do more than save one from scurvy or beri-beri? It's a damned good thing they were discovered, all right, and lives saved thereby. But why must they now feel so embarrassed to admit that vitamins *are* do-gooders?

My very own doctor—the one and same advanced physician who is so forward-thinking by comparison with his contemporaries—said to me recently, as he suggested a vitamin B shot as a possible aid for my writer's exhaustion, "I hate to admit it, but they do work."

Why should he hate to admit it? And why is the FDA, our watchdog of food, so determined to limit our vitamin intake to the minimum? It has taken them this long to limit sleeping pills, amphetamines (and I'll believe that limit when I see it legislated), and the other really dangerous drugs. Why be so determined that we not get the beauty-making, health-giving, healing effects of vitamins? Effects doctors not only discovered, but know are there. They gave us vitamins and now they want to take them away. I will grant you that there are one or two vitamins that ought to be watched. Those are A, D, and, to a certain extent, E, since relatively little is known about it to this date. But that is because these are the oil-soluble vitamins—the ones that can build up in your body to a possible dangerous additive sum. The others, however—those that must be replenished every day, and the ones from which the body can take *only* as much as it needs (the rest goes out with the body wastes)—what can possibly be the harm in those? It's a bit akin to Curie's being embarrassed by X-rays or Thomas Edison's never turning on an electric light.

And if you think you get enough vitamins in your food —well, first check my chart *carefully*. (And that "carefully" is important, because the vitamins are there, all right, but see what you're getting in the amounts of food you eat. You may be surprised, and not pleasantly.) Then listen to two real-life horror stories I am about to relate.

My grandmother's best friend (and this was in the not-so-long-ago twenties) amused herself, and earned a tidy sum on the side, by turning her gourmet-cook talent to catering. This Southern lady was a widow, and so, since Southerners appreciate good cooking, she began to cater parties for her friends, and then for others and soon had a going business—until she became mysteriously ill. Seriously so and, apparently, inexplicably so. She died. Of pellagra, they discovered too late.

For, it seems, she had neglected her own nutrition in favor of being busy. And so she had snacked on those marvelous little goodies that she whipped up as party fare. Well, party fare may be delicious, but it will not suffice for long-term eating. And so this lovely lady died of malnutrition in the 1920s. Incredible.

But there is more. My own cousin was transferred from one city to another and, not wanting to uproot his family in the middle of the children's school year, he took a room in a boardinghouse that served meals . . . just until school was out and his family could join him. Now my cousin was a big eater, and so I am sure he didn't stint on the portions. But boardinghouse cooking can be on the overdone side and, when it comes to vitamins, the more cooking done, the less vitamins left. Pretty soon my cousin was pretty sick. To everyone's disbelief, the doctors found him suffering from beri-beri.

So summer bachelors, beware. And wives who tend to snack instead of lunch. Or working women who hate to eat alone. See for yourself that what you thought were diseases that went out in the dark ages are still right here with us unless we are protected by proper nourishment and—*vitamins*.

Basic and Beautiful B

The B vitamins are so basic, I can't imagine anyone with beautiful expectations going without them. They are the beauty vitamins! They make your hair shining and thick, your skin flawless and luminous, your nails healthy and hard. And they're the calming vitamins—the ones that tame the beauty-killers, strain and stress.

But they're a complex little crowd, and that's just how

they ought to be downed. As a complex. For, just like love and marriage *used* to be, you can't (shouldn't) have one without the other. You see, the beautiful B's work *together* so beautifully (to beautify *you*) that if you take too much of one, you can cause a severe deficiency of another. (Therefore, beware of doctors bearing hypodermics filled with B-12, for example. Unless you want to louse up your complex!)

There's just no dosing about with the beautiful B's. Leave that to the experts. Here's the B-gospel according to Adelle Davis: If your tablet contains two milligrams of B-1, it should contain *equal* amounts of B-2, B-6, and folic acid; ten times more pantothenic acid and niacin (making twenty milligrams of these); twenty times more PABA, or forty milligrams; 500 times more inositol and choline or 1,000 milligrams of each of these B's. And (surprise, surprise) you only need 1 to 3 *micro*grams of B-12. Some proportions. Check your own B-complex vitamin and see if it's anything like that!

Sadly, some of the B vitamins—some of the rarer ones —like B-6, are expensive. While I hate to say it, vitamin manufacturers are out to make a profit, just like everyone else. So what are they going to leave out? The expensive stuff, naturally. B-6 is one that's often missing from that B-complex label. We know what B-6 does for your shape, so shape up and fill in with B-6 if it's missing. As for choline and inositol, they're almost never found in a complex capsule, but we know they're found in lecithin. That's a good enough reason for taking it every day.

Brewer's yeast is one of the very best natural sources of the beautiful B's. I know beautiful creatures who live on it. And grow more beautiful all the while. If you can get it down, then by all means do it. Wrap it in orange juice, or milk, or dream up some marvelous blender concoction. And think, all the while, about B's and beauty.

But *be very careful* not to confuse brewer's yeast with live baker's yeast which is *dangerous*. In fact, to be on the safe side, just get that brewer's yeast at your health-food store where they're not likely to misguide you. (And while you're getting those B vitamins, you'll also be getting powerful protein. Brewer's yeast has protein comparable to that of meat and milk.) And, by the way, if your tummy begins to growl on brewer's yeast—it just means you *really* need it, so carry on, and take that cider vinegar brew all the while.

Another natural source of the B vitamins is desiccated liver—one of my favorite beauty-makers. Here again, you're not only getting protein, you're getting *all* of the B vitamins as well. From a food source. And as easy to swallow as that little liver pill!

Vitamins A and D

Our two beautiful skin vitamins are the *only* two vitamins we're sure that you have to watch, because they're the only two vitamins that are retained in your system. Meaning that if you take too, too much, you get a build-up. And that could be bad. It could be toxic. There is still a great deal of controversy around the subject of just how much is *too* much.

I take 50,000 units of vitamin A each and every day of my life and have for twenty years. If I try to cut down to 25,000 units per day, believe me, it shows in my face all right. And so I don't cut down and I have never seen any ill effects. But I most decidedly wouldn't advise going over that amount *except* under a doctor's care. I read recently an article in which a physician claimed to have cured supposedly incurable psoriasis with enormous doses of vitamin A. But then he was a physician and that life was in his hands. I *do* know, on the other hand, that as with vitamin C, vitamin A can be taken in megadoses of up to 250,000 units per day—*providing* you continue this treatment for *no more than a week*. They say that if megadoses of vitamin C don't work on your common cold, try A. (I'll stick with my 50,000 units, to play it safe.)

As for vitamin D, we all know you can get a lot too much if you sunburn. But vitamin D is another of those tricky vitamins that gets stored up inside, unlike, as I've said, the ones that are simply eliminated when your body has used up its needs. I know people who take 50,000 units of D daily. I don't know why they're living; 20,000 weekly should take care of any lack of sunshine and help you assimilate all that good calcium besides. Because without D, what good is calcium?

Vitamin E

Is it or isn't it? Only *you* can tell for sure whether the so-called sex vitamin is just that for you. Adelle Davis claims it makes you sexier looking! Men look manlier, and women more womanly. I believe that vitamin E can help give you swinging, sexy hair. And that it's a skin plumper-upper *par excellence*. But an aphrodisiac? I say *yes!* I had to cut my own 800 units per day dosage when my amour of the moment begged for surcease. Seems he was just plain tired! Mind you, I didn't cut *out* E. Heavens no! Just down. (I was getting a bit worn out myself.) And I gave *him* some.

I've given this dosage of vitamin E to friends who complained they were too tired even for sex. (And that's too tired!) This megadose of E had the same, immediate sexual-revitalizing effect on them that it had on me. And if that's true, then how great for your shape! Remember those 200 calories you use, every time you take to bed with your mate!

Aphrodisiac or not (and I still say "yes!") vitamin E is, for me, instant *E*nergy. If I'm feeling really tired, I pop an E, 400 units a pop. Because I don't believe in "uppies"—meaning fake energy in the likes of an amphetamine capsule. I'm way up on my own energy most of the time anyway. Tranquillity is what *I* need, and since I don't believe in "downies" (the sedative sort of tranquillity) either, I get it via B vitamins and calcium . . . both great stress-destroyers. We all have our moments of flagging strength, and that's when I run for E. Some of the more vital beauties I know swear by 1200 units of E per day. You should plan your dosage by its obviously best results.

Just remember that the energy that comes from E is the kind that is good, natural, and healthy, not the kind that comes from synthetic stimulants that have the effect of just whipping that tired horse.

Vitamin C

Yes, Dr. Pauling, it *does* cure a common cold. And you can take tons of it. You can take *grams* of C with, apparently, no harmful effects. But C, as we have seen, does much more for your good looks than just cold-curing. It's a great skin-radiance–maker and for that purpose you need a minimum of 1,500 units per day. And never forget that if you're a smoker, or a heavy coffee-drinker, you'd better triple your dosage of C, for these two beauty-killers— caffeine and smoke—eat your C alive.

Just take it and lots of it, and, if your body doesn't want it, well, it will kiss it good-bye with absolutely no harm done.

Keep It Cool!

When it's a matter of nutrition, heat destroys. Heat destroys vitamins. Heat also destroys protein. Heat destroys enzymes. So you can see why there's so much to say for eating your food *raw*. Raw fruits, raw vegetables, raw grains, and meats that have not been cooked to the point of protein-less grayness. Raw sprouts (like bean, alfalfa) are delicious sprinkled over salads. And you can't ask for a healthier way to guarantee a diet full of beauty. And there's one little pointer on heat that I bet you didn't know. *I* didn't, until recently. That is that, once vegetables have been picked, even the sun itself can destroy their vitamin vitality. So all those rows of gorgeous green vegetables you see in those quaint little sidewalk stands—the ones that look so home-grown healthy—well, if I were you, I'd pick the little sidewalk stand on the shady side of the street!

As for cooking, how do you avoid heat? You cook for as short a time as possible and have vegetables *al dente*. Try the French way, which is virtually waterless. Place a couple of lettuce leaves over your vegetables in place of water. These provide extra vitamins and give you just the amount of water to get your vegetables done—crisply and vitamin-full.

Being a Southerner, I am, of course, accustomed to vegetables that have been simmered for hours. I must admit to loving them, for I believe that nothing is better than Southern sun-ripened vegetables. They—plus the heat—are probably one reason people in the South eat more vegetables, less beef. (The cattle-raisers down there are not going to love me, but it's true.) Therefore, I was interested to read in a medical textbook that vegetables cooked the Southern way are as vitamin-vital as any others, for the simple reason that the Southern people always eat the "pot liquor." That means the juice the vegetables were cooked in.

One thing is sure. Never pour that juice, assuming you have any left, down the drain unless that's where you want your vitamins to go.

One more tip on vitamin-cooking before I leave you: Remember that often the vitamins are found closest to the peel—as in potatoes or citrus fruits. If you can eat that part, you're getting what you need. Otherwise, you're needlessly throwing good things into the garbage. Think about it, the next time you peel a potato. Perhaps you will bake it instead and eat it, peel and all.

The Big Bad B's—Beef and Booze

I'm so accustomed to saying "Bully for B"—meaning those beautiful B vitamins, of course—that I forget about the two B's that are *bad!* Bad for your shape, bad for your hair, bad for your skin, bad for your *beauty!* They are booze and (you'll be as surprised as I was) beef. Surely you've gathered by now that there's very little beauty in booze. It may make you feel beautiful—momentarily. But when you check out your mirror the next morning you'll get the real picture. Clearly! Alcohol dries up your hair, wrinkles up your skin, breaks off your nails, ruins your digestion, robs you of your sleep, and wrecks your shape! Do you still want it?

Then let me tell you that it eats up all those beautiful B vitamins as well. (Conversely, B vitamins are a good cure for a hangover, if you don't give a hoot about *how* you look!) If the B vitamins go—well, watch your hair turn white and go thatched-roof on you. Look at the lines under those hung-over eyes.

No matter what manner of shaper-upper diet you've selected, alcohol is a no, no, NO! Although alcohol itself contains zero carbohydrates, it can be *converted* into carbohydrates by your ever-sneaky metabolism. Any low-carbohydrate diet doctor will take away that bottle quick as a wink—the moment your weight stops falling. On a low-calorie diet—well, if you *really* want to drink all your meals, you may feel happy, but you certainly won't be beautiful. If you just *cannot* make do without alcohol, try to limit it to one small glass of wine per day. In case you're interested, *I* gave it up. Beautiful!

As for beef—well, if you're a typical American, you've

no doubt been brainwashed into thinking that beef is diet food. It is, if you're dieting to *gain* weight. But otherwise, that traditional steak-and-salad meal that people *think* is a diet one actually represents approximately a day and a half in the life of a serious dieter. *That's* how many calories are in beef. If you're on the low-carbohydrate–high-protein regimen, beef is high in protein, all right. But you can bet it's one of the first things to go—right along with booze—when weight no longer speeds off.

Just picture beef as one of the most fattening things you can gnaw. If you are really serious about washing away excess bulk, then wash away that steak-as-diet-food picture. You might also consider recent research into all the possibly-cancer-causing things that are injected into beef *before* it gets into your mouth, such as female hormones to fatten up the little steer that's going to market. Consider that the government is presently doing research into just *how much* of this hormone remains in your body. Women might not worry so much, but how about men? Some folk say it's the cause behind the whole fem lib movement! Think on it before you order another steak.

Avoid at All Meals

Since I've been busy telling you what's good for you, perhaps I shouldn't forget to mention things to *avoid*—if beauty's what you're eating for. The list of avoidance foods, unfortunately, reads like the American family's dream menu. For, with all its riches, this country is filled with malnutrition. *That's what we said.* And we're not talking about deprived poverty-pocket Americans. Quite to the contrary. Often the most affluent have the most deprived diets. While they can afford to take off to spas and salons to cover up the damage, or try to—the *healthy* brand of beauty is too long gone.

It has been said that one-half of the American populace suffers from real malnutrition; eighty-five percent is calcium deficient; and more than half of all Americans are deficient in vitamin C. Add to that the horrors of all the additives, preservatives, and empty calories with which we fill up our malnourished bodies, and you'll understand why we're often less than the beautiful people we have every right to be.

Last year alone Americans consumed an average of 2,632 cigarettes apiece! With them went all that vitamin C we're so deficient in. We drank nearly thirty *gallons* of alcohol per person (and there went the beautiful B vitamins) and twenty-five gallons of soft drinks apiece. All in one year!

Dr. Robert Atkins considers the American dream diet of pizzas, hot dogs, hamburgers, French fries, and colas the "killer-diet"—the one responsible for America's being way down at the bottom of the list of healthy nations. He considers that soft drinks, with those colas as the particular villain of this piece, have introduced more harmful sugar into the American diet than any other product.

I hope I've driven home the point.

There is but *no way* you're going to become beautiful on over-processed foods, with all the good things removed and a small token-trace of something put back. Nader's Raiders made a good start when they attacked the empty-calorie cereal industry. Empty calories are certainly not what we're looking for. Wholesome, healthful, vitamin-filled food is. Once you've seen the difference your diet can make, you'll never go the hamburger-soft drink diet route again. Not if I can help it!

Hidden Horrors—Avoid Them!

No matter which diet you've elected to follow—low-carb or low-cal—down the road to skinny, you'll find, lurking along the way, hidden horrors, surprising little things that could trip you up, if you're not aware of them. I don't intend to see that happen. I was hit with a few real surprises on my way to thin, so why not save you from any sad experiences?

If you're on a low-carbohydrate diet, you will quickly remember the vegetables that you are permitted. You'll know that strawberries are your only allowed fruit. But suppose you get in a situation, as I did once, where you're a guest at a dinner where the only non-carbohydrate is the meat course? What to do? Hard to whip out your chart and then tell your hostess you must leave at once! Moral: Make do with the meat in a situation like this. As for fruits—I had the same experience by mistakenly guessing that a piece of watermelon just couldn't hurt me. No re-entry into my clothes.

There are many other hidden carbohydrates as well. Milk has many more than heavy cream. Milk is *forbidden* on the low-carbohydrate diet. So is yogurt. Chewing gum can ruin you, as can catsup, or anything loaded with tomato paste. Even tomato juice. (There's lots of unseen sugar there.) As for diet drinks, read the labels! Many of them now use sugar, and no matter how small the amount it won't mix with low-carb. Ditto for lots of other so-called diet products. You *can*, on the other hand, dive into such gourmet goodies as Quiche Lorraine—providing you ignore the crust. Stay out of Oriental restaurants. Everything in them is sugar-loaded, more often than not. Just think of all those sweet-and-sour sauces and you'll see. Cream soups, of course, usually contain flour, so beware.

As for the low-calorie routine, well, here is where you can really be fooled. Check out steak, for example. Or realize that one tiny rib lamb chop contains approximately 400 calories—and that's just the meat part. If you eat the fat, forget it! Cheese is large on calories, while bread—an average slice of, of course, the good, healthy sort—contains only 63. The diet kind, because it's sliced thinner, has less and usually has the calories listed on the label.

Yogurt is not diet food! Not on anybody's diet. It's great for you, for your digestion, for getting your protein, for keeping your stomach in healthy condition, but it is *not* without calories. And they are plentiful. We're not talking about vanilla yogurt (which another hostess tried to palm off on me as being the "same as plain"—it isn't); we're talking about the *un*flavored kind. If you head for the ones with the gooey preserves at the bottom then you may as well stop eating for the rest of the day. You've blown it!

Did you imagine that black coffee contains 2.3 calories per cup? If you're a heavy coffee drinker (which we hope you're not—unbeautiful), that adds up. Tonic water has 71 calories per glass, and while club soda has 0 calories and 0 carbohydrates just try to remember that *all* carbonated beverages may make *you* bubble up in fat. It's safer to stick to water.

Enzyme Power

No, it's not a plug for a new detergent. Enzymes are those little marvels that digest all the good things you put into your body and get them out there to wherever they're going to do the most beauty good. Without enzymes—that work —nothing else would! Without them, those vitally beautiful vitamins, minerals, proteins, and all the good things we've gotten inside you would never be let out of your (by now) flat little tummy. Apparently the absence of even one enzyme can spell the difference, says enzyme-expert Carlson Wade, between life and health, and death!

That's enough to make us want them. Working.

And they won't, unless you treat them right. Heat kills them instantly. (Not the ones you manufacture inside your stomach—I hope they're in good order—but the ones you eat.) So think of that each and every time you overcook. Remember that no matter how "gourmet" you dish it out, you must have at least *some raw food* each and every day. You might remember that raw wheat kernels are one of the best possible food sources of enzymes. Remember what raw wheat germ does for your hair—and all of you—with its marvelous natural vitamin E store.

Raw vegetables—*crudités*—are standard fare almost anywhere but in this country. They substitute beautifully for the hors d'oeuvres horrors so often served up at cocktail shindigs in this part of the world.

Remember how I told you to chew? Well, chew, chew, and *chew* for your enzymes' sake as well. Because thorough chewing makes more and more enzymes in your digestive tract. Right where you want them and hard at work.

Stress, the great destroyer of virtually *everything*, including happiness, is also a destroyer of enzymes. So for health's sake, relax! Especially when you're eating. Because there is such a thing as indigestion, all right, but it's called "nervous" *not* acid.

There are all sorts of digestive enzymes readily available to you right on the shelves of your health food store. Papaya enzyme is probably one of the best known and most popular. Years ago, when I lived for a time in Cuba, papaya was always being touted as "good for the digestion." Well, apparently, the Cubans knew their papayas all right. There we go again: "civilized" eating is just catching on to "folkways." And believe me, if you feel gut-rumblings, for whatever reason, popping an enzyme tablet is ever so much safer than rushing for that so-called antacid "aid."

Carlson Wade, who's done a whole book on enzymes, in case you want to study up, has devised an "enzyme cocktail" that's bound to be a better kind than Big, Bad Booze. Add four heaping tablespoonsful of fresh brewer's yeast (here's one way to down it) to one glass of papaya juice. Fold in one teaspoon of tupelo honey. (I'd try carob powder—less sucrose.) Stir vigorously and drink the same way. Mr. Wade swears that if you drink *this* kind of cocktail thirty minutes before mealtime, you will discover a different, better digestion for, as he puts it, "instant health." Which is the right road to beauty.

Mining for Beauty—A Magical Mineral Tour

Don't ever imagine you can make beauty without minerals. See what I mean? Everything that makes for beautiful is not only interrelated but interdependent, so that, unless your whole beautiful body machine is well-oiled (literally) and humming along, you won't be the beautiful you we're striving for. As for minerals, they're magic; and you can't make beauty without them. You can't even *live* without them.

Just start with calcium. Make no bones about it. Calcium is good for a lot more than that. Making bones, I mean. Granted, you need it, in abundance, if you're going to have good strong bones, good strong teeth. After all, ninety-nine percent of all your calcium goes for that. (And *not* for your nails! One more old wives' tale down the drain. Those old wives have been hard at talk all these years!) But calcium is the best natural tranquilizer of them all. (When I talked about sleep, I talked about calcium. It's a mineral knockout drop.) Never forget that unnatural tranquilizers can do all sorts of dreadful things to your beauty, like give you wrinkled-crone skin or blow up your stomach to un-beautiful bloat. (It's happened to me, before I knew better. I've seen it happen to others.) So who needs *those* fearsome things when calcium's around? I take my calcium in super-strength, combined with magnesium—

nature's own natural laxative. (You'll soon see how much I *don't* believe in unnatural laxatives either!) In fact, that is the way it occurs in dolomite—a mineral that comes from limestone deposits. Let me assure you, something with a name like dolomite *can* make beautiful people. It, too, can be bought in supplement form at your health food store or your pharmacy. Recently I met an enchanting Southern lady—a friend of my mother's—who is an avowed health-food-and-vitamin (and dolomite) addict. When she left us, my mother asked me to guess her age. Figuring she must be older than she looked, I put her at somewhere around fifty-five. She was over *seventy!* How much over seventy she hadn't told anyone, but it was enough to make me rush right out and stock up on dolomite. I've been taking it ever since.

Potassium, sodium, and chlorine are three little minerals you'd better never forget, for these three, *together*, are responsible for keeping the water in your tissues moving. That is important to staying in shape, for, as you know, water retention is ever the bugaboo of the successful shape-up. (This doesn't mean that you should ever leave off the other natural water-movers, lecithin and vitamin E.) Never fall short on those three little minerals that help keep excess water where it belongs. Out of you!

Potassium, with its natural diuretic benefits, is just one of the very good reasons why doctors who know, like Dr. Robert Atkins, and my own ahead-of-the-pack internist, absolutely refuse to prescribe unnatural diuretics. Diuretics wash out valuable potassium. So forget them and take potassium instead. And sodium. And chlorine.

And if you're wondering how to get them: Well, potassium can be bought as a supplement combined with kelp. That's the way I take mine. And guess where chlorine comes from? Yep. Kelp. As for sodium? Well, sodium chloride is plain old salt, but I always use dehydrated sea water salt. After all, why pass up that valuable iodine from the sea? Speaking of iodine, you should know by now that you simply have to have it. (Kelp helps everything!) Iodine helps your thyroid utilize fats—so that they show up as beautiful, naturally moist skin and shining hair and not as lumps on your shape where they don't belong. Iodine keeps your shape in shape. So never forget that iodine via kelp— or you will certainly need help.

Sulfur is another mineral to consider. Recent research has turned up the interesting fact that nails that are brittle and breaking are almost inevitably lacking in sulfur. Not that the so-called nail experts and researchers have decided what to do about it. But I know what *I'd* do; I'd get more. Remember sulfur-and-molasses tonics? (Well, *I* don't. Here's one I'm not quite old enough for.) This is one old wives' tale that works just fine. Sulfur, it seems, is part of the amino acids, and there we go again. Protein works for nails, too. Well, why shouldn't it? That's what they're made of.

It also works with the B-complex vitamins—a must for beautiful hair, beautiful skin, and, obviously, beautiful nails. Let's just say that sulfur is sometimes called nature's "beauty mineral"; and I would have to concur.

While you're taking sulfur-and-molasses, you'll be getting one more important mineral. Iron. Iron is not just for tired blood. Iron is for red, healthy blood. The kind that gets under your skin and shows. Everybody knows about anemia—not pretty, is it? That sickly gray color. That lack of vitality. Iron will hold it off and keep you healthy. And beautiful.

But while you're getting your iron, make sure you're getting your HCl (hydrochloric acid) as well. It has to be there, that acid, to make use of iron. Perhaps that's where the folk recipe of cider vinegar and blackstrap molasses comes from. But any foods that are *acid*—yogurt, buttermilk, citrus juices—aid in the absorption of iron. Unless it is absorbed, well, it won't make you beautiful just sitting there.

Phosphorus is a mineral that's everywhere in you. It's been called the brain power of the mineral world. It makes lecithin, and we know we need lots of that! Phosphorus *must* be in there if your calcium is going to work properly. White sugar destroys phosphorus—but then white sugar destroys beauty. I told you so. So leave it out! And get phosphorus supplements. And take them.

For the beauty power of minerals is magic, all right. You see?

Eliminate the Negative

Elimination is not a subject that is particularly beautiful to discuss, though from the looks of the cranky-faced folk in the TV commercials it's a national problem. Let's face it: part of what goes in has simply got to come out and surely you'd rather it came out of the normal places than out as repulsive bloated stomachs or acne or something usually unattractive.

For beginnings, I approve of water. Lots of it. If you can latch on to the mineral spring stuff, then great. Minerals are something that we can't get too much of. (Not mineral *oil*. Natural mineral *water!*) When Dr. Stillman recommended his eight glasses of water per day, it seemed to evoke groans from so many of his dieters. I couldn't understand it, since twenty glasses per day is about the norm for me. (And yes—I know the location of every presentable ladies' room in the city of New York. But I don't have a pimple on my skin or a blown-up stomach.)

The body, assuming that all organs are "go," is a pretty remarkable machine. It knows exactly what ought to stay and what ought to get right out. In a recent issue of *Prevention* magazine, the unsavory, albeit *importantissimo* subject of elimination was brought up. (In fact, there was one article that had the arresting title, "The Story Your Bowels Can Tell." I never did quite find out what that story was, since bowels are not my forte and *my* subject is beauty.) And this is a point at which the old-time food habits help out.

First rule: Forget the laxatives. They can be dangerous. They can be a crutch. And they are not the natural way to get rid of anything.

And as for diuretics? Well, my doctor won't hear of it. If you're a chronic water-retainer, as I once was, diuretics are the worst first step to take in getting rid of that water you don't want. They wash away mineral salts, potassium being one of the most important, and can lower mineral content in your body to the danger, even fatal, state.

Besides, there are too many natural ways to get rid of it. Lecithin, for one, our friendly wonder-worker. Lecithin makes everything move, in the right direction, and that includes the water you *don't* want to keep. So does natural vitamin E; its action is uncanny. They're both good, natural diuretics, and they'll make sure that water lands only where it's needed and not on your waistline. And as for that old national malady, constipation—well, luckily, what's good for you is good for your gut, too. First, the things that got you in that shape in the first place are the very things no beauty needs! Like refined foods, processed sugar, white flour. Everything that can destroy your looks, your health, and even you!

Whole grains (full of vitamin E), nuts and seeds (ditto), fresh vegetables and fruits—preferably uncooked —have a laxative action. (In my opinion, *all* fresh vegetables are better uncooked.) And apples. Lately I saw a charming little drawing in *Prevention* magazine. It depicted an old-time apple-bobbing and the caption said, "In the innocent days of our country's youth, bobbing for apples was a favorite party sport. No booze, no pot, and no constipation either." Healthy sport.

Acid Indigestion Is a Myth!

And a potentially dangerous one at that. For, contrary to commercial, and very popular, opinion, your stomach is not just one oversized gas bubble waiting to explode! (That's an ad agency's dream picture.) It is not eaten up with acid, unless you happen to be one of the unlucky folk who has a peptic ulcer—in which case, you're bound to have been informed. The simple truth is that, as with skin, as with hair, as with all of your body, *acid* is the natural state for your stomach to be in. That's what we said, all right. *Acid* inside, as well as outside where it shows beautifully. Acid indigestion is not only a myth, but the myth can be harmful if taken seriously. For those antacids—yes, the very ones you see in those witty little television commercials—actually can *destroy* the acid your stomach must have in order to digest your food. If your food doesn't get digested, then it doesn't get to places like your hair and your skin and your nails, now does it? (Some nutritionists feel that antacids are dangerous enough to be put on the FDA's "dangerous drugs" list.)

The funny part is that the symptoms of too little acid in your stomach are *exactly* like those described in said silly commercials as symptoms of too *much* acid! So how are you to know? Easy. There's a simple test for HCl. Ask your doctor, *before* you reach for that tummy tablet. It has been said, by doctors who do know, that the medium of the stomach is acid, and if it isn't acid you've got some trouble! Apparently you not only need the acid to break down proteins and minerals for digestion, but you need it to kill off bad bacteria as well. According to one physician, a lack of hydrochloric acid can start off a chain of problems from gas, bloating, belching, constipation, and on and on, none of which is going to make you beautiful.

There *is* a tablet which can be found in health food stores these days. It is hydrochloric acid betain plus pepsin. But *I* am not going to recommend that you run out and get HCl tablets until you've gotten that test from your doctor. Which may take some persuasion. Physicians never seem to believe in such simple answers to stomach troubles and so say "Oh, it's only nerves" until it's too late. And you've got *real* stomach troubles.

There is, however, one thing I'll happily recommend. I already have. *Drink your cider vinegar brew!* After every single meal. It's nature's way of making up for any hydrochloric acid you may lack. As my doctor told me, it can't hurt you. You see? Health and beauty go together.

Last year the flying finger of fate landed right on me. On my pancreas, to be exact, with a painful attack of acute pancreatitis. I don't imagine many of you have ever heard of it. My only claim to might-have-been fame is that Harry Houdini died of the disease. Had it not been for my own astute internist, I might have, too, but we found it in time. And I learned a little bit more about the magical thing— the body and its mysterious ways.

Who ever thinks about the pancreas, really? I never had. I'd had trouble with my stomach for years. And years ago I'd been very interested in a passage in one of Linda Clark's books in which she describes the rare things that can happen to one's digestion when there's a lack of HCl. It all sounded too, too familiar. I queried my doctor (he's used to this by now, bless him) and was told that the test for absence of HCl is simple and that we'd do it some time. We never did, to my health's detriment. But, when we finally uncovered the disease and its cure, guess what turned out to make up that cure? Pink pills full of hydrochloric acid and pancreatin, an enzyme that works directly on the pancreas.

As to what caused the disease in the first place, let me say simply that nobody knows. In fact, wherever I looked, in whatever medical textbook, I came up with such immortal lines as, "About pancreatitis, very little is known." Some help. But I'm relieved just to know that those pills of enzymes and HCl will keep me pain-free forever.

Protein Power

We all know about protein power. It's what makes a new you. Completely. Every seven years. There are three *billion* (that's right—that's what I said) cells of *you* that are being rebuilt every minute of your life! And guess what those cells are made of? That's right. Protein. So protein goes in and protein goes on, if you can get those molecules cut down to size. And protein shapes up your body, builds up your hair, and beautifies your skin. What you may not know—and you want to be certain you do—is that *protein cannot be stored in the body*. It must be replenished each and every single day of your life.

Protein is so all-important that you can't even be healthy, much less lovely, unless you get enough every day. And enough, according to Dr. Carlton Fredericks, is a variable. For there's our old friend hydrochloric acid again, and the amount of *it* you have means the amount of your protein that gets digested and therefore used to its powerful advantage. Apparently some of us produce as much as 1,000 times more HCl than others. I would deem it reasonable to overdo protein requirements rather than underdo them. (Watching your HCl all the while via that cider vinegar cocktail after every meal.)

The National Academy of Sciences has set the normal need for protein at .42 grams of protein per pound of body weight, meaning that if you are a man and weigh in at 154 pounds, you need sixty-five grams of protein per day, minimum. A woman at 128 pounds needs fifty-four. (I'd go for more!) That should give you enough to go on and my explicit chart will give you the rest.

Just never forget that protein makes skin. Protein makes hair. Protein makes nails. And more protein can make a whole new you.

B Is for Balance—The Key to All Beauty

My bout with pancreatitis had one beautiful side effect. It taught me a lot about the balance of nature when it comes to beauty. If all of your vitamins and minerals and enzymes and metabolic system and odd-organs (like pancreases) are in there working in beautiful rhythm, then you're in beautifully for you. When it doesn't, it's usually because we humans have mucked up somewhere along the way, by dosing ourselves with unnecessary, though well-advertised, medications, or by eating improperly—possibly through lack of information rather than through intention.

Since my pink-pill pancreas cure I have, of late, been flirting with fat. A kind of diet-roulette, if you will. And I've been eating more than I want, really. It's a dangerous game, all right, and certainly not one that I'd suggest for you. But I think that, in the back of my mind, I'm still testing. Testing to see whether now all cylinders are kicking in perfect harmony. For once. Recently, for example, I had not one, but four, helpings of lima beans, liberally doused in (no, not butter) my favorite safflower margarine. I've been eating like that for a while now and deliberately staying away from the scales. Finally, I had the nerve to step on them and I had actually lost a pound.

Again, let me assure you that I am *not* suggesting that you have a go at this sort of lustful eating. As I have already said, it's dangerous. Maybe soon I'll show up as three hundred pounds of blubber. But somehow I don't think so. Because I believe that, with the discovery of what *my* problem was—namely the lack of sufficient hydrochloric acid and pancreatic enzymes to digest my food properly—my own diet problem has been solved. And, as you have seen, my other beauty problems are well under my own control.

And now, with my enzymes, hormones, proteins, minerals, vitamins, carbohydrates, and all those things that matter seemingly working for me, in a harmonious manner, I think my shape is together as well. I have not forgotten to think fat. I always watch all parts carefully, for the body is like any other delicate piece of machinery. When one part goes, the rest shows the strain. So watch yourself, have your doctor watch over you, and above all, stick to the pattern of good beauty-living you've set for yourself. It should be good for a lifetime.

In Praise of Medical Men

One last thing I'd like to say before you set off to get gorgeous: that is that I *do* believe in doctors, although you might not think so from the way I've ticked off some of them. I don't believe in embarking on *any* program that might affect your health without first checking with a good physician. And I mean a good physician, for there are plenty of bad ones about, too. In a profession as vast as medicine, there'd have to be.

You will notice that throughout this book I have suggested that you keep a firm check on your general health through your general physician. I think it's a must and I think it should be done relatively often. I think, considering how little everyone knows—including the medical profession—about blood chemistry, that a test called a blood profile should be done on everyone as a matter of course. It would help tell whether some obscure organ (such as my pancreas) is not working just as it should be. And it could save a lot of agony later.

My only beef with some physicians is that they tend to scoff at what they don't understand. They can't understand everything since the world is always on its way to newer scientific discoveries. Otherwise, we'd still be seeing that world as flat. I wish their minds were more open and that, if they really don't understand, they would find out.

But there's where money rears its head. Research money. Very few philanthropists, it seems, wish to give money for beauty research, even though it might mean a psychological salvation for someone. They prefer more severe-sounding causes such as research for cancer, or other deadly diseases. Those are certainly causes well undertaken, one cannot argue that. But I believe, and I believe completely, that one day preventive medicine will be upon us, and perhaps deadly diseases won't even exist.

Until that day arrives, I hope the doctors will keep their minds open to fresh ideas, and I hope that you will always and forever keep in close touch with your own doctor.

Here's to *healthy* beauty!

Other Authors I Have Known

Believe me, when you read as much on the health subject as I have, you quickly learn to separate the knowledgeables from the fashionables. And some of the best comes from some of the least well known, whether it be books or authors. There are, of course, the big three. There is Adelle Davis, probably number one health food authority, and the one whose books ought to be in every library for ready reference. Miss Davis is so full of expert information that her books have become encyclopedic. It would be practically impossible for the average mind—like mine—to digest and retain every piece of information she has to offer. But her books should be always readily available for looking up any food questions that come to mind.

Linda Clark is a different breed of food-thinker. She combines it with beauty—I don't see how you can avoid it—and her books are not only chock-full of information but are easily-readable as well.

Possibly my very favorite of the big three is Carlton Fredericks—not only because of what he knows, which seems to be everything, but because of his humor—a quality too often lacking in this field. Reading his books is not only educational, but chuckle-making as well, and the world needs more of that. (Remember what I said about having humor?)

Frances Moore Lappé has written the authoritative book on vegetable protein in her *Diet for a Small Planet*. It takes some real chewing, but it's worth it to your diet. One of the best little pamphlets I've come across—and how lucky for me that I did—was written by an English nutritionist and beauty expert, Charles Perry. Its title is "New Beauty," and if your health-food shop has a copy, grab it. You're sure to learn plenty. Health-food shops have practically become book-and-beauty stalls as well, these days, and in them you'll find racks of these books on virtually every vitamin, every mineral, every subject. Almost all are worth reading, though I am not convinced that all are worth believing. For I remain a cynic at heart—it's the reporter in me, ever questioning. And so I suggest you check them against what you have learned here and begin to learn to ask your own questions. Even of the so-called experts.

Rodale Press publishes a magazine called *Prevention* and

I consider it one of the most important publications to which I subscribe. Try it and see whether you feel the same way. *Consumer Reports* is another good one at letting you know just what some of the government agencies are allowing manufacturers of food and cosmetics to get away with. On the other hand, *Consumer Reports* seems to have an inordinate fear of anything that smacks of "health." I can't imagine why unless their staff isn't up to health snuff.

Colette Dowling's *The Skin Game* is a must to read if you want to find out just who isn't protecting your skin. It was a revelation to me, all right, and will be to you as well, I am sure. It will give you plenty of pause before you plunge into some of the well-advertised skin remedies.

The point is, the material is endless and will go on being so as long as there is life. For, as we have already pointed out, life's continuation also means progress. I hope that, in the world of health and beauty, *that* progress will be the happy sort.

The Summa Cum Chart—Everything You Need to Know About Everything You Eat

The chart that you are going to find at the very end of this book is, in fact, the heart and soul of the book. It is there because I needed it. And, therefore, I figured you needed it just as much. And deserved it. For there's nothing more frustrating than being told what you ought to get for the way you want to look—and then not being able to find out how to get it. This isn't just another chart, so, chart-haters, don't leave. This is *everything* you need to know about all the things I've told you you ought to have. It is the result of months and months of painstaking searching. Search for research, because the minds behind the beauties didn't bother in this case. Neither did the U.S. Department of Agriculture—whose food charts are the basis for most food charts found in most nutrition books. And who freely admit that they take their so-called facts from whatever sources they can find. And also have no explanation for the unlikely fact that some of their charts don't check out against others. Unnerving it is, if your will is unswerving and you really want to do right by your diet, for whatever result you've got your sights on—shape, or skin, or whatever.

Well, my chart is accurate to the *n*th degree. But, not only are its figures accurate, its servings are normal and consistent. You won't find, for example, unsweetened applesauce given by the cupful while sweetened applesauce is given by the gallon. Oh, no! To be perfectly honest, math is not my forte. And why should a reader be forced to do the higher math hurdles just to find out what she's had for lunch? And what about restaurant eating? How can you possibly outguess the calories or carbohydrates or vitamin or protein content of the slab of fish set before you? Well, if your eye is good (and it soon gets size-adjusted), you'll be able to tell, for I've often given measurements of portions as well. Get it in your mind what the piece would look like. (If you've got the nerve, take your tapemeasure when you go out to eat, so you needn't, like my intrepid researcher, have to take your food scale out to dinner.)

I have tried and tried and then gone back and tried even harder to make this chart as readable and easy to understand as it is humanly possible to do. It must be *used*. For, if you're going to take the advice I've given and eat all those things that are guaranteed good for hair, skin, shape —then you'll have to keep accurate tabs on what's going into you. You'll know the calories, the carbohydrates, the protein, the unsaturated and saturated fatty acids, all the B vitamins, C, D, E, plus some important minerals. You'll also get, with each chapter, a reprise of what works for what. Then you look it up in the chart to find just what's in your favorite dish.

If, on occasion, I swerve on servings, it's because I found consistency didn't always make for common sense. You may eat a handful, or cupful, of salted peanuts, but would you eat the same amount of hickory nuts? I thought about all this. Seriously. And long. And then made the decision as to what seemed normal to me. If a serving doesn't seem normal to you and you want to eat, say, a dozen hickory nuts at a gulp—multiply the serving by the number given for one. Easy does it.

If, in some cases, you find the letters DNA ("data not available"), this means that no research of any kind has been done to discover the amount of that particular nutrient in this particular food. It should give you some idea as to how much scientists, medical men, the government agencies, and all those who ought to care really *do* care about what you get in your diet. And shouldn't they be the ones who would want to know?

Unfortunately, I have no laboratory of my own. And, in any case, it might take years, and certainly more millions in money than I possess, to find the missing numbers. But I want you to know how I tried—enough so that virtually every single bit of information that *can* be found has been found and is in this chart. The dashes (−) mean that traces of a nutrient have been found but not counted. Or perhaps the numbers turned up so small that you wouldn't want to know in any case. Just remember, − means it's there but not in amounts you can count on.

I think when you look the chart over you'll be as amazed as I was by the minute amounts of vitamins available in the average servings of food. Take spinach, that old health favorite, which some nutritionists are already having a second nutritional thought about. It seems that you may fight to the finish when you eat your spinach, but while you're at it, you'd best make sure you're supplementing it with equal amounts of calcium. Spinach gobbles up calcium at a Popeye-kind of clip! Spinach is one of the big vitamin vegetables. A one-cup serving will give you 14,580 units of vitamin A, and that's swell. But then there's frozen brussels sprouts, and the one cup yield there is only 108 I.U. of A per cup, with A being the largest vitamin content of the lovely little vegetable. Fresh brussels sprouts in a cup will give you 810 I.U.'s of the same vitamin, and that, too, is good. But notice that some of the other nutrients may be numbers like .076. Meaning that, if you want that particular vitamin or mineral to fatten up your hair, for example, you're going to have to get it elsewhere. That elsewhere will be in supplement form. Again—*don't* forget to check that supplement's label just as carefully as you would any other. Just because something comes from a health-food shop doesn't mean it's necessarily worthwhile. In many cases you would admittedly have to swallow some thirty or forty capsules of certain supplements to have any benefit whatsoever. I don't know about you, but my water capacity isn't big enough for that much pill-taking.

This chart has taken into account the loss of nutrients in cooking, plus the loss of size—shrinkage and all that. So if sometimes a cup of spinach raw (back to spinach) seems to have less of something than a cup of spinach cooked, the answer is simple. You can get more cooked spinach into a cup. Get the picture?

Trust me. The chart is real. It is accurate. You will be able to know exactly what you and your family have just eaten, and then be able to supplement accordingly if need be. Who knows? With a little help from your friendly chart, you may work out meals that supply everything. Just don't get fat trying to get your vitamins by the food road alone.

While we're at it, there's a point I must make again with regard to cooking. Nutrients are lost in the process. There's simply no getting around that fact. The less you cook, the better. The more raw fruits and vegetables you get, the better. Try to have something raw each and every day of your life. You'll learn to love it. Raw cauliflower is one of my favorites. Raw carrots are an old trick. Even raw meat—as in steak tartare—is considered a delicacy. When you cook, try your best to avoid aluminum. Aluminum is a vitamin enemy. Try glass. Sounds delicate, but preserves vitamins best and therefore is worth the care. Above all, never overcook. And *never* pour off the liquid in which you've cooked vegetables unless you want to pour your health down the drain as well. Learn to eat the skins of fruits and vegetables. Often the nutrients that matter lie in the skin. The skin of citrus fruits is one example; potatoes, another. I, personally, like *only* the skin of a baked potato. Somebody else gets the fattening rest.

Learn not to equate protein with meat. If you look carefully at the chart, you will see that some of the very best protein comes from vegetables. Beans—just have a look at them. A cup of cooked, dried lentils will give you 33.3 grams of protein. If 60 grams of protein—which ought to be your very minimum daily intake—is your goal, then you're halfway home.

I'm not suggesting you become vegetarians, one and all, but I've already lectured you on overdoing the meat-eating routine. I've given up beef altogether and feel the better for it, but you must use your own judgment. Anyway, beef is too caloric for my body.

There are some rather obscure vitamins and minerals that you may point out have been omitted. And you're right. For charts will hold only so much and I've given you every single thing I thought you needed for that beautiful you you want to become. Choline and inositol, two relatively obscure B vitamins (and the B-vitamin complex is expanding every day that scientists are at work isolating new components), are two very important vitamins for your hair. Mostly for your hair. And so there's a chart on choline and inositol (with another obscure B vitamin, biotin, included) on page 245. To me, it made sense. I hope you will find it not only sensible, but simple. And that you will use it.

You'll find something else in the chart that I disapprove of. Alcoholic beverages, soft drinks, desserts. But I know you can't change human nature, so it's best to show you how little you're getting in the way of beauty-making nutrients, how much you're getting in calories and carbohydrates. It may be enough to make you stop. I can hope, can't I? For a more beautiful, naturally, you!

SOME IMPORTANT SOURCES OF CALCIUM AND MAGNESIUM

CALCIUM

Buttermilk	Canned smelt
Brick cheese	Dates
Cheddar cheese	Rhubarb
Swiss cheese	Whole-grain buckwheat
American cheese	Cottonseed flour
Cheese soufflé	Farina, enriched
Whipping cream	Almonds
Sour cream	Almond meal
Ice milk	Peanuts
Whole milk, all forms	Pigeon peas, mature, dry
Skim milk, all forms	Safflower seed meal
Whey	Mature, dry, raw soybeans
Yogurt	Soybean curd
Black sea bass	Soybean flour
Dried, salted cod	Sunflower seed flour
Canned herring	Blackstrap molasses
Canned mackerel	Brown sugar
Mussels	Raw common beans, all
Canned salmon	types
Sardines, canned	Raw mung beans
Steamed scallops	Beet greens

CALCIUM

Broccoli
Spoon cabbage (pakchoy)
Chickpeas
Collards
Dandelion greens
Kale

Mustard greens
Raw, mature, dry peas
Spinach
Turnip greens
Kelp

MAGNESIUM

Dry whole milk
Dry skim milk
Dried, uncooked apricots
Avocados
Banana flakes
Dates
Whole-grain buckwheat
Whole-ground cornmeal
Cottonseed flour
Whole-grain millet
Whole-grain rye
Whole-grain wheat
Wholewheat flour
Wild rice
Almonds
Cashew nuts

Peanuts
Defatted peanut flour
Pecans
Pigeon peas, mature seeds,
  dry
Mature, dry, raw soybeans
Soybean curd
Soybean flour
Walnuts
Raw common beans
Lima beans
Beet greens
Cowpeas (including black-
  eyed peas)
Mature, dry peas

Lesser Known Vitamins in Foods*:
Biotin, choline, and inositol content
of foods, edible portion

Food	Portion		Biotin		Choline		Inositol	
	Amt.	Wt. Gm.	Mcg./ portion	Mcg./ 100 Gm.	Mg./ portion	Mg./ 100 Gm.	Mg./ portion	Mg./ 100 Gm.
Cereals and Bread Products								
Cereals, cooked, whole								
Barley, whole.........	½ c.	30 (dry)	9.3	31.0	41.7	139.0	117.6	392.0
Corn, yellow..........	½ c.	20 (dry)	4.2	21.0	12.2	61.0	10.0	50.0
Oats.................	½ c.	20 (dry)	4.8	24.0	31.2	156.0	53.8	269.0
Rice, brown...........	½ c.	30 (dry)	3.6	12.0	33.6	112.0	35.7	119.0
Wheat, whole.........	½ c.	30 (dry)	4.8	16.0	28.2	94.0	110.0	370.0
Cereals, refined, cooked								
Cornmeal								
White.............	½ c.	20 (dry)	1.3	6.6	..	..	10.2	51
Yellow.............	½ c.	20 (dry)	..	..	2.0	10.0	..	..
Hominy grits..........	½ c.	20 (dry)	0.1	0.7	..	..	0.6	3
Rice								
Converted..........	½ c.	30 (dry)	2.4	8.0	26.7	89.0	6.0	20
Parboiled..........	½ c.	30 (dry)	3.0	10.0	29.4	98.0	7.5	25
White.............	½ c.	30 (dry)	1.5	5.0	17.7	59.0	3.0	10
Cereal concentrates, raw								
Rice								
Bran..............	1 oz.	30 (dry)	18.0	60.0	51.0	170.0	138.9	463
Germ.............	1 oz.	30 (dry)	17.4	58.0	90.0	300.0	111.6	372
Polishings..........	1 oz.	30 (dry)	17.1	57.0	30.6	102.0	136.2	454
Wheat								
Bran..............	1 oz.	30 (dry)	4.2	14.0	42.9	143.0	..	..
Germ.............	1 oz.	30 (dry)	..	..	121.8	406.0	231.0	770
Ready-to-eat, dark cereal								
Corn soya............	1 c.	30	..	..	..	..	..	..
Oats.................	1 c.	25	..	..	..	..	..	..
Wheat								
Bran..............	1 c.	35	..	..	..	..	..	..
Flakes.............	1 c.	35	..	..	..	..	..	..
Shredded Wheat......	1 bisc.	30	..	..	..	..	..	..
Ready-to-eat, white cereal								
Corn flakes..........	1 c.	25	..	..	..	..	..	..
Rice.................	1 c.	30	0.4	1.3	..	..	5.7	19
Bread								
White...............	1 sl.	23	0.3	1.1	..	..	11.7	51
Whole wheat.........	1 sl.	23	0.4	1.9	..	..	15.4	67
Flour								
White...............	1 c.	110	1.1	1.0	57.2	52	51.7	47
Whole wheat........	1 c.	120	10.8	9.0	..	..	132.0	110
Dairy Products								
Cheese								
Cheddar.............	1 oz.	30	1.0	3.6	13.6	48	7.0	25
Cottage.............	1 oz.	30	..	..	..	..	..	..
Processed............	1 oz.	30	1.3	4.6	..	..	..	..
Egg								
Whole...............	1 med.	50	11.2	22.5	252.0	504	16.5	33
Yolk...............	1 med.	17	8.8	52.0	253.3	1490	..	..
White...............	1 med.	31	2.2	7.0	0.6	2	..	..

* Table adapted from Hardinge, M. G. and Crooks, H., J. Am. Dietet. A. 38:240, 1961, by permission of the authors and the Journal.

Food	Portion Amt.	Portion Wt. Gm.	Biotin Mcg./portion	Biotin Mcg./100 Gm.	Choline Mg./portion	Choline Mg./100 Gm.	Inositol Mg./portion	Inositol Mg./100 Gm.
Dairy Products (Continued)								
Milk								
Whole................	1 c.	244	11.5	4.7	36.6	15	31.7	13
Evaporated reconstituted	1 c.	244	11.0	4.5	36.6	15	..	..
Nonfat dry reconstituted	1 c.	244	8.3	3.4	25.4	10.4	..	..
Fats, Oils, and Oily Foods								
Butter.................	1 tbsp.	14	..	..	0.7	5	..	..
Lard..................	1 tbsp.	14	..	..	0.7	5	..	..
Margarine.............	1 tbsp.	14	..	..	0.7	5	..	..
Vegetable oils..........	1 tbsp.	14	..	..	0.7	5	..	..
Fruits								
Fruits, fresh or frozen								
Apples, medium.......	1	130	1.2	0.9	..	..	31.2	24
Apricots.............	3 med.	100	..	..	..	..	..	..
Bananas..............	1 med.	100	4.4	4.4	..	..	34.0	34
Berries								
Blackberry..........	⅔ c.	100	..	..	..	..	..	..
Blueberry...........	⅔ c.	100	..	..	..	..	..	..
Raspberry, sweetened	¾ c.	100	..	..	..	..	..	..
Strawberry, sweetened	⅔ c.	100	4.0	4.0	..	..	60.0	60
Cantaloupe, diced.....	⅔ c.	100	3.1	3.1	..	..	120.0	120
Cherries, sour, red, pitted	⅔ c.	100	..	..	..	..	..	..
Figs, small..........	3	114	..	..	..	..	..	..
Grapefruit, small.....	½	120	3.6	3.0	..	..	180.0	150
Grapes, 1 bunch.....	3½ ozs.	100	1.6	1.6	..	..	..	..
Oranges, small........	1	100	1.9	1.9	..	..	210.0	210
Peaches, sweetened...	½ c.	100	1.7	1.7	..	..	96.0	96
Pineapple............	3½ ozs.	100	..	..	..	..	..	..
Rhubarb, sweetened...	3½ ozs.	100	..	..	..	..	..	..
Watermelon, diced....	1 c.	150	5.4	3.6	..	..	96.0	64
Fruits, canned								
Apricots.............	½ c.	125	..	..	..	..	..	..
Blackberries..........	½ c.	125	..	..	..	..	..	..
Blueberries..........	½ c.	125	..	..	..	..	..	..
Cherries, sweet.......	½ c.	125	..	..	..	..	..	..
Peaches..............	½ c.	125	0.3	0.2	..	..	..	..
Pineapple............	½ c.	125	..	..	..	..	..	..
Plums, purple.........	½ c.	125	..	..	..	..	..	..
Fruit, dried								
Apricots, small........	6 halves	30	..	..	..	..	..	..
Dates, pitted..........	5	45	..	..	..	..	..	..
Figs, large...........	2	40	..	..	..	..	..	..
Prunes..............	5 med.	35	..	..	..	..	..	..
Raisins, seedless.......	3 tbsp.	30	1.4	4.5	..	..	36.0	120
Fruit Juices								
Canned fruit juice								
Apple...............	½ c.	120	..	..	..	..	..	..
Grapefruit............	½ c.	120	1.0	0.8	..	..	120.0	100
Lemon...............	½ c.	120	..	..	..	..	..	..
Orange..............	½ c.	120	1.0	0.8	..	..	169.0	141
Pineapple............	½ c.	120	..	..	..	..	..	..
Frozen or fresh								
Apple...............	½ c.	120	0.5	0.4	0.7	0.6	28.8	24
Grape...............	½ c.	120	0.4	0.3	..	..	..	..

Food	Portion		Biotin		Choline		Inositol	
	Amt.	Wt. Gm.	Mcg./ portion	Mcg./ 100 Gm.	Mg./ portion	Mg./ 100 Gm.	Mg./ portion	Mg./ 100 Gm.
Fruit Juices (Continued)								
Grapefruit........	½ c.	120	0.8	0.7	..	..	120.0	100
Lemon, single........	½ c.	120	..	..	..	..	..	..
Orange, fresh........	½ c.	120	0.4	0.3	14.4	12	141.6	118
Orange, frozen........	½ c.	120	0.4	0.3	14.4	12	110.4	92
Pineapple............	½ c.	120	..	..	..	..	..	..
Legumes, cooked								
Mung bean............	½ c.	32 (dry)	2.4	7.5	66.9	209	22.4	70
Cowpeas..............	½ c.	32 (dry)	6.7	21.0	82.2	257	76.9	240
Garbanzos............	½ c.	32 (dry)	3.2	10.0	78.4	245	76.8	240
Lentils..............	½ c.	32 (dry)	4.2	13.2	71.4	223	41.6	130
Lima beans....	½ c.	32 (dry)	3.1	9.8	..	..	54.4	130
Navy beans...........	½ c.	32 (dry)	..	..	..	..	160.0	500
Kidney beans..........	½ c.	32 (dry)	..	..	..	..	..	..
Split peas............	½ c.	32 (dry)	5.9	18.4	64.3	201	48.0	150
Soy beans............	½ c.	32 (dry)	19.5	61.0	108.8	340	64.0	200
Soy flour.............	1 c.	90 (dry)	63.0	70.0	202.5	225	184.5	205
Meat and Poultry†								
Beef								
Ground...........	3½ ozs.	100	..	..	..	..	29.1	51
Liver..............	2 ozs.	57	54.7	96.0	290.7	510	29.1	51
Rib roast, lean.../.....	3 ozs.	100	3.4	3.4	82.0	82	..	..
Round.............	3 ozs.	100	2.6	2.6	68.0	68	11.5	11.5
Lamb								
Leg...............	3 ozs.	100	5.9	5.9	84.0	84	58.0	58
Liver..............	2 ozs.	57	72.4	127.0	..	..	..	..
Loin chop..........	3 ozs.	100	..	..	76.0	76	..	..
Veal								
Chop..............	3½ ozs.	100	2.0	2.0	96.0	96	33.0	33
Leg...............	3½ ozs.	100	..	..	132.0	132	..	..
Shoulder...........	3½ ozs.	100	..	..	93.0	93	..	..
Stew meat..........	3½ ozs.	100	..	..	96.0	96	..	..
Pork								
Bacon.............	2 sl.	16	1.2	7.6	12.8	80	6.9	43
Ham...............	3½ ozs.	100	5.0	5.0	122.0	122	31.0	31
Liver..............	2 ozs.	57	57.0	100.0	314.6	552	..	..
Loin..............	3½ ozs.	100	5.2	5.2	77.0	77	45.0	45
Poultry								
Chicken								
Dark meat........	3½ ozs.	100	10.0	10.0	..	..	47.0	47
White meat.......	3½ ozs.	100	11.3	11.3	..	..	48.0	48
Turkey.............	3½ ozs.	100	..	..	..	..	..	..
Bologna, A. & P........	2 ozs.	57	..	..	34.2	60	..	..
Frankfurter, A. & P......	1	50	..	..	28.5	57	..	..
Sausage, pork, A. & P....	2 ozs.	57	..	..	27.4	48	..	..
Fish and Shellfish								
Fish								
Halibut, canned.......	3½ ozs.	100	8.0	8.0	..	..	17.0	17
Mackerel, Pacific, canned	3½ ozs.	100	18.0	18.0	..	..	..	..
Salmon, canned........	3½ ozs.	100	15.0	15.0	..	..	17.0	17
Tuna, canned.........	3½ ozs.	100	3.0	3.0	..	..	..	..
Sardines, Pacific, canned	3½ ozs.	100	24.0	24.0	..	..	..	..
Shellfish, canned								
Clams..............	3½ ozs.	100	..	..	..	..	..	..
Crabs..............	3½ ozs.	100	..	..	..	..	..	..
Oysters............	3½ ozs.	100	8.7	8.7	..	..	44.0	44

Food	Portion		Biotin		Choline		Inositol	
	Amt.	Wt. Gm.	Mcg./ portion	Mcg./ 100 Gm.	Mg./ portion	Mg./ 100 Gm.	Mg./ portion	Mg./ 100 Gm.
Fish and Shellfish (Continued)								
Shrimp..............	3½ ozs.	100	..	..	..	..	..	..
Nuts and Oily Fruits								
Almonds.............	12–15	15	2.7	18.0	..	..	..	..
Brazil nuts...........	2 med.	15	..	..	..	..	..	..
Cashews.............	6–8	15	..	..	..	..	..	..
Coconut, fresh........	½ oz.	15	..	..	..	..	..	..
Filbert..............	10–12	15	..	..	..	..	..	..
Peanuts, roasted.......	15–17	15	5.1	34.0	24.3	162	27.0	180
Pecan halves.........	12	15	4.0	27.0	7.5	50	..	..
Walnut halves........	8–15	15	5.5	37.0	..	..	..	..
Peanut butter..........	1 tbsp.	16	6.2	39.0	23.2	145	28.8	180
Fruits, oily								
Avocado, Fuerte....... (cubed)	½ c.	75	4.1	5.5	..	..	..	..
Olive, ripe, mammoth...	6	40	..	..	..	..	..	..
Vegetables								
Fresh or frozen								
Asparagus...........	3½ ozs.	100	..	..	10.0	10.0	..	..
Beans, Lima..........	3½ ozs.	100	..	..	..	..	..	..
Beans, snap, green.....	3½ ozs.	100	..	..	42.0	42.0	..	..
Beets (diced).........	⅔ c.	100	1.9	1.9	..	..	21.0	21
Broccoli.............	⅔ c.	100	..	..	..	..	..	..
Brussels sprouts.......	3½ ozs.	100	..	..	..	..	..	..
Cabbage (fine shreds)..	1 c.	100	2.4	2.4	23.0	23.0	95.0	95
Carrots (grated).......	½ c.	55	1.4	2.5	7.0	13.4	26.4	48
Cauliflower (buds).....	1 c.	100	17.0	17.0	..	..	95.0	95
Celery (diced)........	1 c.	100	..	..	..	..	..	..
Corn...............	3½ ozs.	100	6.0	6.0	..	..	..	..
Lettuce.............	¼ hd.	100	3.1	3.1	..	..	55.0	55
Mixed vegetables.....	3½ ozs.	100	..	..	..	..	..	..
Onion (2½ in.).......	1	110	3.8	3.5	..	..	96.8	88
Peas, cow...........	3½ ozs.	100	21.0	21.0	97.0	97.0	240.0	240
Peas, green..........	3½ ozs.	100	9.4	9.4	75.0	75.0	162.0	162
Potatoes, peeled......	1 med.	100	..	..	29.0	29.0	29.0	29
Potatoes, sweet.......	½ med.	100	4.3	4.3	11.5	11.5	66.0	66
Squash, winter........	3½ ozs.	100	..	..	..	..	..	..
Squash, yellow........	3½ ozs.	100	..	..	..	..	..	..
Tomato.............	1 small	110	4.4	4.0	..	..	50.6	46
Mushrooms, fresh......	2 ozs.	60	9.6	16.0	..	..	10.2	17
Greens								
Beet...............	3½ ozs.	100	2.7	2.7	..	..	21.0	21
Kale...............	3½ ozs.	100	..	..	..	..	..	0
Mustard............	3½ ozs.	100	..	..	22.0	22.0	..	..
Spinach.............	3½ ozs.	100	6.9	6.9	22.0	22.0	27.0	27
Turnip.............	3½ ozs.	100	..	..	27.0	27.0	46.0	46
Canned with liquid								
Asparagus, green.......	½ c.	120	2.0	1.7	..	..	..	
Beans								
Lima..............	½ c.	120	..	..	..	..	..	
Green string........	½ c.	120	1.5	1.3	..	..	..	
Beets (diced).........	½ c.	125	..	..	..	..	..	..
Carrots (diced).......	½ c.	125	1.9	1.5	..	..	..	..
Corn...............	½ c.	125	2.7	2.2	..	..	..	..
Mushrooms...........	½ c.	120	8.7	7.3	..	..	20.4	17

Food	Portion		Biotin		Choline		Inositol	
	Amt.	Wt. Gm.	Mcg./ portion	Mcg./ 100 Gm.	Mg./ portion	Mg./ 100 Gm.	Mg./ portion	Mg./ 100 Gm.
Vegetables (Continued)								
Peas								
Cow................	½ c.	125	..	..	..	..	..	..
Green..............	½ c.	125	2.6	2.1	..	..	..	..
Spinach..............	½ c.	120	2.8	2.3	..	..	..	..
Tomatoes............	½ c.	120	2.2	1.8	..	..	..	..
Tomato juice..........	½ c.	120	..	..	..	..	..	..
Miscellaneous								
Chocolate......	1 oz.	28.4	9.0	32.0	..	..	24.1	85
Molasses..............	1 tbsp.	20	1.8	9.0	17.2	86	30.0	150
Yeast, brewer's..........	1 tbsp.	8	16.0	200.0	19.2	240	..	..
Food yeast, torula........	1 tbsp.	8	8.0	100.0	20.0	250	21.6	270
Honey.................	1 tbsp.	20	..	..	..	..	..	..

Dots indicate that no representative value was found in the literature for particular constituent.

Raw values, except where indicated.

† Cooked values.

Supplementary References

Bunnell, R. H., et al.: "Alpha-tocopherol content of foods." Am. J. Clin. Nutr., 17:1, 1965.

Dicks-Bushnell, M. W., and Davis, K. C.: "Vitamin E content of infant formulas and cereals." Am. J. Clin. Nutr., 20:262, 1967.

Polansky, M. M., and Murphy, E. W.: "Vitamin B₆ components in fruits and nuts." J. Am. Dietet. A., 48:109, 1966.

Roels, O. A.: "Present knowledge of vitamin E." Nutr. Rev., 25:33, 1967.

The Everything Chart

CONTENTS

KEY:

— Means believed present in measurable amounts but un-
measured.

Iodine—locale of food source given where available because amount of iodine varies with local soil conditions.

NA—Data not available.

Food and Amount	Calories	Carbo-hydrate gm.	Protein gm.	Sat. Fatty Acids gm.	Unsat. Fatty Acids gm.	Vitamin A IU	Thiamin B₁ mg.
Ale—1 large glass, 8 fl. oz., 230 gm.	98	8	1.1	---	---	0	trace
Beer—1 large glass, 8 fl. oz., 240 gm.	114	10.6	1.4	---	---	0	trace
Champagne—1 wine glass, 4 fl. oz., 120 gm.	84	3	.2	NA	NA	NA	NA
Cocktail, Bloody Mary—1 cocktail, 3½ fl. oz., 100 gm.	130	5.7	NA	NA	NA	NA	NA
Cocktail, Daiquiri—1 cocktail glass, 3½ fl. oz., 100 gm.	122	5.2	.1	NA	NA	0	.014
Cocktail, Manhattan—1 cocktail, 3½ fl. oz., 100 gm.	164	7.9	trace	NA	NA	35	.003
Cocktail, Martini—1 cocktail, 3½ fl. oz., 100 gm.	140	.3	.1	NA	NA	4	trace
Cocktail, Old Fashioned—1 glass, 4 fl. oz., 100 gm.	179	3.5	NA	NA	NA	NA	NA
Cocktail, Tom Collins—1 tall glass, 10 fl. oz., 300 gm.	180	9	.3	NA	NA	0	.03
Cocktail, Whiskey Sour—1 cocktail, 3½ fl. oz., 100 gm.	175	17	NA	NA	NA	NA	NA
Cognac—1 brandy pony, 30 gm.	73	NA	NA	NA	NA	NA	NA
Distilled liquors,* unflavored, 80 proof —1 jigger, 42 gm.	100	trace	---	---	---	---	---
Distilled liquors,* unflavored, 86 proof —1 jigger, 42 gm.	105	trace	---	---	---	---	---
Distilled liquors,* unflavored, 90 proof —1 jigger, 42 gm.	110	trace	---	---	---	---	---
Distilled liquors,* unflavored, 94 proof —1 jigger, 42 gm.	115	trace	---	---	---	---	---
Distilled liquors,* unflavored, 100 proof —1 jigger, 42 gm.	125	trace	---	---	---	---	---
Liqueur, Anisette—1 cordial glass, 20 gm.	74	7	NA	NA	NA	NA	NA
Liqueur, Benedictine—1 cordial glass, 20 gm.	69	6.6	NA	NA	NA	NA	NA
Liqueur, Creme de Menthe—1 cordial glass, 20 gm.	67	6	NA	NA	NA	NA	NA
Red wine, sweet—1 glass, 3½ fl. oz., 100 gm.	88	6.3	NA	NA	NA	NA	NA
Red wine, dry—1 glass, 3½ fl. oz., 100 gm.	81	4.3	NA	NA	NA	NA	NA
Sherry, cream—1 glass, 3½ fl. oz., 100 gm.	148	8.4	NA	NA	NA	NA	NA
Sherry, dry—1 glass, 3½ fl. oz., 100 gm.	120	4.5	NA	NA	NA	NA	NA
Vermouth, dry—1 wine glass, 3½ fl. oz., 100 gm.	105	1	NA	NA	NA	NA	NA
Vermouth, sweet—1 wine glass, 3½ fl. oz., 100 gm.	167	12	NA	NA	NA	NA	NA
White wine, sweet—1 glass, 3½ fl. oz., 100 gm.	64	6.1	NA	NA	NA	NA	NA
White wine, dry—1 glass, 3½ fl. oz., 100 gm.	74	2.1	NA	NA	NA	NA	NA
Wines, dessert—1 wine glass, 3½ fl. oz., 103 gm.	140	8	trace	---	---	---	.01
Wines, table—1 wine glass, 3½ fl. oz., 102 gm.	85	4	trace	---	---	---	trace

*Includes bourbon, brandy, Canadian whiskey, gin, Irish whiskey, rum, rye whiskey, Scotch whiskey, tequila, and vodka.

Ribo-flavin B₂ mg.	Niacin mg.	B₆ mg.	Folic Acid mg.	PABA mg.	Panto-thenic Acid mg.	B₁₂ mcg.	Vitamin C mg.	Vitamin D IU	Vitamin E IU	Calcium mg.	Iodine mg.
.069	.5	NA	NA	NA	NA	0	0	0	0	30	NA
.072	.5	.0144	NA	NA	.0192	0	0	0	0	10	NA
NA	NA	NA	NA	NA	NA	0	NA	NA	NA	NA	NA
NA	NA	NA	NA	NA	NA	NA	NA	NA	NA	NA	NA
.001	trace	NA	NA	NA	NA	0	8	0	0	4	NA
.002	trace	NA	NA	NA	NA	0	0	NA	0	1	NA
trace	trace	NA	NA	NA	NA	0	0	NA	0	5	NA
NA	NA	NA	NA	NA	NA	NA	NA	NA	NA	NA	NA
trace	trace	NA	NA	NA	NA	0	21	0	0	6	NA
NA	NA	NA	NA	NA	NA	NA	NA	NA	NA	NA	NA
NA	NA	NA	NA	NA	NA	NA	NA	NA	NA	NA	NA
...	...	NA	NA	NA	NA	0	...	NA	0	...	NA
...	...	NA	NA	NA	NA	0	...	NA	0	...	NA
...	...	NA	NA	NA	NA	0	...	NA	0	...	NA
...	...	NA	NA	NA	NA	0	...	NA	0	...	NA
...	...	NA	NA	NA	NA	0	...	NA	0	...	NA
NA	NA	NA	NA	NA	NA	0	NA	NA	0	NA	NA
NA	NA	NA	NA	NA	NA	0	NA	NA	0	NA	NA
NA	NA	NA	NA	NA	NA	0	NA	NA	0	NA	NA
NA	NA	NA	NA	NA	NA	NA	NA	NA	NA	NA	NA
NA	NA	NA	NA	NA	NA	NA	NA	NA	NA	NA	NA
NA	NA	NA	NA	NA	NA	NA	NA	NA	NA	NA	NA
NA	NA	NA	NA	NA	NA	NA	NA	NA	NA	NA	NA
NA	NA	NA	NA	NA	NA	0	NA	NA	0	NA	NA
NA	NA	NA	NA	NA	NA	0	NA	NA	0	NA	NA
NA	NA	NA	NA	NA	NA	NA	NA	NA	NA	NA	NA
NA	NA	NA	NA	NA	NA	NA	NA	NA	NA	NA	NA
.02	.2	NA	NA	NA	NA	0	...	NA	0	8	NA
.01	.1	.00408	NA	NA	.00306	0	...	NA	0	9	NA

Food and Amount	Iron mg.	Magnesium mg.	Phosphorus mg.	Potassium mg.	Sodium mg.
Ale—1 large glass, 8 fl. oz., 230 gm.	.2	NA	41	NA	NA
Beer—1 large glass, 8 fl. oz., 240 gm.	0	NA	62	46	8
Champagne—1 wine glass, 4 fl. oz., 120 gm.	NA	NA	NA	NA	NA
Cocktail, Bloody Mary—1 cocktail, 3½ fl. oz., 100 gm.	NA	NA	NA	NA	NA
Cocktail, Daiquiri—1 cocktail glass, 3½ fl. oz., 100 gm.	.1	NA	3	NA	NA
Cocktail, Manhattan—1 cocktail, 3½ fl. oz., 100 gm.	trace	NA	1	NA	NA
Cocktail, Martini—1 cocktail, 3½ fl. oz., 100 gm.	.1	NA	1	NA	NA
Cocktail, Old Fashioned—1 glass, 4 fl. oz., 100 gm.	NA	NA	NA	NA	NA
Cocktail, Tom Collins—1 tall glass, 10 fl. oz., 300 gm.	trace	NA	6	NA	NA
Cocktail, Whiskey Sour—1 cocktail, 3½ fl. oz., 100 gm.	NA	NA	NA	NA	NA
Cognac—1 brandy pony, 30 gm.	NA	NA	NA	NA	NA
Distilled liquors,* unflavored, 80 proof —1 jigger, 42 gm.	---	NA	---	.84	.42
Distilled liquors,* unflavored, 86 proof —1 jigger, 42 gm.	---	NA	---	.84	.42
Distilled liquors,* unflavored, 90 proof —1 jigger, 42 gm.	---	NA	---	.84	.42
Distilled liquors,* unflavored, 94 proof —1 jigger, 42 gm.	---	NA	---	.84	.42
Distilled liquors,* unflavored, 100 proof —1 jigger, 42 gm.	---	NA	---	.84	.42
Liqueur, Anisette—1 cordial glass, 20 gm.	NA	NA	NA	NA	NA
Liqueur, Benedictine—1 cordial glass, 20 gm.	NA	NA	NA	NA	NA
Liqueur, Creme de Menthe—1 cordial glass, 20 gm.	NA	NA	NA	NA	NA
Red wine, sweet—1 glass, 3½ fl. oz., 100 gm.	NA	NA	NA	NA	NA
Red wine, dry—1 glass, 3½ fl. oz., 100 gm.	NA	NA	NA	NA	NA
Sherry, cream—1 glass, 3½ fl. oz., 100 gm.	NA	NA	NA	NA	NA
Sherry, dry—1 glass, 3½ fl. oz., 100 gm.	NA	NA	NA	NA	NA
Vermouth, dry—1 wine glass, 3½ fl. oz., 100 gm.	NA	10	NA	NA	NA
Vermouth, sweet—1 wine glass, 3½ fl. oz., 100 gm.	NA	10	NA	NA	NA
White wine, sweet—1 glass, 3½ fl. oz., 100 gm.	NA	NA	NA	NA	NA
White wine, dry—1 glass, 3½ fl. oz., 100 gm.	NA	NA	NA	NA	NA
Wines, dessert—1 wine glass, 3½ fl. oz., 103 gm.	---	NA	---	77	4.12
Wines, table—1 wine glass, 3½ fl. oz., 102 gm.	.4	NA	10.2	93.8	5.1

* Includes bourbon, brandy, Canadian whiskey, gin, Irish whiskey, rum, rye whiskey, Scotch whiskey, tequila, and vodka.

Food and Amount	Calories	Carbohydrate gm.	Protein gm.	Sat. Fatty Acids gm.	Unsat. Fatty Acids gm.	Vitamin A IU	Thiamin B₁ mg.
Butter—see Fats and Oils							
Buttermilk, fluid, made from skim milk —1 cup, 245 gm.	90	12	9	...	...	10	.10
Cheese, Bleu or Roquefort—1 cubic inch, 17 gm.	65	trace	4	3	2	210	.01
Cheese, Brick—1 cubic inch, 18 gm.	66.6	.34	3.99	NA	NA	223.2	...
Cheese, Camembert (domestic)— 1 wedge, 3 wedges per 4 oz. package, 38 gm.	115	1	7	5	3	380	.02
Cheese, Cheddar (domestic)—1 cubic inch, 17 gm.	70	trace	4	3	2	230	.01
Cheese, Cottage, large or small curd, creamed—1 scoop, 65 gm.	69	1.88	8.84	1.3	.65	110	.01
Cheese, Cottage, large or small curd, uncreamed—1 scoop, 58 gm.	50	1.56	9.86	NA	NA	5	.01
Cheese, Cream—1 cubic inch, 16 gm.	60	trace	1	3	2	250	trace
Cheese, Limburger—1 cubic inch, 16 gm.	55.2	.35	3.39	NA	NA	182.4	.01
Cheese, Parmesan—1 tbsp., 5 gm.	25	trace	2	1.3	trace	60	trace
Cheese, Swiss (domestic)—1 slice, ⅛"x 3" sq., 25 gm.	68	trace	5	2.6	1.3	205	trace
Cheese, Pasteurized process, American, 1 slice, ⅛"x 3" sq., 20 gm.	67	trace	4.1	3.1	2	221	trace
Cheese, Pasteurized process, Pimento (American)—1 cubic inch, 18 gm.	66	.32	4	NA	NA	...	...
Cheese, Pasteurized process, Swiss— 1 cubic inch, 18 gm.	65	trace	5	3	2	200	trace
Cheese, Pasteurized process cheese food, American—1 cubic inch, 18 gm.	60	1	4	2	1	170	trace
Cheese, Pasteurized process cheese food spread, American—1 tbsp., 8 gm.	23	.65	1	1.44	.009	69	trace
Cheese fondue, from home recipe— 1 tbsp., 16 gm.	42.4	1.6	2.36	...	...	140.8	.009
Cheese soufflé, from home recipe— 1 cup, 190 gm.	414.2	11.78	18.81	...	...	1520	.09
Cheese straws—1 piece, 2"x ½", 12 gm.	54.36	4.14	1.34	...	...	46.8	.002
Cottage Cheese, 1 tbsp. (level)—22 gm.	21	.621	2.95	.42	.22	36.6	.003
Cream Cheese—1 oz., 28 gm.	104.72	.588	16.8	5.4	3.8	431.2	.0056
Cream, sour—1 tbsp., 15 gm.	30.3	.625	.4375	1.625	1.06	120.625	.00437
Cream, fluid, half and half—1 tbsp., 15 gm.	20	1	1	1	1	70	trace
Cream, fluid, light, coffee or table— 1 tbsp., 15 gm.	30	1	1	2	1	130	trace
Cream, fluid, light whipping (volume doubled when whipped)—1 cup, 239 gm.	715	9	6	41	27	3,060	.05
Cream, fluid, heavy whipping (volume doubled when whipped)—1 cup, 238 gm.	840	7	5	50	33	3,670	.05
Cream, sour—1 cup, 230 gm.	485	10	7	26	17	1,930	.07
Cream, whipped topping (pressurized) —1 tbsp., 3 gm.	10	trace	trace	trace	trace	30	...

Food and Amount	Ribo-flavin B₂ mg.	Niacin mg.	B₆ mg.	Folic Acid mg.	PABA mg.	Panto-thenic Acid mg.	B₁₂ mcg.
Butter—see Fats and Oils							
Buttermilk, fluid, made from skim milk —1 cup, 245 gm.	.44	2	.0882	.02695	NA	.75215	.53
Cheese, Bleu or Roquefort—1 cubic inch, 17 gm.	.11	.2	NA	NA	NA	NA	NA
Cheese, Brick—1 cubic inch, 18 gm.	.08	.01	NA	NA	NA	NA	NA
Cheese, Camembert (domestic)— 1 wedge, 3 wedges per 4 oz. package, 38 gm.	.29	.3	NA	NA	NA	NA	NA
Cheese, Cheddar (domestic)—1 cubic inch, 17 gm.	.08	trace	.0136	.00272	NA	.085	.17
Cheese, Cottage, large or small curd, creamed—1 scoop, 65 gm.	.16	.06	.026	.02015	NA	.143	.65
Cheese, Cottage, large or small curd, uncreamed—1 scoop, 58 gm.	.16	.05	---	---	NA	---	---
Cheese, Cream—1 cubic inch, 16 gm.	.04	trace	.0088	NA	NA	.0432	.03
Cheese, Limburger—1 cubic inch, 16 gm.	.08	.03	NA	NA	NA	NA	NA
Cheese, Parmesan—1 tbsp., 5 gm.	.04	trace	.0048	NA	NA	.0265	---
Cheese, Swiss (domestic)—1 slice, ⅛″ x 3″ sq., 25 gm.	.08	trace	.00113	NA	NA	.056	.31
Cheese, Pasteurized process, American, 1 slice, ⅛″ x 3″ sq., 20 gm.	.078	trace	.01446	.00198	NA	.0724	.147
Cheese, Pasteurized process, Pimento (American)—1 cubic inch, 18 gm.	---	---	---	---	NA	---	---
Cheese, Pasteurized process, Swiss— 1 cubic inch, 18 gm.	.07	trace	NA	NA	NA	NA	---
Cheese, Pasteurized process cheese food, American—1 cubic inch, 18 gm.	.10	trace	---	---	NA	---	---
Cheese, Pasteurized process cheese food spread, American—1 tbsp., 8 gm.	.04	trace	---	---	NA	---	---
Cheese fondue, from home recipe— 1 tbsp., 16 gm.	.05	.03	NA	NA	NA	NA	NA
Cheese soufflé, from home recipe— 1 cup, 190 gm.	.45	.38	NA	NA	NA	NA	NA
Cheese straws—1 piece, 2″ x ½″, 12 gm.	.01	.03	NA	NA	NA	NA	NA
Cottage Cheese, 1 tbsp. (level)—22 gm.	.051	.02	.008	.00671	NA	.048	.22
Cream Cheese—1 oz., 28 gm.	.0672	.028	.0142	NA	NA	.078	.054
Cream, sour—1 tbsp., 15 gm.	.0218	.00625	NA	NA	NA	NA	NA
Cream, fluid, half and half—1 tbsp., 15 gm.	.02	trace	NA	NA	NA	NA	NA
Cream, fluid, light, coffee or table— 1 tbsp., 15 gm.	.02	trace	.00495	NA	NA	.04815	.03
Cream, fluid, light whipping (volume doubled when whipped)—1 cup, 239 gm.	.29	.1	.06931	NA	NA	---	.47
Cream, fluid, heavy whipping (volume doubled when whipped)—1 cup, 238 gm.	.26	.1	---	NA	NA	---	---
Cream, sour—1 cup, 230 gm.	.35	.1	NA	NA	NA	NA	NA
Cream, whipped topping (pressurized) —1 tbsp., 3 gm.	trace	---	NA	NA	NA	NA	NA

Vitamin C mg.	Vitamin D IU	Vitamin E IU	Calcium mg.	Iodine mg.	Iron mg.	Magnesium mg.	Phosphorus mg.	Potassium mg.	Sodium mg.
2	NA	NA	296	NA	.1	34.3	232	343	318
0	NA	NA	54	NA	.1	NA	57.63	---	---
0	NA	NA	131.4	NA	.16	NA	81.9	---	---
0	NA	NA	40	NA	.2	NA	70	42	---
0	NA	NA	129	NA	.2	7.65	81	14	119
0	NA	NA	61	.00397 Ohio	.2	---	99	55	149
0	NA	NA	52	.00354 Ohio	.2	---	101	41	168
0	NA	NA	10	NA	trace	---	15	12	40
0	NA	NA	94.4	NA	.09	NA	62.88	---	---
0	NA	NA	68	NA	trace	2.4	39	7	36
0	NA	NA	161	NA	.18	---	101	25	136
0	NA	NA	129	NA	.22	---	151	16	219
---	NA	NA	---	NA	---	NA	---	---	---
0	NA	NA	159	NA	.2	NA	156	18	210
0	NA	NA	100	NA	.1	NA	135	---	---
0	NA	NA	45	NA	.04	NA	70	19	130
trace	NA	NA	50.72	NA	.19	NA	47.04	26.4	86.72
trace	NA	NA	381.9	NA	1.9	NA	370.5	229.9	691.6
0	NA	NA	31.08	NA	.07	NA	24.72	7.56	86.52
0	NA	NA	20.3	.00132 Ohio	.066	---	33	18.3	49.6
0	NA	NA	17.36	NA	.056	---	26.6	20.72	70
.125	NA	NA	14.687	---	.006	NA	NA	NA	NA
trace	trace	NA	16	---	trace	---	12	19	7
trace	trace	NA	15	.00086 Ohio	trace	1.65	12	18	6
2	trace	NA	203	---	.1	21.5	160	243	86
2	trace	NA	179	---	.1	19.0	140	211	76
2	NA	NA	235	---	.1	NA	NA	NA	NA
---	NA	NA	3	.00022 Ohio	---	NA	NA	NA	NA

Food and Amount	Calories	Carbo-hydrate gm.	Protein gm.	Sat. Fatty Acids gm.	Unsat. Fatty Acids gm.	Vitamin A IU	Thiamin B₁ mg.
Cream substitute, dried, w/skim milk (calcium reduced) and lactose—1 cup, 94 gm.	477	57	8	14.1	9.4	902	.04
Cream substitute, dried, w/skim milk, lactose, and sodium hexametaphosphate—1 cup, 94 gm.	478	50	13	14.1	9.4	488	.13
Cream, imitation product (w/vegetable fats), powdered creamer—1 teaspoon, 2 gm.	10	1	trace	trace	trace	trace	---
Cream, imitation (w/vegetable fat, frozen) liquid creamer—1 tbsp., 15 gm.	20	2	trace	1	trace	10	0
Cream, imitation (w/vegetable fat). Sour dressing (imitation sour cream)—1 cup, 235 gm.	440	17	9	35	1	10	.07
Cream, imitation (w/vegetable fat, pressurized whipped topping—1 tbsp., 4 gm.	10	trace	trace	1	trace	20	---
Cream, imitation (w/vegetable fat, frozen), whipped topping—1 tbsp., 4 gm.	10	1	trace	1	trace	30	---
Cream, imitation (w/vegetable fat), powdered, whipped topping, w/whole milk—1 tbsp., 4 gm.	10	1	trace	1	trace	20	trace
Eggs, chicken, whole, fresh, raw—1 egg, large, 50 gm.	80	trace	7	2	3	590	.05
Eggs, chicken, whites, fresh, raw—1 white, large, 33 gm.	15	trace	4	---	---	0	trace
Eggs, chicken, yolks, fresh, raw—1 yolk, large, 17 gm.	60	trace	3	2	2	580	.04
Eggs, cooked, fried—1 medium w/1 tsp. margarine, 50 gm.	108	.4	6.2	3	4	710	.05
Eggs, cooked, hard-cooked—1 medium egg, 48 gm.	78	.4	6.2	1.92	2.88	570	.04
Eggs, cooked, omelet—1 large egg, 62 gm.	107	1.5	7.2	2.48	3.72	670	.05
Eggs, cooked, poached—1 medium egg, 48 gm.	78	.4	6.1	1.92	2.88	560	.04
Eggs, cooked, scrambled—1 large egg, 64 gm.	110	1	7	3	3	690	.05
Egg, Guinea 1 egg, 30 gm.	50	---	4.1	NA	NA	NA	NA
Frozen custard—see Ice Cream							
Goat's milk—see Milk, goat							
Ice cream and frozen custard, 10% fat—1 cup, 133 gm.	255	28	6	8	5	590	.05
Ice cream and frozen custard, 12% fat—1 cup, 140 gm.	290	29	5.6	9.8	5.6	728	.05
Ice cream and frozen custard, rich: 16% fat—1 cup, 148 gm.	330	27	4	13	9	980	.03
Ice milk, hardened—1 cup, 131 gm.	200	29	6	4	2	280	.07
Milk, cow, fluid, whole, fresh, 3.7% fat—1 cup, 244 gm.	161	12	8.4	5	3	370	.07
Milk, cow, fluid, fresh, skim—1 cup, 245 gm.	90	12	9	---	---	10	.09
Milk, cow, fluid, fresh, partially skimmed, w/2% nonfat milk solids—1 cup, 246 gm.	145	15	10	3	2	200	.10

Riboflavin B₂ mg.	Niacin mg.	B₆ mg.	Folic Acid mg.	PABA mg.	Pantothenic Acid mg.	B₁₂ mcg.	Vitamin C mg.	Vitamin D IU	Vitamin E IU	Calcium mg.	Iodine mg.
1.09	.09	NA	NA	NA	NA	NA	---	NA	NA	77	NA
.66	.28	NA	NA	NA	NA	NA	---	NA	NA	465	NA
---	---	NA	NA	NA	NA	NA	---	NA	NA	1	NA
0	---	NA	NA	NA	NA	NA	---	NA	NA	2	NA
.38	.2	NA	NA	NA	NA	NA	1	NA	NA	277	NA
0	---	NA	NA	NA	NA	NA	---	NA	NA	trace	NA
0	---	NA	NA	NA	NA	NA	---	NA	NA	trace	NA
trace	trace	NA	NA	NA	NA	NA	trace	NA	NA	3	NA
.15	trace	.055	.0025	.15	.8	1	0	27	1.5	27	.0108 Ohio
.09	trace	.00066	.00033	---	.066	.03	0	0	NA	3	NA
.07	trace	.051	.00221	---	.748	1.02	0	27	---	24	NA
.15	.1	---	---	NA	---	---	0	27	---	30	NA
.13	trace	---	---	NA	---	---	0	23	---	26	NA
.17	.1	---	---	NA	---	---	0	31	---	50	NA
.12	trace	---	---	NA	---	---	0	27	---	26	NA
.18	trace	---	---	NA	---	---	0	31	---	51	NA
NA	NA	NA	NA	NA	NA	NA	NA	NA	NA	NA	NA
.28	.1	---	NA	NA	---	---	1	NA	---	194	NA
.26	.1	---	NA	NA	.6888	---	1	NA	.08	172	NA
.16	.1	---	NA	NA	---	---	1	NA	---	115	NA
.29	.1	NA	NA	NA	NA	NA	1	NA	NA	204	NA
.42	.2	.0976	.00244	1.68	.8296	.97	10	100 added	.09	285	.00805 Ohio
.44	.2	.1029	trace	.011	.9065	.98	2	100 added	NA	296	---
.52	.2	---	---	---	---	---	2	100 added	NA	352	---

Food and Amount	Iron mg.	Magnesium mg.	Phosphorus mg.	Potassium mg.	Sodium mg.
Cream substitute, dried, w/skim milk (calcium reduced) and lactose—1 cup, 94 gm.	.18	•••	•••	•••	540
Cream substitute, dried, w/skim milk, lactose, and sodium hexametaphosphate—1 cup, 94 gm.	.28	•••	•••	•••	•••
Cream, imitation product (w/vegetable fats),powdered creamer—1 teaspoon, 2 gm.	trace	NA	NA	NA	NA
Cream, imitation (w/vegetable fat, frozen) liquid creamer—1 tbsp., 15 gm.	•••	NA	NA	NA	NA
Cream, imitation (w/vegetable fat), Sour dressing (imitation sour cream)—1 cup, 235 gm.	.1	NA	NA	NA	NA
Cream, imitation (w/vegetable fat), pressurized whipped topping—1 tbsp., 4 gm.	•••	NA	NA	NA	NA
Cream, imitation (w/vegetable fat, frozen), whipped topping—1 tbsp., 4 gm.	•••	NA	NA	NA	NA
Cream, imitation (w/vegetable fat), powdered, whipped topping, w/whole milk—1 tbsp., 4 gm.	trace	NA	NA	NA	NA
Eggs, chicken, whole, fresh, raw—1 egg, large, 50 gm.	1.1	5.5	102	64	61
Eggs, chicken, whites, fresh, raw—1 white, large, 33 gm.	trace	2.97	5	45	48
Eggs, chicken, yolks, fresh, raw—1 yolk, large, 17 gm.	.9	2.72	97	16	9
Eggs, cooked, fried—1 medium w/1 tsp. margarine, 50 gm.	1.2	5	111	70	169
Eggs, cooked, hard-cooked—1 medium egg, 48 gm.	1.1	5	98	62	59
Eggs, cooked, omelet—1 large egg, 62 gm.	1	7	117	91	160
Eggs, cooked, poached—1 medium egg, 48 gm.	1.1	5	98	62	130
Eggs, cooked, scrambled—1 large egg, 64 gm.	1.1	7	123	95	167
Egg, Guinea—1 egg, 30 gm.	NA	NA	NA	NA	NA
Frozen custard—see Ice Cream					
Goat's milk—see Milk, goat					
Ice cream and frozen custard, 10% fat—1 cup, 133 gm.	.1	•••	153	240	83
Ice cream and frozen custard, 12% fat—1 cup, 140 gm.	.14	19.6	138	157	56
Ice cream and frozen custard, rich: 16% fat—1 cup, 148 gm.	trace	•••	90	140	49
Ice milk, hardened—1 cup, 131 gm.	.1	•••	162	255	89
Milk, cow, fluid, whole, fresh, 3.7% fat—1 cup, 244 gm.	trace	37	224	342	122
Milk, cow, fluid, fresh, skim—1 cup, 245 gm.	.1	34.3	232	355	127
Milk, cow, fluid, fresh, partially skimmed, w/2% nonfat milk solids—1 cup, 246 gm.	.1	•••	275	430	150

Food and Amount	Calories	Carbohydrate gm.	Protein gm.	Sat. Fatty Acids gm.	Unsat. Fatty Acids gm.	Vitamin A IU	Thiamin B₁ mg.
Milk, cow, canned, evaporated, unsweetened—1 cup, 252 gm.	345	24	18	11	8	810	.10
Milk, cow, canned, condensed, sweetened—1 cup, 306 gm.	980	166	25	15	10	1,100	.24
Milk, cow, dry, whole—1 cup, 245 gm. (liquid)†	1,230	93	64	36.75	24.5	2.768	.71
Milk, cow, dry, skim, regular—1 cup, 245 gm; (liquid)	889	128	88	NA	NA	73	.85
Milk, cow, dry, skim, instant—1 cup, 245 gm (liquid)†	879	126	87	NA	NA	73	.85
Milk, malted, beverage (malt and milk)—1 cup, 235 gm.	245	28	11	---	---	590	.14
Milk, chocolate drink, fluid, commercial, made w/whole milk—1 cup, 250 gm.	212	27	8.5	2.5	2.5	325	.07
Milk beverage, homemade, hot chocolate—1 cup, 220 gm.	209	23	7.2	6.6	4.4	308	.06
Milk beverage, homemade, hot cocoa—1 cup, 250 gm.	245	27	10	7	4	400	.10
Milk, buttermilk—see Buttermilk							
Milk, goat, fluid—1 cup, 244 gm.	163	11.2	7.8	4.88	2.44	390	.10
Oleomargarine—see Fats and Oils—Margarine							
Yogurt,** made from partially skimmed milk—1 cup, 245 gm.	125	13	8	2	1	170	.10
Yogurt,** made from whole milk—1 cup, 245 gm.	150	12	7	6	3	340	.07
Yogurt,** from partially skimmed milk—1 tbsp., 15 gm.	7.8	.8	.5	.125	.0625	10.6	.00625
Yogurt,** from whole milk—1 tbsp., 15 gm.	9.375	.75	.4375	.3125	.1875	21.25	.00438
Whey, fluid—1 cup, 225 gm.	58	11.4	2	NA	NA	22	.06
Welsh rarebit—1 cup, 280 gm.	501	17.64	22.68	---	---	1484	.112

*If fortified, amount of vitamin D listed on can.   † Mixed according to package directions.

FATS AND OILS

Food and Amount	Calories	Carbohydrate gm.	Protein gm.	Sat. Fatty Acids gm.	Unsat. Fatty Acids gm.	Vitamin A IU	Thiamin B₁ mg.
Butter, regular—1 stick, ½ cup, 113 gm.	810	1	1	51	33	3,750	---
Butter, regular—1 tbsp., 14 gm.	100	trace	trace	6	4	470	---
Butter, whipped—1 pat, 1¼" sq. x ⅓", 5 gm.	35	trace	trace	2	1	170	---
Butter, whipped—1 stick, ½ cup, 76 gm.	540	trace	1	34	22	2,500	---
Butter, whipped—1 tbsp., 9 gm.	65	trace	trace	4	3	310	---
Butter, whipped—1 pat, 1¼" sq. x ⅓", 4 gm.	25	trace	trace	2	1	130	---
Cooking oil—see Oils							

Food and Amount	Ribo-flavin B₂ mg.	Niacin mg.	B₆ mg.	Folic Acid mg.	PABA mg.	Panto-thenic Acid mg.	B₁₂ mcg.
Milk, cow, canned, evaporated, un-sweetened—1 cup, 252 gm.	.86	.5	.05544	.00176	NA	.83	---
Milk, cow, canned, condensed, sweet-ened—1 cup, 306 gm.	1.16	.6	---	---	NA	---	---
Milk, cow, dry, whole—1 cup, 245 gm. (liquid)†	3.57	1.71	---	---	NA	---	---
Milk, cow, dry, skim, regular—1 cup, 245 gm. (liquid)	4.41	2.2	.08085	.00049	NA	.83	---
Milk, cow, dry, skim, instant—1 cup, 245 gm. (liquid)†	4.36	2.2	---	---	NA	---	---
Milk, malted, beverage (malt and milk)—1 cup, 235 gm.	.49	.2	NA	NA	NA	NA	NA
Milk, chocolate drink, fluid, commercial, made w/whole milk—1 cup, 250 gm.	.40	.25	NA	NA	NA	NA	NA
Milk beverage, homemade, hot choco-late—1 cup, 220 gm.	.35	.2	NA	NA	NA	NA	NA
Milk beverage, homemade, hot cocoa—1 cup, 250 gm.	.45	.5	NA	NA	NA	NA	NA
Milk, buttermilk—see Buttermilk							
Milk, goat, fluid—1 cup, 244 gm.	.27	.7	.1098	NA	NA	.7808	.19
Oleomargarine—see Fats and Oils—Margarine							
Yogurt,** made from partially skimmed milk—1 cup, 245 gm.	.44	.2	.1127	NA	NA	.76685	.26
Yogurt,** made from whole milk—1 cup, 245 gm.	.39	.2	---	NA	NA	---	---
Yogurt,** from partially skimmed milk—1 tbsp., 15 gm.	.0275	.0125	.007	NA	NA	.0479	.016
Yogurt,** from whole milk—1 tbsp., 15 gm.	.02438	.0125	---	NA	NA	---	---
Whey, fluid—1 cup, 225 gm.	.31	.2	NA	NA	NA	NA	NA
Welsh rarebit—1 cup, 280 gm.	.644	.28	NA	NA	NA	NA	NA

* If fortified, amount of vitamin D listed on can.
** Yogurt—see also page 372.
† Mixed according to package directions.

FATS AND OILS

Food and Amount	Ribo-flavin B₂ mg.	Niacin mg.	B₆ mg.	Folic Acid mg.	PABA mg.	Panto-thenic Acid mg.	B₁₂ mcg.
Butter, regular—1 stick, ½ cup, 113 gm.	---	---	.00339	---	NA	---	trace
Butter, regular—1 tbsp., 14 gm.	---	---	.00042	---	NA	---	trace
Butter, whipped—1 pat, 1¼" sq. x ½", 5 gm.	---	---	.00015	---	NA	---	trace
Butter, whipped—1 stick, ½ cup, 76 gm.	---	---	.00228	---	NA	---	trace
Butter, whipped—1 tbsp., 9 gm.	---	---	.00027	---	NA	---	trace
Butter, whipped—1 pat, 1¼" sq. x ⅓", 4 gm.	---	---	.00012	---	NA	---	trace
Cooking oil—see Oils							

* Values for unsalted butter and margarine.

Vitamin C mg.	Vitamin D IU	Vitamin E IU	Calcium mg.	Iodine mg.	Iron mg.	Magnesium mg.	Phosphorus mg.	Potassium mg.	Sodium mg.
3	7.56	NA	635	NA	.3	63	516	763	297
3	NA*	NA	802	NA	.3	76.5	630	960	342
14	NA*	NA	2,227	.01641 Md.	1.2	240	1,734	3,258	992
17	NA*	NA	3,204	.02230 Md.	1.4	350	2,489	4,275	1,303
17	NA*	NA	3,168	---	1.4	348	2,462	4,226	1,288
2	NA	NA	317	.01974 Ohio	.7	---	286	470	214
2	NA	NA	277	NA	.5	NA	235	365	117
2	NA	NA	229	NA	.4	NA	206	125	105
3	NA	NA	295	NA	1	NA	282	362	127
2	NA	NA	'315	NA	.2	41	259	439	83
2	NA	NA	294	NA	.1	---	230	350	125
2	NA	NA	272	NA	.1	---	213	323	115
.125	NA	NA	18.38	NA	.00625	---	14.375	21.875	7.8
.125	NA	NA	17	NA	.00625	---	13.3	20.1875	7.1875
---	NA	NA	114	NA	NA	NA	.119	---	---
trace	NA	NA	702.8	NA	.84	NA	520.8	386.4	929.6

FATS AND OILS

Vitamin C mg.	Vitamin D IU	Vitamin E IU	Calcium mg.	Iodine mg.	Iron mg.	Magnesium mg.	Phosphorus mg.	Potassium mg.	Sodium mg.
0	90.4	1.13	23	.01661 Ohio	0	2	18.08	26	11*
0	11.2	.14	3	.00206 Ohio	0	.25	2.24	3.22	1.32*
0	4	.05	1	.00074 Ohio	0	.09	.80	1.15	.49*
0	60.8	.76	15	.01117 Ohio	0	1.52	12.16	17.48	7.6*
0	7.2	.09	2	.00132 Ohio	0	.18	1.44	2.07	.9*
0	3.2	.04	1	.00059 Ohio	0	.08	.64	.92	.4*

Food and Amount	Calories	Carbo-hydrate gm.	Protein gm.	Sat. Fatty Acids gm.	Unsat. Fatty Acids gm.	Vitamin A IU	Thiamin B₁ mg.
Corn oil—see Oils							
Cottonseed oil—see Oils							
Fats, cooking, lard—1 cup, 205 gm.	1,850	0	0	78	114	0	0
Fats, cooking, lard—1 tbsp., 13 gm.	115	0	0	5	7	0	0
Fats, cooking, vegetable fats—1 cup, 200 gm.	1,770	0	0	50	144	---	0
Fats, cooking, vegetable fats—1 tbsp., 13 gm.	110	0	0	3	9	---	0
Lecithin—granular, 1 tbsp., 7.5 gm.	68	0		.75	4.5	(also Choline, 250 mg.,	
Lecithin—liquid, 1 tbsp., 16 gm.	25	0		---	6.2	(also Choline, 64 mg.,	
Margarine, regular—1 stick, ½ cup, 113 gm.	815	1	1	17	71	3,750	---
Margarine, regular—1 tbsp., 14 gm.	100	trace	trace	2	9	470	---
Margarine, regular—1 pat, 1″ sq. x ⅓″, 5 gm.	35	trace	trace	1	3	170	---
Margarine, whipped—1 pat, 1″ sq. x ⅓″, 1.1 gm.	7.2	trace	.013	.113	.64	33.33	---
Margarine, whipped—1 stick, ½ cup, 76 gm.	545	trace	1	11	48	2,500	---
Margarine, whipped, soft—1 tub† (2 tubs equal 1 lb.), 227 gm.	1,635	1	1	34	136	7,500	---
Margarine, whipped, soft—1 tbsp., 14 gm.	100	trace	trace	2	8	470	---
Mayonnaise—see Salad dressing							
Oils, cooking and salad, Corn—1 cup, 220 gm.	1,945	0	0	22	179	---	0
Oils, cooking and salad, Corn—1 tbsp., 14 gm.	125	0	0	1	11	---	0
Oils, cooking and salad, Cottonseed—1 cup, 220 gm.	1,945	0	0	55	156	---	0
Oils, cooking and salad, Cottonseed—1 tbsp., 14 gm.	125	0	0	4	10	---	0
Oils, cooking and salad, Olive—1 cup, 220 gm.	1,945	0	0	24	182	---	0
Oils, cooking and salad, Olive—1 tbsp., 14 gm.	125	0	0	2	12	---	0
Oils, cooking and salad, Palm—1 tbsp., 14 gm.	124	0	0	11.9	2.1	NA	0
Oils, cooking and salad, Peanut—1 cup, 220 gm.	1,945	0	0	40	167	---	0
Oils, cooking and salad, Peanut—1 tbsp., 14 gm.	125	0	0	3	11	---	0
Oils, cooking and salad, Safflower—1 cup, 220 gm.	1,945	0	0	18	202	---	0
Oils, cooking and salad, Safflower—1 tbsp., 14 gm.	125	0	0	1	12	---	0
Oils, cooking and salad, Soybean—1 cup, 220 gm.	1,945	0	0	33	158	---	0
Oils, cooking and salad, Soybean—1 tbsp., 14 gm.	125	0	0	1	12	---	0
Oils, cooking and salad, Sunflower—1 cup, 220 gm.	1,945	0	0	26.4	193.6	---	0

† 1 tub equals 1 cup.

Riboflavin B₂ mg.	Niacin mg.	B₆ mg.	Folic Acid mg.	PABA mg.	Pantothenic Acid mg.	B₁₂ mcg.	Vitamin C mg.	Vitamin D IU	Vitamin E IU	Calcium mg.	Iodine mg.
0	0	.041	---	NA	---	0	0	0	0	0	NA
0	0	.0026	---	NA	---	0	0	0	0	0	NA
0	0	NA	NA	NA	NA	0	0	NA	NA	0	NA
0	0	NA	NA	NA	NA	0	0	NA	NA	0	NA
and Inositol, 250 mg.)									10		
and Inositol, 292 mg.)									10		
---	---	NA	---	NA	NA	0	0	---	14.69	23	NA
---	---	NA	---	NA	NA	0	0	---	1.82	3	NA
---	---	NA	---	NA	NA	0	0	---	.65	1	NA
---	---	NA	---	NA	NA	0	0	---	.13	.2	NA
---	---	NA	---	NA	NA	0	0	---	9.88	15	NA
---'	---	NA	---	NA	NA	0	0	---	29.51	45	NA
---	---	NA	---	NA	NA	0	0	---	1.82	3	NA
0	0	NA	---	NA	NA	0	0	0	79.2	0	NA
0	0	NA	---	NA	NA	0	0	0	5.04	0	NA
0	0	NA	---	NA	NA	0	0	0	133.1	0	NA
0	0	NA	---	NA	NA	0	0	0	8.47	0	NA
0	0	NA	---	NA	NA	0	0	NA	147.4	0	.01452 (dried)
0	0	NA	---	NA	NA	0	0	NA	9.38	0	.00092 (dried)
0	0	NA	---	NA	NA	0	0	NA	15.4	0	NA
0	0	NA	---	NA	NA	0	0	NA	134.2	0	NA
0	0	NA	---	NA	NA	0	0	NA	8.54	0	NA
0	0	NA	---	NA	NA	0	0	NA	198	0	NA
0	0	NA	---	NA	NA	0	0	NA	12.6	0	NA
0	0	NA	---	NA	NA	0	0	NA	46.2	0	NA
0	0	NA	---	NA	NA	0	0	NA	2.94	0	NA
0	0	NA	NA	NA	NA	0	0	NA	NA	0	NA

Food and Amount	Iron mg.	Mag-nesium mg.	Phos-phorus mg.	Potas-sium mg.	Sodium mg.
Corn oil—see Oils					
Cottonseed oil—see Oils					
Fats, cooking, lard—1 cup, 205 gm.	0	0	0	0	0
Fats, cooking, lard—1 tbsp., 13 gm.	0	0	0	0	0
Fats, cooking, vegetable fats—1 cup, 200 gm.	0	0	0	0	0
Fats, cooking, vegetable fats—1 tbsp., 13 gm.	0	0	0	0	0
Lecithin—granular, 1 tbsp., 7.5 gm.			225		
Lecithin—liquid, 1 tbsp., 16 gm.			267		
Margarine, regular—1 stick, ½ cup, 113 gm.	0	16.94	18.08	25.99	11*
Margarine, regular—1 tbsp., 14 gm.	0	2	2.24	3.22	1.32*
Margarine, regular—1 pat, 1″ sq. x ⅓″, 5 gm.	0	.65	.80	1.15	.49*
Margarine, whipped—1 pat, 1″ sq. x ⅓″, 1.1 gm.	0	.1447	.162	.233	.11*
Margarine, whipped—1 stick, ½ cup, 76 gm.	0	10.8528	12.16	17.48	7.6*
Margarine, whipped, soft—1 tub† (2 tubs equal 1 lb.), 227 gm.	0	32.4156	36.32	52.21	22.7*
Margarine, whipped, soft—1 tbsp., 14 gm.	0	2	2.24	3.22	1.32*
Mayonnaise—see Salad dressing					
Oils, cooking and salad, Corn—1 cup, 220 gm.	0	NA	NA	.22	.44
Oils, cooking and salad, Corn—1 tbsp., 14 gm.	0	NA	NA	.01	.02
Oils, cooking and salad, Cottonseed—1 cup, 220 gm.	0	NA	NA	NA	NA
Oils, cooking and salad, Cottonseed—1 tbsp., 14 gm.	0	NA	NA	NA	NA
Oils, cooking and salad, Olive—1 cup, 220 gm.	0	NA	NA	.44	.44
Oils, cooking and salad, Olive—1 tbsp., 14 gm.	0	NA	NA	.02	.02
Oils, cooking and salad, Palm—1 tbsp., 14 gm.	0	NA	NA	NA	NA
Oils, cooking and salad, Peanut—1 cup, 220 gm.	0	NA	NA	.22	.44
Oils, cooking and salad, Peanut—1 tbsp., 14 gm.	0	NA	NA	.01	.02
Oils, cooking and salad, Safflower—1 cup, 220 gm.	0	NA	NA	NA	NA
Oils, cooking and salad, Safflower—1 tbsp., 14 gm.	0	NA	NA	NA	NA
Oils, cooking and salad, Soybean—1 cup, 220 gm.	0	NA	NA	NA	NA
Oils, cooking and salad, Soybean—1 tbsp., 14 gm.	0	NA	NA	NA	NA
Oils, cooking and salad, Sunflower—1 cup, 220 gm.	0	NA	NA	NA	NA

† 1 tub equals 1 cup.

Food and Amount	Calories	Carbo-hydrate gm.	Protein gm.	Sat. Fatty Acids gm.	Unsat. Fatty Acids gm.	Vitamin A IU	Thiamin B₁ mg.
Oils, cooking and salad, Sunflower— 1 tbsp., 14 gm.	125	0	0	1.68	12.32	---	0
Oils, Wheat germ—1 tbsp., 14 gm.	124	0	0	NA	NA	---	0
Salad dressing, Bleu or Roquefort cheese, regular commercial— 1 tbsp., 14 gm.	71	1	.7	2	6	29	.0014
Shortening, vegetable—1 tbsp., 14 gm.	123	NA	NA	5.62	7.62	0	0
Salad dressing, French, regular commercial—1 tbsp., 14 gm.	57	2.4	.08	1	4	---	---
Salad dressing, Italian, regular commercial—1 tbsp., 14 gm.	77	1	.03	1.4	6.16	trace	trace
Salad dressing, Mayonnaise—1 tbsp., 14 gm.	101	.3	.15	2	8	39	.003
Salad dressing, Mayonnaise type, regular commercial—1 tbsp., 14 gm.	61	2	.14	1	4	31	.001
Salad dressing, Russian regular commercial—1 tbsp., 14 gm.	69	1.45	.22	1.26	5.18	96	.007
Salad dressing, Thousand Island, regular commercial—1 tbsp., 14 gm.	70	2.2	.11	1	6	45	.003
Salad dressing, French, home recipe— 1 tbsp., 14 gm.	88	.5	.04	.98	7.98	---	---
Salad dressing, Cooked, home recipe— 1 tbsp., 14 gm.	23	2.1	.62	1	1	69	.007

FISH, SHELLFISH, SEAFOOD, ETC.

Food and Amount	Calories	Carbo-hydrate gm.	Protein gm.	Sat. Fatty Acids gm.	Unsat. Fatty Acids gm.	Vitamin A IU	Thiamin B₁ mg.
Abalone, canned—1 cup, 130 gm.	104	3	20.8	NA	NA	---	.15
Albacore, raw—1 piece, 2″ x 2″ x ¼″, 68 gm.	120.36	0	17.2	2.04	.68	---	---
Anchovy, pickled, lightly salted, canned—1 fillet, 4 gm.	7	.01	.76	NA	NA	---	---
Anchovy paste—1 teaspoon, 7 gm.	14	.3	1.4	NA	NA	---	---
Bass, black sea, raw—3¼″ x 4″ x ¾″, 150 gm.	139	0	28.8	NA	NA	---	---
Bass, black sea, baked—1 serving, 3″ x 4″ x ½″, 160 gm.	427	4.4	33.7	NA	NA	141.9	.1
Bass, striped, cooked— 3″ x 3″ x ½″, 110 gm.	215.6	7.37	23.65	NA	NA	---	---
Bluefish, baked or broiled—1 serving, ½ fish (3¼″ x 3½″ x ⅞″), 122 gm.	194	0	32	NA	NA	61	.13
Butterfish, cooked, fried—1 fish, 6¼″ long, 50 gm.	211	0	9.1	NA	NA	---	.027
Carp, raw—1 piece, 3″ x 2¾″ x ½″, 100 gm.	115	0	18	NA	NA	170	.01
Catfish, fresh water, raw—5″ x 3″ x ½″, 242 gm.	249.26	0	42.58	NA	NA	---	.08
Caviar, sturgeon (Beluga), canned, pressed—1 rd. tbsp., 10 gm.	32	.5	3.4	NA	NA	---	---

* Where values for "raw" fish or shellfish are given, no information was available on the cooked foods.

Food and Amount	Riboflavin B_2 mg.	Niacin mg.	B_6 mg.	Folic Acid mg.	PABA mg.	Pantothenic Acid mg.	B_{12} mcg.
Oils, cooking and salad, Sunflower—1 tbsp., 14 gm.	0	0	NA	NA	NA	NA	0
Oils, Wheat germ—1 tbsp., 14 gm.	0	0	NA	NA	NA	NA	0
Salad dressing, Bleu or Roquefort cheese, regular commercial—1 tbsp., 14 gm.	.014	.91	NA	NA	NA	NA	NA
Shortening, vegetable—1 tbsp., 14 gm.	0	0	NA	NA	NA	NA	0
Salad dressing, French, regular commercial—1 tbsp., 14 gm.	---	---	NA	NA	NA	NA	NA
Salad dressing, Italian, regular commercial—1 tbsp., 14 gm.	trace	trace	NA	NA	NA	NA	NA
Salad dressing, Mayonnaise—1 tbsp., 14 gm.	.006	trace	NA	NA	NA	NA	NA
Salad dressing, Mayonnaise type, regular commercial—1 tbsp., 14 gm.	.004	trace	NA	NA	NA	NA	NA
Salad dressing, Russian regular commercial—1 tbsp., 14 gm.	.007	.08	NA	NA	NA	NA	NA
Salad dressing, Thousand Island, regular commercial—1 tbsp., 14 gm.	.004	.03	NA	NA	NA	NA	NA
Salad dressing, French, home recipe—1 tbsp., 14 gm.	---	---	NA	NA	NA	NA	NA
Salad dressing, Cooked, home recipe—1 tbsp., 14 gm.	.022	.03	NA	NA	NA	NA	NA

FISH, SHELLFISH, SEAFOOD, ETC.

Food and Amount	Riboflavin B_2 mg.	Niacin mg.	B_6 mg.	Folic Acid mg.	PABA mg.	Pantothenic Acid mg.	B_{12} mcg.
Abalone, canned—1 cup, 130 gm.	---	---	NA	NA	NA	NA	NA
Albacore, raw—1 piece, 2″ x 2″ x ¼″, 68 gm.	---	---	NA	NA	NA	NA	NA
Anchovy, pickled, lightly salted, canned—1 fillet, 4 gm.	---	---	NA	NA	NA	NA	NA
Anchovy paste—1 teaspoon, 7 gm.	---	---	NA	NA	NA	NA	NA
Bass, black sea, raw—3¼″ x 4″ x ¾″, 150 gm.	---	---	---	NA	NA	.768	---
Bass, black sea, baked—1 serving, 3″ x 4″ x ½″, 160 gm.	.22	5.1	---	NA	NA	---	---
Bass, striped, cooked—3″ x 3″ x ½″, 110 gm.	---	---	NA	NA	NA	NA	NA
Bluefish, baked or broiled—1 serving, ½ fish (3¼″ x 3½″ x ⅞″), 122 gm.	.12	2.3	NA	NA	NA	NA	NA
Butterfish, cooked, fried—1 fish, 6¼″ long, 50 gm.	.032	2	NA	NA	NA	NA	NA
Carp, raw—1 piece, 3″ x 2¾″ x ½″, 100 gm.	.04	1.5	NA	NA	NA	NA	NA
Catfish, fresh water, raw—5″ x 3″ x ½″, 242 gm.	.06	4.1	NA	NA	NA	NA	NA
Caviar, sturgeon (Beluga), canned, pressed—1 rd. tbsp., 10 gm.	---	---	NA	NA	NA	NA	NA

* Where values for "raw" fish or shellfish are given, no information was available on the cooked foods.

Vitamin C mg.	Vitamin D IU	Vitamin E IU	Calcium mg.	Iodine mg.	Iron mg.	Magnesium mg.	Phosphorus mg.	Potassium mg.	Sodium mg.
0	NA	NA	0	NA	0	NA	NA	NA	NA
0	NA	10	0	NA	0	NA	NA	NA	NA
.3	NA	---	11	NA	.03	NA	10	5	153
0	NA	NA	0	NA	0	NA	0	NA	NA
---	NA	---	2	NA	.06	1.4	2	11	192
NA	NA	---	2	NA	.03	NA	1	2	293
NA	NA	3.4	3	.00379 Ohio	.01	.28	4	5	84
---	NA	---	2	NA	.03	NA	4	1	82
.8	NA	---	2	NA	.08	NA	5	22	121
.4	NA	---	2	NA	.08	NA	2	16	98
---	NA	---	1	NA	.01	NA	1	4	92
trace	NA	---	12	NA	.08	NA	13	16	102

FISH, SHELLFISH, SEAFOOD, ETC.

Vitamin C mg.	Vitamin D IU	Vitamin E IU	Calcium mg.	Iodine mg.	Iron mg.	Magnesium mg.	Phosphorus mg.	Potassium mg.	Sodium mg.
---	NA	NA	18	.13689 (fresh) Pacif.	---	NA	166	---	---
3.4	NA	NA	17.68	.03026 Pacif.	---	NA	---	199.24	27.2
---	NA	NA	6.7	NA	---	NA	8.4	---	---
---	NA	NA	---	NA	---	NA	---	---	---
0	---	NA	---	.0267 Wash.	---	---	---	384	102
0	1.4	NA	141.1	---	1.7	---	401.8	383.4	101
---	NA	NA	---	NA	---	NA	---	---	---
---	NA	NA	35	.03172	.85	---	350	---	126
---	NA	NA	10	NA	NA	NA	104	NA	NA
1	NA	NA	50	.0012 Wash.	.9	NA	253	286	50
---	NA	NA	---	.101614 S. Car.	.96	NA	---	498.6	145.2
---	---	NA	---	NA	---	NA	---	18	22

Food and Amount	Calories	Carbohydrate gm.	Protein gm.	Sat. Fatty Acids gm.	Unsat. Fatty Acids gm.	Vitamin A IU	Thiamin B_1 mg.
Caviar, sturgeon (Beluga), granular—1 rd. tbsp., 10 gm.	26	.33	2.7	NA	NA	---	---
Clam Chowder—see Miscellaneous—Soups							
Clam juice (liquid)—½ cup, 125 gm.	23	2.6	2.87	NA	NA	---	---
Clams, raw; hard, soft, and unspecified; meat and liquid—½ cup, 120 gm.	63	3	9.7	NA	NA	---	---
Clams, raw; hard, soft, and unspecified; meat only—½ cup, 110 gm.	83	2.2	13.8	NA	NA	110	.11
Clams, canned, all types, solids and liquid—½ cup, 100 gm.	52	2.8	7.9	NA	NA	---	.01
Clams, canned, all types, drained solids—½ cup, 100 gm.	98	1.9	15.8	NA	NA	---	---
Cod, canned—½ cup, 110 gm.	93.5	0	21.12	NA	NA	---	---
Cod, cooked, broiled—1 piece, 3″ x 4″ x ¾″, 130 gm.	215	0	36	NA	NA	228	.09
Cod dried, salted—2½″ x 2½″ x ⅜″, 56 gm.	72.8	0	16.24	NA	NA	---	---
Codfish cakes—see Fishcakes							
Crab, rock and king (incl. blue, Dungeness), cooked, steamed—½ cup, 85 gm.	79	.42	14	NA	NA	1844	.13
Crab, canned—½ cup flakes, 85 gm.	85	.93	14	NA	NA	---	.06
Crab, deviled—1 tbsp. (rounded), 12 gm.	22.56	1.59	1.36	NA	NA	---	.009
Crab, deviled, 1 shell, approx. 6 tbsp., 72 gm.	135.36	9.54	8.16	NA	NA	---	.054
Crab, softshell, fried—1 piece, 3″ x 2″, 65 gm.	185	8.6	10.7	---	---	---	---
Crappie, white, raw—1 piece, 4″ x 3″ x ½″, 150 gm.	118.5	0	25.2	NA	NA	---	trace
Crayfish, freshwater, and spiny lobster, raw—4″ x 2″ x ½″, 118 gm.	84.96	1.41	17.22	NA	NA	---	.01
Croaker, Atlantic, cooked, baked, 1 serving, 4″ x 3″ x ¾″, 130 gm.	177.3	0	32.4	NA	NA	93.3	.173
Croaker, white, raw—3″ x 3½″ x ¾″, 120 gm.	100.8	0	21.6	NA	NA	---	---
Croaker, yellowfin, raw—3½″ x 3″ x ¾″, 120 gm.	106.8	0	23.04	NA	NA	---	---
Drum, freshwater, raw—3″ x 5″ x 1⅟₁₆″, 200 gm.	242	0	34.6	NA	NA	---	---
Drum, red (redfish), raw—4″ x 2″ x ½″, 60 gm.	48	0	10.8	NA	NA	---	.09
Eel, smoked—1 piece, 2″ sq. x ½″, 50 gm.	165	0	9.3	3	5	---	---
Finnan haddie (smoked haddock)—1 piece, 2½″ x 2½″ x ¼″, 100 gm.	103	0	23.2	NA	NA	---	.06
Fishcakes, cooked, fried—1 cake, 2½″ diam., 44 gm.	75.68	4.09	6.46	NA	NA	---	---
Fishcakes, cooked, frozen, fried, reheated—2″ diam., 44 gm.	118.8	7.56	4.04	NA	NA	---	---
Fish flour, from whole fish—1 cup, 120 gm.	403.2	0	93.6	NA	NA	---	.08

* Where values for "raw" fish or shellfish are given, no information was available on the cooked foods.

Ribo-flavin B₂ mg.	Niacin mg.	B₆ mg.	Folic Acid mg.	PABA mg.	Panto-thenic Acid mg.	B₁₂ mcg.	Vitamin C mg.	Vitamin D IU	Vitamin E IU	Calcium mg.	Iodine mg.
•••	•••	NA	NA	NA	NA	NA	•••	•••	NA	28	NA
•••	•••	NA	NA	NA	NA	NA	•••	NA	NA	•••	•••
•••	•••	•••	•••	NA	•••	•••	•••	NA	NA	•••	.09996 Amer.
.19	1.43	•••	•••	NA	•••	•••	11	NA	NA	76	.09163 Amer.
.11	1.0	.083	.002	NA	.59	•••	•••	NA	NA	55	•••
•••	•••	•••	•••	NA	•••	•••	•••	NA	NA	•••	•••
.08	•••	NA	NA	NA	NA	NA	•••	•••	NA	•••	•••
.13	5.8	NA	NA	NA	NA	NA	•••	65.9	NA	38.6	•••
•••	•••	NA	NA	NA	NA	NA	•••	•••	NA	126	.0672
.06	2.38	•••	•••	NA	•••	•••	1.7	NA	NA	36	.02312 Pacif.
.06	1.61	.255	trace	NA	.51	8.5	•••	NA	NA	38	.0357 Va.
.01	.18	•••	•••	NA	•••	•••	.72	NA	NA	5.64	•••
.06	1.08	•••	•••	NA	•••	•••	4.32	NA	NA	33.84	•••
•••	•••	NA	NA	NA	NA	NA	•••	NA	NA	•••	•••
.04	2.1	NA	NA	NA	NA	NA	•••	NA	NA	•••	NA
.04	2.24	NA	NA	NA	NA	NA	•••	NA	NA	90.86	NA
.13	8.66	NA	NA	NA	NA	NA	•••	NA	NA	•••	NA
•••	•••	NA	NA	NA	NA	NA	•••	NA	NA	•••	NA
•••	•••	NA	NA	NA	NA	NA	•••	NA	NA	•••	NA
•••	•••	NA	NA	NA	NA	NA	•••	NA	NA	•••	NA
.03	2.1	NA	NA	NA	NA	NA	•••	NA	NA	•••	NA
•••	•••	NA	NA	NA	NA	NA	•••	NA	NA	•••	.04 (dry)
.05	2.1	NA	NA	NA	NA	NA	•••	NA	NA	•••	.023 (canned)
•••	•••	NA	NA	NA	NA	NA	•••	NA	NA	•••	.01496 (raw)
•••	•••	NA	NA	NA	NA	NA	•••	NA	NA	•••	.01496 (raw)
.74	2.64	NA	NA	NA	NA	NA	•••	NA	NA	5,532	NA

Food and Amount	Iron mg.	Mag-nesium mg.	Phos-phorus mg.	Potas-sium mg.	Sodium mg.
Caviar, sturgeon (Beluga), granular—1 rd. tbsp., 10 gm.	1.2	NA	36	18	220
Clam Chowder—see Miscellaneous—Soups					
Clam juice (liquid)—½ cup, 125 gm.	---	NA	---	---	---
Clams, raw; hard, soft, and unspecified; meat and liquid—½ cup, 120 gm.	---	---	236	---	---
Clams, raw; hard, soft, and unspecified; meat only—½ cup, 110 gm.	6.7	---	178	199	132
Clams, canned, all types, solids and liquid—½ cup, 100 gm.	4.1	---	137	140	---
Clams, canned, all types, drained solids—½ cup, 100 gm.	---	---	---	---	---
Cod, canned—½ cup, 110 gm.	---	---	---	---	---
Cod, cooked, broiled—1 piece, 3″ x 4″ x ¾″, 130 gm.	1.3	---	346.6	514.6	138.6
Cod dried, salted—2½″ x 2½″ x ⅜″, 56 gm.	---	---	---	---	---
Codfish cakes—see Fishcakes					
Crab, rock and king (incl. blue, Dungeness), cooked, steamed—½ cup, 85 gm.	.68	28.9	148	---	---
Crab, canned—½ cup flakes, 85 gm.	.68	28.9	154	93	850
Crab, deviled—1 tbsp. (rounded), 12 gm.	.14	---	16.44	19.92	104.04
Crab, deviled, 1 shell, approx. 6 tbsp., 72 gm.	.84	---	98.64	119.52	624.24
Crab, softshell, fried—1 piece, 3″ x 2″, 65 gm.	---	---	---	---	---
Crappie, white, raw—1 piece, 4″ x 3″ x ½″, 150 gm.	---	NA	---	---	---
Crayfish, freshwater, and spiny lobster, raw—4″ x 2″ x ½″, 118 gm.	1.77	NA	237.18	---	---
Croaker, Atlantic, cooked, baked, 1 serving, 4″ x 3″ x ¾″, 130 gm.	---	NA	---	430.6	160
Croaker, white, raw—3″ x 3½″ x ¾″, 120 gm.	---	NA	---	---	---
Croaker, yellowfin, raw—3½″ x 3″ x ¾″, 120 gm.	---	NA	---	---	---
Drum, freshwater, raw—3″ x 5″ x 11/16″, 200 gm.	---	NA	---	572	140
Drum, red (redfish), raw—4″ x 2″ x ½″, 60 gm.	---	NA	---	163.8	33
Eel, smoked—1 piece, 2″ sq. x ½″, 50 gm.	---	NA	---	---	---
Finnan haddie (smoked haddock)—1 piece, 2½″ x 2½″ x ¼″, 100 gm.	---	NA	---	---	---
Fishcakes, cooked, fried—1 cake, 2½″ diam., 44 gm.	---	NA	---	---	---
Fishcakes, cooked, frozen, fried, reheated—2″ diam., 44 gm.	---	NA	---	---	---
Fish flour, from whole fish—1 cup, 120 gm.	49.2	NA	3,720	516	204

*Where values for "raw" fish or shellfish are given, no information was available on the cooked foods.

Food and Amount	Calories	Carbo-hydrate gm.	Protein gm.	Sat. Fatty Acids gm.	Unsat. Fatty Acids gm.	Vitamin A IU	Thiamin B_1 mg.
Fish sticks, frozen, cooked—3″ x 1″ diam., 51 gm.	89.76	3.31	8.46	NA	NA	0	.02
Flatfishes, raw (flounder, sole, sand dab)—1 piece, 3″ x 4″ x ⅜″, 135 gm.	105.3	0	22.26	NA	NA	---	.06
Flounder, cooked, baked—1 piece, 3″ x 3″ x ⅜″, 100 gm.	202	0	30	NA	NA	---	.07
Frogs' legs, cooked, fried—1 large leg, 28.8 gm.	83.6	2.44	5.16	NA	NA	0	.0336
Frogs' legs, raw—4 large legs, 100 gm.	73	0	16.4	NA	NA	0	.14
Grouper, incl. red, black, and speckled kind, raw—4″ x 2″ x ½″, 140 gm.	121.8	0	17.02	NA	NA	---	.22
Haddock, cooked fried—1 filet, 3″ x 3″ x ½″, 100 gm.	165	5.8	19.6	NA	NA	---	.04
Haddock, raw—1 filet, 3″ x 3″ x ½″, 100 gm.	79	0	18.3	NA	NA	---	.04
Haddock, smoked, canned or not canned —1 piece, 2½″ x 2½″ x ¼″, 100 gm.	103	0	23.2	NA	NA	---	.06
Halibut, Atlantic and Pacific, cooked, broiled—3″ x 4″ x 1″, 250 gm.	426	0	63	NA	NA	1,700	.12
Halibut, Atlantic and Pacific, raw—1 piece, 3″ x 4″ x 1″, 200 gm.	200	0	41.8	NA	NA	880	.14
Halibut, Atlantic and Pacific, smoked—1 piece, 3″ x 3½″ x ½″, 115 gm.	257	0	24	NA	NA	---	---
Herring, Atlantic or Pacific, canned, solids and liquid—1 cup, 230 gm.	478.4	0	45.77	4.6	4.6	---	---
Herring, canned in tomato sauce—1 cup, 240 gm.	422.4	8.88	37.92	4.8	4.8	---	---
Herring, pickled, Bismarck type—6″ x 2½″ x ¼″, 62 gm.	138.26	0	12.64	1.24	1.24	---	---
Herring, salted or brined—1 piece, 2¼″ x 2¼″ x ⅝″, 88 gm.	191.84	0	16.72	1.76	1.76	---	---
Herring, smoked, Kippered—1 piece, 5½″ x 1″ x ¼″, 31 gm.	65.41	0	6.88	.62	.62	9.30	---
Kingfish, Southern, gulf, and Northern (whiting), raw—3″ x 4″ x ½″, 98 gm.	102.9	0	17.82	NA	NA	---	---
Lake herring (Cisco), raw—1 small, (7″ long), 100 gm.	96	0	17.7	NA	NA	---	.09
Lake trout, raw—3″ x 2½″ (widest part) x ½″, 48 gm.	80.64	0	8.78	NA	NA	---	.04
Lobster, northern, broiled w/2 tbsp. butter—1 lobster, 9″ length, 12 oz. (approx. ¾ lb.), 334 gm.	308	.8	20	NA	NA	920	.110
Lobster, northern, canned—½ cup, 85 gm.	80	.25	15.9	NA	NA	---	.08
Lobster Newburg—½ cup, 112 gm.	217.28	5.71	20.72	NA	NA	---	.07
Lobster paste—1 teaspoon, 7 gm.	12.6	.10	1.45	NA	NA	---	---
Lobster salad—1 cup, 200 gm.	220	4.6	20.2	NA	NA	---	.18
Lobster salad—1 scoop, 50 gm.	55	1.65	5.55	NA	NA	---	.045
Lobster, spiny—see Crayfish							
Mackerel, Atlantic, canned, solids and liquid—½ cup, 100 gm.	183·	0	19.3	NA	NA	430	.06

* Where values for "raw" fish or shellfish are given, no information was available on the cooked foods.

Food and Amount	Ribo-flavin B₂ mg.	Niacin mg.	B₆ mg.	Folic Acid mg.	PABA mg.	Panto-thenic Acid mg.	B₁₂ mcg.
Fish sticks, frozen, cooked—3" x 1" diam., 51 gm.	.03	.81	NA	NA	NA	NA	NA
Flatfishes, raw (flounder, sole, sand dab)—1 piece, 3" x 4" x ⅜", 135 gm.	.06	.56	---	NA	NA	---	---
Flounder, cooked, baked—1 piece, 3" x 3" x ⅜", 100 gm.	.08	2.5	---	NA	NA	---	---
Frogs' legs, cooked, fried—1 large leg, 28.8 gm.	.0704	.36	NA	NA	NA	NA	NA
Frogs' legs, raw—4 large legs, 100 gm.	.25	1.2	NA	NA	NA	NA	NA
Grouper, incl. red, black, and speckled kind, raw—4" x 2" x ½", 140 gm.	---	---	NA	NA	NA	NA	NA
Haddock, cooked fried—1 filet, 3" x 3" x ½", 100 gm.	.07	3.2	---	NA	NA	---	---
Haddock, raw—1 filet, 3" x 3" x ½", 100 gm.	.07	3.0	.18	NA	NA	.13	1.3
Haddock, smoked, canned or not canned —1 piece, 2½" x 2½" x ¼", 100 gm.	.05	2.1	---	NA	NA	---	---
Halibut, Atlantic and Pacific, cooked, broiled—3" x 4" x 1", 250 gm.	.16	20.6	NA	NA	NA	NA	NA
Halibut, Atlantic and Pacific, raw— 1 piece, 3" x 4" x 1", 200 gm.	.14	16.6	NA	NA	NA	NA	NA
Halibut, Atlantic and Pacific, smoked— 1 piece, 3" x 3½" x ½", 115 gm.	---	---	NA	NA	NA	NA	NA
Herring, Atlantic or Pacific, canned, solids and liquid—1 cup, 230 gm.	.41	---	---	NA	NA	---	4.6 (fresh)
Herring, canned in tomato sauce— 1 cup, 240 gm.	.26	8.4	---	NA	NA	---	---
Herring, pickled, Bismarck type— 6" x 2½" x ¼", 62 gm.	---	---	---	NA	NA	---	---
Herring, salted or brined—1 piece, 2¼" x 2¾" x ⅝", 88 gm.	.16	---	---	NA	NA	---	---
Herring, smoked, Kippered—1 piece, 5½" x 1" x ¼", 31 gm.	.08	1.02	---	NA	NA	---	---
Kingfish, Southern, gulf, and Northern (whiting), raw—3" x 4" x ½", 98 gm.	---	---	NA	NA	NA	NA	NA
Lake herring (Cisco), raw—1 small, (7" long), 100 gm.	.10	3.3	NA	NA	NA	NA	NA
Lake trout, raw—3" x 2½" (widest part) x ½", 48 gm.	.05	1.29	NA	NA	NA	NA	NA
Lobster, northern, broiled w/2 tbsp. butter—1 lobster, 9" length, 12 oz. (approx. ¾ lb.), 334 gm.	.06	2.3	---	NA	NA	---	---
Lobster, northern, canned—½ cup, 85 gm.	.05	---	---	NA	NA	1.275	.42
Lobster Newburg—½ cup, 112 gm.	.12	---	---	NA	NA	---	---
Lobster paste—1 teaspoon, 7 gm.	.01	---	---	NA	NA	---	---
Lobster salad—1 cup, 200 gm.	.16	---	---	NA	NA	---	---
Lobster salad—1 scoop, 50 gm.	.04	---	---	NA	NA	---	---
Lobster, spiny—see Crayfish							
Mackerel, Atlantic, canned, solids and liquid—½ cup, 100 gm.	.21	5.8	---	---	NA	---	NA

* Where values for "raw" fish or shellfish are given, no information was available on the cooked foods.

Vitamin C mg.	Vitamin D IU	Vitamin E IU	Calcium mg.	Iodine mg.	Iron mg.	Magnesium mg.	Phosphorus mg.	Potassium mg.	Sodium mg.
---	NA	NA	5.61	NA	.2	NA	85.17	---	---
---	NA	NA	16	NA	1.06	---	260	456	104
2	NA	NA	23	.029 Atlan.	1.4	30 (raw)	344	587	237
---	NA	NA	5.6	NA	.4	NA	46.2	---	---
---	NA	NA	18	NA	1.5	NA	147	---	---
---	NA	NA	---	NA	---	NA	---	---	---
2	NA	---	40	---	1.2	24	247	348	177
---	NA	.6 (broiled)	23	.1647 N.Y.	.7	24	197	304	61
---	NA	---	---	---	---	---	---	---	---
---	NA	NA	40	---	2	---	620	1,312	334
---	NA	NA	26	.0608 Wash.	1.4	---	422	898	108
---	NA	NA	---	---	---	---	---	---	---
---	NA	NA	338.1	---	4.14	NA	683.1	---	---
---	NA	NA	---	---	---	NA	583.2	---	---
---	NA	NA	---	---	---	NA	---	---	---
---	NA	NA	---	---	---	NA	---	---	---
---	NA	NA	20.46	.0164	.43	NA	78.74	---	---
---	NA	NA	---	NA	---	NA	---	245	81.34
---	NA	NA	12	NA	.5	17	206	319	47
---	NA	NA	---	NA	.38	NA	114.24	---	---
0	NA	NA	80	.46092 (raw)	.7	---	229	180	210
---	NA	NA	55	.11305	.68	18.7	163	153	178
---	NA	NA	97.44	---	1	---	215.04	191.52	256.48
---	NA	NA	---	---	---	---	---	---	---
36	NA	NA	72	---	1.8	---	190	528	248
9	NA	NA	18	---	.45	---	48	132	62
---	165	---	185	---	2.1	---	274	---	---

Food and Amount	Calories	Carbo-hydrate gm.	Protein gm.	Sat. Fatty Acids gm.	Unsat. Fatty Acids gm.	Vitamin A IU	Thiamin B_1 mg.
Mackerel, Atlantic, cooked, broiled w/butter or margarine—5″ x 3″ x ½″, 176 gm.	415.2	0	38.36	NA	NA	932.8	.26
Mackerel, Pacific, canned—½ cup, 100 gm.	180	0	21.1	NA	NA	30	.03
Mackerel, salted—2″ x 1½″ x ½″, 35 gm.	106.75	0	6.47	NA	NA	•••	•••
Mullet, striped, raw—3″ x 4″ x ½″, 116 gm.	169.36	0	22.72	NA	NA	•••	.08
Mussels, Atlantic and Pacific, raw, meat and liquid—1 cup, 168 gm.	110.88	5.2	16.12	NA	NA	•••	•••
Mussels, Atlantic and Pacific, raw, meat only—1 cup, 180 gm.	171	5.94	25.92	NA	NA	•••	.28
Mussels, Pacific, canned, drained solids—½ cup, 110 gm.	125	1.65	20	NA	NA	•••	•••
Ocean perch, Atlantic (redfish), broiled —5″ x 1¼″ x ⅜″, 40 gm:	NA	NA	NA	NA	NA	NA	NA
Ocean perch, Atlantic (redfish), cooked, fried—4″ x 1¼″ x ⅜″, 35 gm.	79.45	2.38	6.65	NA	NA	•••	.03
Ocean perch, Atlantic (redfish), frozen, breaded, fried, reheated—4″ x 1½″ x ⅜″, 42 gm.	133.98	6.93	7.93	NA	NA	•••	•••
Ocean perch, Pacific, raw—5″ x 2″ (widest part) x ⅜″, 52 gm.	49.4	0	9.88	NA	NA	•••	•••
Octopus, raw—1¼″ sq. x ½″, 26 gm.	18.98	0	3.97	NA	NA	•••	.005
Oyster stew, commercial, frozen, prepared w/equal volume water—1 cup, 260 gm.	132.6	8.84	5.98	NA	NA	260	.07
Oyster stew, commercial, frozen, prepared w/equal volume milk—1 cup, 265 gm.	222.6	15.63	11.13	NA	NA	450.5	.13
Oyster stew, homemade, 1 pt. oysters, 2 pt. milk—1 cup, 260 gm.	252.2	11.7	13.52	NA	NA	884	.15
•Oyster stew, homemade, 1 pt. oysters, 3 pt. milk—1 cup, 260 gm.	223.6	12.22	12.74	NA	NA	728	.15
Oysters, raw, meat only, Eastern—6 med. oysters (1″ diam.), 80 gm.	52	2.72	6.7	NA	NA	248	.11
Oysters, raw, meat only, Pacific and Western—4 oysters, 100 gm.	91	6.4	10.6	NA	NA	•••	.12
Oysters, cooked, fried (w/egg, milk, breadcrumbs)—1 oyster, 1¼″ diam., 18 gm.	43.02	3.34	1.54	NA	NA	79.2	.03
Oysters, canned, solids and liquid—1 cup, 180 gm.	136	8.82	15.3	NA	NA	•••	.03
Oysters, frozen, solids and liquid—1 cup, 170 gm.	•••	•••	10.37	NA	NA	527	.23
Perch, white, raw—5″ x 1½″ x ¼″, 40 gm.	47.2	0	7.72	NA	NA	•••	•••
Perch, yellow, raw—5″ x 1½″ x ¼″, 40 gm.	36.4	0	7.8	NA	NA	•••	.02
Pickerel, raw—3″ x 4″ x ⅜″, 90 gm.	75.6	0	16.82	NA	NA	•••	•••
Pike, blue, raw—6″ x 2″ x ¼″, 92 gm.	82.8	0	17.57	NA	NA	•••	•••
Pike, northern, raw—6″ x 2½″ x ¼″, 115 gm.	101.2	0	21.04	NA	NA	•••	•••

* Where values for "raw" fish or shellfish are given, no information was available on the cooked foods.

Riboflavin B_2 mg.	Niacin mg.	B_8 mg.	Folic Acid mg.	PABA mg.	Pantothenic Acid mg.	B_{12} mcg.	Vitamin C mg.	Vitamin D IU	Vitamin E IU	Calcium mg.	Iodine mg.
.46	13.36	---	---	NA	---	NA	---	---	---	10.56	.05328 (raw) Mass.
.33	8.8	.27	.0006	NA	.47	NA	---	250	---	260	---
---	---	---	---	NA	---	NA	---	NA	---	---	.014
.08	6.02	NA	NA	NA	NA	NA	---	NA	NA	30.16	.5626 Fla.
---	---	NA	NA	NA	NA	NA	---	NA	NA	---	.1347 Pacif.
.37	---	NA	NA	NA	NA	NA	---	NA	NA	158.4	.1443 Pacif.
.14	---	NA	NA	NA	NA	NA	---	NA	NA	---	.1067
NA	NA	NA	NA	NA	NA	NA	NA	NA	NA	NA	NA
.03	.63	NA	NA	NA	NA	NA	---	NA	NA	11.55	---
---	---	NA	NA	NA	NA	NA	---	NA	NA	---	---
---	---	NA	NA	NA	NA	NA	---	NA	NA	---	.0091 Pacif.
.01	.46	NA	NA	NA	NA	NA	---	NA	NA	7.54	NA
.2	.52	NA	NA	NA	NA	NA	---	NA	NA	171.6	---
.45	.53	NA	NA	NA	NA	NA	trace	NA	NA	336.5	---
.46	2.34	---	---	NA	---	NA	---	NA	NA	296.4	---
.46	1.82	---	---	NA	---	NA	---	NA	NA	304.2	---
.14	2	.04	.0088 (canned)	NA	.2	14.4	---	4	NA	75	NA
---	1.3	NA	NA	NA	NA	NA	30	5	NA	85	.0935 Pacif.
.05	.57	NA	NA	NA	NA	NA	---	NA	NA	27.36	---
.36	1.44	.0666	.0198	NA	.88	---	---	---	NA	50	.063
.3	4.25	---	---	NA	---	NA	---	---	NA	---	---
---	---	NA	NA	NA	NA	NA	---	NA	NA	---	.0168
.06	.68	NA	NA	NA	NA	NA	---	NA	NA	---	.0008 Potomac R.
---	---	NA	NA	NA	NA	NA	---	NA	NA	---	.0063 Potomac R.
---	---	---	NA	NA	---	---	---	NA	NA	---	NA
---	---	---	NA	NA	---	---	---	NA	NA	---	NA

Food and Amount	Iron mg.	Magnesium mg.	Phosphorus mg.	Potassium mg.	Sodium mg.
Mackerel, Atlantic, cooked, broiled w/butter or margarine—5″ x 3″ x ½″, 176 gm.	2.1	29.28 (raw)	492.8	...	...
Mackerel, Pacific, canned—½ cup, 100 gm.	2.2	NA	288	...	...
Mackerel, salted—2″ x 1½″ x ½″, 35 gm.	...	NA	...	...	...
Mullet, striped, raw—3″ x 4″ x ½″, 116 gm.	2.08	37.12	255.2	338.72	93.96
Mussels, Atlantic and Pacific, raw, meat and liquid—1 cup, 168 gm.	...	38.64	...	...	...
Mussels, Atlantic and Pacific, raw, meat only—1 cup, 180 gm.	6.12	...	424.8	567	520.2
Mussels, Pacific, canned, drained solids—½ cup, 110 gm.	...	...	...	...	...
Ocean perch, Atlantic (redfish), broiled —5″ x 1¼″ x ⅜″, 40 gm.	NA	NA	NA	NA	NA
Ocean perch, Atlantic (redfish), cooked, fried—4″ x 1¼″ x ⅜″, 35 gm.	.45	...	79.1	99.4	53.55
Ocean perch, Atlantic (redfish), frozen, breaded, fried, reheated—4″ x 1½″ x ⅜″, 42 gm.	...	...	...	...	...
Ocean perch, Pacific, raw—5″ x 2″ (widest part) x ⅜″, 52 gm.	...	...	...	202.8	32.76
Octopus, raw—1¼″ sq. x ½″, 26 gm.	...	NA	44.98	...	...
Oyster stew, commercial, frozen, prepared w/equal volume water—1 cup, 260 gm.	1.56	NA	150.8	265.2	884
Oyster stew, commercial, frozen, prepared w/equal volume milk—1 cup, 265 gm.	1.59	NA	280.9	466.4	969.9
Oyster stew, homemade, 1 pt. oysters, 2 pt. milk—1 cup, 260 gm.	4.94	NA	288.6	345.8	881.4
Oyster stew, homemade, 1 pt. oysters, 3 pt. milk—1 cup, 260 gm.	3.64	NA	283.4	358.8	527.8
Oysters, raw, meat only, Eastern—6 med. oysters (1″ diam.), 80 gm.	4.4	25.6	114	96	58
Oysters, raw, meat only, Pacific and Western—4 oysters, 100 gm.	7.2	24	153	...	...
Oysters, cooked, fried (w/egg, milk, breadcrumbs)—1 oyster, 1¼″ diam., 18 gm.	1.45	...	43.38	36.54	37.08
Oysters, canned, solids and liquid—1 cup, 180 gm.	10.08	...	223	126	10
Oysters, frozen, solids and liquid—1 cup, 170 gm.	...	...	...	357	646
Perch, white, raw—5″ x 1½″ x ¼″, 40 gm.	...	NA	76.8	...	...
Perch, yellow, raw—5″ x 1½″ x ¼″, 40 gm.	.24	NA	72	92	27.2
Pickerel, raw—3″ x 4″ x ⅜″, 90 gm.	.62	NA	...	...	...
Pike, blue, raw—6″ x 2″ x ¼″, 92 gm.	...	...	...	...	...
Pike, northern, raw—6″ x 2½″ x ¼″, 115 gm.	...	...	...	...	...

* Where values for "raw" fish or shellfish are given, no information was available on the cooked foods.

Food and Amount	Calories	Carbo-hydrate gm.	Protein gm.	Sat. Fatty Acids gm.	Unsat. Fatty Acids gm.	Vitamin A IU	Thiamin B₁ mg.
Pike, walleye, raw—7" x 2½" x ¼", 125 gm.	116.25	0	24.12	NA	NA	•••	.31
Pompano, raw—1 piece, 6" x 3" x ¾", 200 gm.	332	0	37.6	NA	NA	•••	.82
Porgy or scup, cooked, fried—1 piece, 3" x 2½" x ¾", 93 gm.	279	10.8	22.7	NA	NA	75	.073
Raja fish—see Skate							
Red and Gray Snapper, raw— 2" x 4" x ½", 96 gm.	89.29	0	19	NA	NA	•••	.16
Redfish—see Drum, red, and Ocean Perch, Atlantic							
Roe, canned, solids and liquid, incl. cod, haddock, herring—1 tbsp., 10 gm.	11.8	.03	2.15	NA	NA	•••	•••
Roe, cooked, baked, or broiled, cod, and shad—3" x 1½", 50 gm.	63	.95	11	NA	NA	•••	•••
Roe, cooked, baked or broiled, cod, and shad—1 tbsp., 10 gm.	12.6	.19	2.2	NA	NA	•••	•••
Salmon, Atlantic, canned, solids and liquid—½ cup, 100 gm.	203	0	21.7	•••	•••	•••	•••
Salmon, Atlantic, raw—2" x 3" x ¾", 50 gm.	108.5	0	11.25	•••	•••	•••	•••
Salmon, Chinook (king), canned, solids and liquid—1 cup, 250 gm.	525	0	49	10	10	575	.07
Salmon, Chinook (king), raw— 2" x 2" x ¾", 35 gm.	77.7	0	6.68	•••	•••	108.5	.03
Salmon, Chum, canned, solids and liquid—½ cup, 100 gm.	139	0	21.5	•••	•••	60	.02
Salmon, Chum, raw—2" x 3" x ¾", 55 gm.	•••	0	•••	•••	•••	•••	.05
Salmon, Coho (silver), canned, solids and liquid—½ cup, 100 gm.	153	0	20.8	•••	•••	80	.03
Salmon, Coho (silver), raw— 2" x 3" x ¾", 50 gm.	•••	0	•••	•••	•••	•••	.04
Salmon, Pink (humpback), canned, solids and liquid—1 cup, 250 gm.	352	0	51.2	5	2.5	175	.07
Salmon, Pink (humpback), raw— 2" x 2" x ¾", 35 gm.	41.65	0	7	•••	•••	•••	.04
Salmon, Sockeye (red), canned, solids and liquid—1 cup, 250 gm.	427	0	50.75	•••	•••	575	.10
Salmon, Sockeye (red), raw— 2" x 2½" x ¾", 45 gm.	•••	0	•••	•••	•••	67.5	.06
Salmon, cooked, broiled or baked— 1 piece, 4" x 3" x ½", 115 gm.	209	0	31	•••	•••	186	.18
Salmon, smoked—1 slice, 3" x 1" x ⅛", 12 gm.	21.12	0	2.59	NA	NA	•••	•••
Salmon salad—1 cup, 200 gm.	296	1.8	20.8	NA	NA	NA	NA
Salmon salad—1 scoop, 55 gm.	81.4	.49	5.72	NA	NA	NA	NA
Sand dab—see Flatfishes							
Sardines, Atlantic, canned in oil, solids and liquid—3, 3¼" long, 75 gm.	233	.45	15.45	NA	NA	135	.01
Sardines, Atlantic, canned in oil, drained solids—1 sardine, 3", 10 gm.	20.3	•••	2.4	NA	NA	22	.003

* Where values for "raw" fish or shellfish are given, no information was available on the cooked foods.

Food and Amount	Ribo-flavin B₂ mg.	Niacin mg.	B₆ mg.	Folic Acid mg.	PABA mg.	Panto-thenic Acid mg.	B₁₂ mcg.
Pike, walleye, raw—7" x 2½" x ¼", 125 gm.	.2	2.87	•••	NA	NA	•••	•••
Pompano, raw—1 piece, 6" x 3" x ¾", 200 gm.	.44	•••	NA	NA	NA	NA	NA
Porgy or scup, cooked, fried—1 piece, 3" x 2½" x ¾", 93 gm.	.082	3.7	NA	NA	NA	NA	NA
Raja fish—see Skate							
Red and Gray Snapper, raw— 2" x 4" x ½", 96 gm.	.013	•••	NA	NA	NA	NA	NA
Redfish—see Drum, red, and Ocean Perch, Atlantic							
Roe, canned, solids and liquid, incl. cod, haddock, herring—1 tbsp., 10 gm.	•••	•••	NA	NA	NA	NA	NA
Roe, cooked, baked, or broiled, cod, and shad—3" x 1½", 50 gm.	•••	•••	NA	NA	NA	NA	NA
Roe, cooked, baked or broiled, cod, and shad—1 tbsp., 10 gm.	•••	•••	NA	NA	NA	NA	NA
Salmon, Atlantic, canned, solids and liquid—½ cup, 100 gm.	•••	•••	.45	.0005	NA	.58	NA
Salmon, Atlantic, raw—2" x 3" x ¾", 50 gm.	.04	3.6	NA	NA	NA	NA	NA
Salmon, Chinook (king), canned, solids and liquid—1 cup, 250 gm.	.35	18.25	•••	•••	NA	•••	NA
Salmon, Chinook (king), raw— 2" x 2" x ¾", 35 gm.	.08	•••	NA	NA	NA	NA	NA
Salmon, Chum, canned, solids and liquid—½ cup, 100 gm.	.16	7.1	•••	•••	NA	•••	NA
Salmon, Chum, raw—2" x 3" x ¾", 55 gm.	.03	•••	NA	NA	NA	NA	NA
Salmon, Coho (silver), canned, solids and liquid—½ cup, 100 gm.	.18	7.4	•••	•••	NA	•••	NA
Salmon, Coho (silver), raw— 2" x 3" x ¾", 50 gm.	.05	•••	NA	NA	NA	NA	NA
Salmon, Pink (humpback), canned, solids and liquid—1 cup, 250 gm.	.45	20.00	•••	•••	NA	•••	•••
Salmon, Pink (humpback), raw— 2" x 2" x ¾", 35 gm.	.01	•••	NA	NA	NA	NA	NA
Salmon, Sockeye (red), canned, solids and liquid—1 cup, 250 gm.	.40	18.25	•••	•••	NA	•••	NA
Salmon, Sockeye (red), raw— 2" x 2½" x ¾", 45 gm.	.03	•••	NA	NA	NA	NA	NA
Salmon, cooked, broiled or baked— 1 piece, 4" x 3" x ½", 115 gm.	.06	11.27	NA	NA	NA	NA	NA
Salmon, smoked—1 slice, 3" x 1" x ⅛", 12 gm.	•••	•••	NA	NA	NA	NA	NA
Salmon salad—1 cup, 200 gm.	NA	NA	NA	NA	NA	NA	NA
Salmon salad—1 scoop, 55 gm.	NA	NA	NA	NA	NA	NA	NA
Sand dab—see Flatfishes							
Sardines, Atlantic, canned in oil, solids and liquid—3, 3¼" long, 75 gm.	.12	3.30	•••	•••	NA	•••	•••
Sardines, Atlantic, canned in oil, drained solids—1 sardine, 3", 10 gm.	.02	.54	•••	•••	NA	•••	•••

* Where values for "raw" fish or shellfish are given, no information was available on the cooked foods.

Vitamin C mg.	Vitamin D IU	Vitamin E IU	Calcium mg.	Iodine mg.	Iron mg.	Magnesium mg.	Phosphorus mg.	Potassium mg.	Sodium mg.
•••	NA	NA	•••	NA	.5	•••	26.75	398.75	63.75
•••	NA	NA	•••	.016	•••	NA	•••	382	94
0	NA	NA	24	.0279	1.5	NA	258	266	58
•••	NA	NA	15.36	.02688 Fla.	.76	26.88	205.44	310.08	64.32
.2	NA	NA	1.5	.0151	.12	NA	34.6	•••	•••
•••	NA	NA	6.5	•••	1.15	NA	201	66	36.5
•••	NA	NA	1.3	•••	.23	NA	40.2	13.2	7.3
•••	500	NA	•••	•••	•••	NA	•••	•••	•••
4.5	NA	•••	39.5	•••	.45	NA	93	•••	•••
•••	687.5	NA	385	.1675 Alas.	2.25	67.5	722	915	••
•••	NA	•••	•••	.01274 Wash.	•••	NA	105.35	139.65	15.75
•••	225	NA	249	.022 Alas.	.7	30	352	336	•••
•••	NA	•••	•••	.0133 Wash.	•••	NA	•••	235.95	29.15
•••	NA	NA	244	•••	.9	30	288	339	351
.5	NA	•••	87.5	.0103	•••	NA	115.5	210.5	24
•••	1,562.5	•••	490	.0525 Alas.	2.0	75	715	902	967
•••	NA	•••	•••	.0092 Wash.	•••	NA	•••	107.1	22.4
•••	2,000	NA	647	.1325 Alas.	3.0	72.5	860	860	1,305
•••	NA	•••	•••	.0182 Wash.	•••	NA	•••	175.95	21.6
•••	•••	1.55	•••	•••	1.38	•••	476	509	133
•••	NA	NA	1.68	•••	•••	NA	29.4	•••	•••
NA	NA	NA	68	•••	.6	22.4	196	281	648
NA	NA	NA	18.7	•••	.16	6.16	53.9	77.27	178.2
•••	249.75	NA	265	•••	2.62	•••	325	420	382
•••	29.4	NA	43.7	•••	.29	NA	49.9	59	82.3

Food and Amount	Calories	Carbo-hydrate gm.	Protein gm.	Sat. Fatty Acids gm.	Unsat. Fatty Acids gm.	Vitamin A IU	Thiamin B_1 mg.
Sardines, Pacific, canned, in brine or mustard, solids and liquid—1 fish, 2½″ long, 15 gm.	29.4	.25	2.82	NA	NA	4.5	---
Sardines, Pacific, canned, in oil, drained solids—1 fish, 2½″, 17 gm.	---	---	---	NA	NA	---	.001
Sardines, Pacific, canned, in tomato sauce, solids and liquid—1, 5″ long, 95 gm.	187	1.6	17.7	NA	NA	28	.009
Sardines, Pacific, raw—4, 2½″ long, 50 gm.	80	0	9.6	NA	NA	---	---
Scallops, bay and sea, raw—1 cup, 210 gm.	170	6.9	32	NA	NA	---	---
Scallops, bay and sea, cooked, steamed—1 cup, 100 gm.	112	---	23.2	NA	NA	---	---
Scallops, bay and sea, frozen, breaded, fried, reheated—1 cup, 145 gm.	281.3	15.22	26.1	NA	NA	---	---
Sea bass, white, raw—1 piece, 4″ x 3″ x ½″, 120 gm.	115.2	0	25.68	NA	NA	---	---
Shad or American shad, canned, solids and liquid—1 cup, 210 gm.	319.2	0	35.49	NA	NA	---	---
Shad or American shad, cooked, baked —1 piece, 3″ x 3″ x ¾″, 95 gm.	191	0	22	NA	NA	28.5	.12
Shad or American shad, raw—1 piece, 3″ x 3″ x ¾″, 100 gm.	170	0	18.6	NA	NA	---	.15
Sheepshead, freshwater—see Drum							
Shrimp, canned, dry pack or drained, solids—8 med. (1½″ x ½″), 65 gm.	75	.45	15.7	NA	NA	39	.006
Shrimp, canned, wet pack, solids and liquid—½ cup, 100 gm.	80	.8	16.2	NA	NA	50	.01
Shrimp, cooked, broiled—1½″ x ¾″, 28 gm.	NA	NA	NA	NA	NA	NA	NA
Shrimp, cooked, french-fried—1 shrimp, 1½″ x ½″, 18 gm.	40.5	1.8	3.65	NA	NA	---	.007
Shrimp, frozen, breaded, raw, not more than 50% breading—1 shrimp, 1¼″ x ½″, 23 gm.	31.97	4.57	2.82	NA	NA	---	.006
Shrimp, raw—1 shrimp, 1½″ x ½″, 20 gm.	18.2	.3	3.62	NA	NA	---	.004
Shrimp paste, canned—1 tbsp., 7 gm.	12.6	.10	1.45	NA	NA	---	---
Smelt, Atlantic, jack and bay, canned, solids and liquid—1 fish, 5¾″ long, 40 gm.	80	0	7.36	NA	NA	---	---
Smelt, Atlantic, jack and bay, raw—1 fish, 5¾″ long, 40 gm.	39.2	0	7.44	NA	NA	---	.004
Snail, raw—1 snail, ¾″ diam., 10 gm.	9	.2	1.61	NA	NA	---	---
Snapper, red or gray—see Red and Gray Snapper							
Sole—see Flatfishes							
Spanish Mackerel, raw—1 piece, 3″ x 3″ x ¾″, 100 gm.	177	0	19.5	NA	NA	---	.13
Spot, cooked, baked—3″ x 4″ x ½″, 135 gm.	393.3	0	30.4	NA	NA	---	---
Squid, raw—8½″ long x 1¾″ diam., 72 gm.	60.48	1.08	11.8	NA	NA	---	.01

* Where values for "raw" fish or shellfish are given, no information was available on the cooked foods.

Riboflavin B₂ mg.	Niacin mg.	B₆ mg.	Folic Acid mg.	PABA mg.	Pantothenic Acid mg.	B₁₂ mcg.	Vitamin C mg.	Vitamin D IU	Vitamin E IU	Calcium mg.	Iodine mg.
•••	•••	•••	•••	NA	•••	•••	•••	NA	NA	45.45	•••
.05	1.25	•••	•••	NA	•••	•••	•••	NA	NA	•••	•••
.25	5.03	.152	.00095	NA	.665	9.5	•••	NA	NA	426	•••
•••	•••	•••	•••	NA	•••	•••	•••	NA	NA	16.5	•••
.12	2.71	•••	NA	NA	.2772	2.52	•••	NA	•••	54	.16779 Pacif.
•••	•••	•••	NA	NA	•••	•••	•••	NA	•••	115	•••
•••	•••	NA	NA	NA	NA	NA	•••	NA	.87	•••	•••
•••	•••	NA	NA	NA	NA	NA	•••	NA	•••	•••	NA
.33	•••	•••	NA	NA	•••	•••	•••	NA	NA	•••	•••
.24	8.17	•••	NA	NA	•••	•••	•••	NA	NA	22	•••
.24	8.4	•••	NA	NA	.608	•••	•••	NA	NA	20	.0306 Wash.
.019	1.17	.039	.0013	NA	.1365	•••	•••	•••	NA	74	•••
.03	1.5	.111	.0018	NA	.21	•••	•••	•••	NA	59	.038
NA	NA	NA	NA	NA	NA	NA	NA	NA	NA	NA	NA
.01	.48	•••	•••	NA	•••	•••	•••	NA	.1	12.96	•••
.006	.46	•••	•••	NA	•••	•••	•••	NA	.13	8.74	•••
.006	.64	•••	•••	NA	•••	•••	•••	NA	NA	12.6	.0075 Pacif.
.01	•••	•••	•••	NA	•••	•••	•••	NA	NA	•••	•••
•••	•••	NA	NA	NA	NA	NA	•••	NA	NA	143	•••
.04	.56	NA	NA	NA	NA	NA	•••	NA	NA	•••	.0004
•••	•••	NA	NA	NA	NA	NA	•••	NA	NA	•••	NA
.14	4.8	NA	NA	NA	NA	NA	•••	NA	NA	71	.0316
•••	•••	NA	NA	NA	NA	NA	•••	NA	NA	•••	NA
.08	•••	NA	NA	NA	NA	NA	•••	NA	NA	8.64	.015 Pacif.

Food and Amount	Iron mg.	Mag- nesium mg.	Phos- phorus mg.	Potas- sium mg.	Sodium mg.
Sardines, Pacific, canned, in brine or mustard, solids and liquid—1 fish, 2½″ long, 15 gm.	.78	---	53.1	39	114
Sardines, Pacific, canned, in oil, drained solids—1 fish, 2½″, 17 gm.	---	NA	---	---	---
Sardines, Pacific, canned, in tomato sauce, solids and liquid—1, 5″ long, 95 gm.	3.89	22.8	454	304	380
Sardines, Pacific, raw—4, 2½″ long, 50 gm.	.9	12	107	---	---
Scallops, bay and sea, raw—1 cup, 210 gm.	3.78	---	436	831	535
Scallops, bay and sea, cooked, steamed—1 cup, 100 gm.	3.0	---	338	476	265
Scallops, bay and sea, frozen, breaded, fried, reheated—1 cup, 145 gm.	---	NA	---	---	---
Sea bass, white, raw—1 piece, 4″ x 3″ x ½″, 120 gm.	---	NA	---	---	---
Shad or American shad, canned, solids and liquid—1 cup, 210 gm.	1.47	---	---	---	---
Shad or American shad, cooked, baked —1 piece, 3″ x 3″ x ¾″, 95 gm.	.57	---	297	358	75
Shad or American shad, raw—1 piece, 3″ x 3″ x ¾″, 100 gm.	.5	---	260	330	54
Sheepshead, freshwater—see Drum					
Shrimp, canned, dry pack or drained, solids—8 med. (1½″ x ½″), 65 gm.	2.01	33.15	171	79	---
Shrimp, canned, wet pack, solids and liquid—½ cup, 100 gm.	1.8	---	152	---	---
Shrimp, cooked, broiled—1½″ x ¾″, 28 gm.	NA	NA	NA	NA	NA
Shrimp, cooked, french-fried—1 shrimp, 1½″ x ½″, 18 gm.	.36	---	34.38	41.22	33.48
Shrimp, frozen, breaded, raw, not more than 50% breading—1 shrimp, 1¼″ x ½″, 23 gm.	.23	---	25.53	---	---
Shrimp, raw—1 shrimp, 1½″ x ½″, 20 gm.	.32	8.4	33.2	44	28
Shrimp paste, canned—1 tbsp., 7 gm.	---	---	---	---	---
Smelt, Atlantic, jack and bay, canned, solids and liquid—1 fish, 5¼″ long, 40 gm.	.68	NA	148	---	---
Smelt, Atlantic, jack and bay, raw— 1 fish, 5¼″ long, 40 gm.	.16	NA	108	---	---
Snail, raw—1 snail, ¾″ diam., 10 gm.	.35	NA	---	---	---
Snapper, red or gray—see Red and Gray Snapper					
Sole—see Flatfishes					
Spanish Mackerel, raw—1 piece, 3″ x 3″ x ¾″, 100 gm.	1.0	NA	249	264	68
Spot, cooked, baked—3″ x 4″ x ½″, 135 gm.	---	NA	---	---	416
Squid, raw—8½″ long x 1¼″ diam., 72 gm.	.36	NA	85.68	---	---

* Where values for "raw" fish or shellfish are given, no information was available on the cooked foods.

Food and Amount	Calories	Carbo-hydrate gm.	Protein gm.	Sat. Fatty Acids gm.	Unsat. Fatty Acids gm.	Vitamin A IU	Thiamin B1 mg.
Sturgeon, cooked, steamed—1 piece, 2½" sq. x ⅝", 82 gm.	131.2	0	20.82	NA	NA	•••	•••
Sturgeon, raw—1 piece, 3"x 3"x ¾", 100 gm.	94	0	18.1	NA	NA	•••	•••
Sturgeon, smoked—1 slice, 3"x 2"x ⅛", 14 gm.	20.86	0	4.36	NA	NA	•••	•••
Swordfish, cooked, broiled—1 piece, 3"x 3"x ½", 125 gm.	217	0	35	NA	NA	2,562	.05
Swordfish, raw—1 piece, 3"x 3"x ¾", 100 gm.	118	0	19.2	NA	NA	1,580	.05
Trout—see Lake Trout							
Trout, brook, raw—6"x 2"x ½", 120 gm.	121.2	0	23.04	NA	NA	•••	•••
Trout, rainbow or steelhead, canned—2½"x 1¾"x ½", 49 gm.	102.41	0	10.09	1.47	.98	•••	•••
Trout, rainbow or steelhead, raw—1 pc., 5"x 2"x ½", 116 gm.	226.2	0	24.94	3.48	2.32	•••	.08
Tuna, bluefin, raw—1 piece, 3"x 4"x ½", 120 gm.	174	0	30.24	.12	.12	•••	•••
Tuna, canned, in oil, solids and liquid—1 cup, 130 gm.	374	0	31.4	6.5	15.6	117	.05
Tuna, canned, in oil, drained solids—1 cup, 160 gm.	315	0	46.08	4.8	6.4	128	.08
Tuna, canned, in water, solids and liquid—1 cup, 200 gm.	254	0	56	•••	•••	•••	•••
Tuna Casserole w/noodles—1 cup, 292 gm.	420	37	26.2	NA	NA	•••	•••
Tuna salad—1 cup, 205 gm.	348	7.17	30	6.15	12.30	594	.08
Tuna salad—1 scoop, 60 gm.	102	2.10	8.76	1.8	3.60	174	.02
Tuna, yellowfin, raw—3"x 4"x ½", 120 gm.	159.6	0	29.64	.12	.12	•••	•••
Turtle Soup—1 cup, 246 gm.	56	8.2	2.9	NA	NA	•••	•••
Whitefish, Lake, raw (meat only)—1 piece, 6"x 3"x ⅞", 200 gm.	310	0	37.8	NA	NA	4,520	.28
Whitefish, Lake, smoked (meat only)—1 piece, 6"x 3"x ⅞", 178 gm.	275.8	0	37.2	NA	NA	•••	•••

* Where values for "raw" fish or shellfish are given, no information was available on the cooked foods.

FRUITS AND FRUIT PRODUCTS

Food and Amount	Calories	Carbo-hydrate gm.	Protein gm.	Sat. Fatty Acids gm.	Unsat. Fatty Acids gm.	Vitamin A IU	Thiamin B1 mg.
Acerola juice, raw—1 cup, 245 gm.	56.35	11.76	.98	•••	•••	•••	.04
Apple, dried, cooked w/o sugar—½ cup, 156 gm.	122	31.7	.47	•••	•••	•••	.016
Apple, dried, uncooked—1 cup, 114 gm.	313	81.8	1.14	•••	•••	•••	.069
*Apple, raw, eaten w/skin—1 apple, 2½" diam., 171 gm.	90	22.6	.32	•••	•••	144	.048

* Measure and weight apply to whole fruit, including parts not usually eaten; nutritive value given for edible portions only.

Food and Amount	Riboflavin B2 mg.	Niacin mg.	B6 mg.	Folic Acid mg.	PABA mg.	Pantothenic Acid mg.	B12 mcg.
Sturgeon, cooked, steamed—1 piece, 2½" sq. x ⅝", 82 gm.	---	---	NA	NA	NA	NA	NA
Sturgeon, raw—1 piece, 3" x 3" x ¾", 100 gm.	---	---	NA	NA	NA	NA	NA
Sturgeon, smoked—1 slice, 3" x 2" x ⅛", 14 gm.	---	---	NA	NA	NA	NA	NA
Swordfish, cooked, broiled—1 piece, 3" x 3" x ½", 125 gm.	.06	13.62	NA	NA	NA	NA	NA
Swordfish, raw—1 piece, 3" x 3" x ¾", 100 gm.	.05	8.0	NA	NA	NA	NA	NA
Trout—see Lake Trout							
Trout, brook, raw—6" x 2" x ½", 120 gm.	.08	---	NA	NA	NA	NA	NA
Trout, rainbow or steelhead, canned—2½" x 1¾" x ½", 49 gm.	---	---	NA	NA	NA	NA	NA
Trout, rainbow or steelhead, raw—1 pc., 5" x 2" x ½", 116 gm.	.22	9.74	NA	NA	NA	NA	NA
Tuna, bluefin, raw—1 piece, 3" x 4" x ½", 120 gm.	---	---	---	---	NA	---	---
Tuna, canned, in oil, solids and liquid—1 cup, 130 gm.	.11	13.13	.5525	.0026	NA	.416	2.86
Tuna, canned, in oil, drained solids—1 cup, 160 gm.	.19	19.04	---	---	NA	---	---
Tuna, canned, in water, solids and liquid—1 cup, 200 gm.	.20	26.3	NA	NA	NA	NA	NA
Tuna Casserole w/noodles—1 cup, 292 gm.	---	---	NA	NA	NA	NA	NA
Tuna salad—1 cup, 205 gm.	.22	10.25	---	---	NA	---	---
Tuna salad—1 scoop, 60 gm.	.06	3.0	---	---	NA	---	---
Tuna, yellowfin, raw—3" x 4" x ½", 120 gm.	---	---	---	---	NA	---	---
Turtle Soup—1 cup, 246 gm.	---	---	NA	NA	NA	NA	NA
Whitefish, Lake, raw (meat only)—1 piece, 6" x 3" x ⅞", 200 gm.	.24	6	NA	NA	NA	NA	NA
Whitefish, Lake, smoked (meat only)—1 piece, 6" x 3" x ⅞", 178 gm.	---	---	NA	NA	NA	NA	NA

* Where values for "raw" fish or shellfish are given, no information was available on the cooked foods.

FRUITS AND FRUIT PRODUCTS

Food and Amount	Riboflavin B2 mg.	Niacin mg.	B6 mg.	Folic Acid mg.	PABA mg.	Pantothenic Acid mg.	B12 mcg.
Acerola juice, raw—1 cup, 245 gm.	.14	.98	NA	NA	NA	NA	0
Apple, dried, cooked w/o sugar—½ cup, 156 gm.	.05	.156	NA	NA	NA	NA	0
Apple, dried, uncooked—1 cup, 114 gm.	.14	.57	NA	NA	NA	NA	0
*Apple, raw, eaten w/skin—1 apple, 2½" diam., 171 gm.	.032	.16	.048	.0032	NA	.168	0

* Measure and weight apply to whole fruit, including parts not usually eaten; nutritive value given for edible portions only.

Vitamin C mg.	Vitamin D IU	Vitamin E IU	Calcium mg.	Iodine mg.	Iron mg.	Magnesium mg.	Phosphorus mg.	Potassium mg.	Sodium mg.
...	NA	NA	32.8	...	1.64	NA	215.66	192.7	88.56
...	NA	NA	...	.0629 Wash.	...	NA	...	...	...
...	NA	NA	...	...	...	NA	...	...	...
...	NA	NA	33	NA	1.62	NA	343	...	...
...	NA	NA	19	NA	.9	NA	195	...	...
...	NA	NA	...	.002 Wash.	...	NA	319.2	...	...
...	NA	NA	...	...	...	NA	...	...	...
...	NA	NA	...	.028 Wash.	...	NA	...	...	...
...	NA	NA	...	.0456 Pacif.	.156	NA	...	...	...
...	429	NA	7.8	.0208	1.43	...	382	391	1,040
...	392	NA	12.8	.0256	3.04	...	374	...	...
...	470	NA	32	.032	3.02	...	380	558	82
...	NA	NA	...	...	...	NA	...	...	...
2.05	...	NA	41	...	2.66	...	291	...	...
.60	...	NA	12	...	.78	...	85	...	...
...	NA	NA	...	.0408 Pacif.	...	NA	...	...	44.4
...	NA	NA	18	NA	1.3	NA	29	NA	1,098
...	NA	NA	...	.006 L. Erie	.8	NA	540	598	104
...	NA	NA	39.16	NA	...	NA	487.72	...	...

FRUITS AND FRUIT PRODUCTS

Vitamin C mg.	Vitamin D IU	Vitamin E IU	Calcium mg.	Iodine mg.	Iron mg.	Magnesium mg.	Phosphorus mg.	Potassium mg.	Sodium mg.
3,920	0	NA	24.5	NA	1.22	•NA	22.05	...	7.35
trace	0	NA	14	NA	.78	9.36	23.4	252.7	1.56
11.4	0	NA	37	.0010146 Neb.	1.82	25.08	59.3	648.7	5.7
5.7	0	.497	11.2	.0273	.48	12.8	16	176	1.6

Food and Amount	Calories	Carbo-hydrate gm.	Protein gm.	Sat. Fatty Acids gm.	Unsat. Fatty Acids gm.	Vitamin A IU	Thiamin B₁ mg.
*Apple, raw, eaten w/o skin—1 apple, 2½″ diam., 171 gm.	84	22.3	.32	•••	•••	64	.048
Apple butter, canned—1 tablespoon, 20 gm.	37	9.1	.1	•••	•••	0	.002
Apple cider—1 cup, 249 gm.	124	34.4	.2	•••	•••	90	.05
Apple jelly, sweetened—see Sweets, Sugars, Desserts, and Related Products							
Apple juice—1 cup, 248 gm.	120	30	trace	•••	•••	•••	.02
Applesauce, canned, unsweetened—1 cup, 244 gm.	100	26	1	•••	•••	100	.05
Applesauce, canned, w/sugar added—1 cup, 255 gm.	230	61	1	•••	•••	100	.05
Apricot nectar, canned—1 cup, 251 gm.	132.5	36.5	.75	•••	•••	2,375	.025
Apricots, candied—1 avg. (15 to a lb.), 30 gm.	101	26.0	.2	•••	•••	370	trace
Apricots, canned, halves, solids and liquid, heavy syrup—1 cup, 259 gm.	220	57	2	•••	•••	4,510	.05
Apricots, canned, halves, solids and liquid, water pack—1 cup, 240 gm.	91.2	23.04	1.68	•••	•••	4,392	.04
Apricots, dried, uncooked—1 cup (approx. 40 halves), 150 gm.	390	100	8	•••	•••	16,350	.02
Apricots, dried, cooked, solids and liquid, unsweetened—1 cup, 285 gm.	240	62	5	•••	•••	8,550	.01
Apricots, raw—1 apricot, 1¼″ diam., 38 gm.	18.3	4.6	.3	•••	•••	963.3	.01
*Avocado, raw, California variety—1 avocado, 3⅛″ diam., 284 gm.	370	13	5	8.52	39.76	630	.24
*Avocado, raw, Florida variety—1 avocado, 3⅝″ diam., 454 gm.	390	27	4	9.08	40.86	·880	.33
Banana flakes—1 cup, 100 gm.	340	89	4	•••	•••	760	.18
*Bananas, raw, common, 1 banana, medium size, 6½″ x 1½″, 175 gm.	100	26	1	•••	•••	230	.06
Blackberry jam, sweetened—see Sweets, Sugars, Desserts, and Related Products							
Blackberries, canned, solids and liquid, water pack—1 cup, 250 gm.	100	22.5	2	•••	•••	350	.05
Blackberries, canned, solids and liquid, heavy syrup pack—1 cup, 250 gm.	227.5	55.5	2	•••	•••	325	.025
Blackberries, raw (incl. boysenberries, dewberries, youngberries)—½ cup, 75 gm.	42.5	9.5	1	•••	•••	145	.025
Blueberries, canned, solids and liquid, water pack—½ cup, 121 gm.	47	11.9	.6	•••	•••	50	.01
Blueberries, canned, solids and liquid, heavy syrup pack—½ cup, 120 gm.	121	31.2	.5	•••	•••	48	.01
Blueberries, frozen, not thawed, unsweetened—½ cup, 80 gm.	44	10.88	.56	•••	•••	56	.024
Blueberries, raw—½ cup, approx. 75 gm.	42.5	10.5	.5	•••	•••	70	.02
Boysenberries (also blackberries), frozen, not thawed, unsweetened—1 cup, 150 gm.	72	17.1	1.8	•••	•••	255	.03
Boysenberries, raw—see Blackberries, raw							

* Measure and weight apply to whole fruit, including parts not usually eaten; nutritive value given for edible portions only.

Ribo-flavin B_2 mg.	Niacin mg.	B_6 mg.	Folic Acid mg.	PABA mg.	Panto-thenic Acid mg.	B_{12} mcg.	Vitamin C mg.	Vitamin D IU	Vitamin E IU	Calcium mg.	Iodine mg.
.032	.16	NA	NA	NA	NA	0	3.2	0	.497	9.6	NA
.004	.04	NA	NA	NA	NA	0	trace	0	NA	3	NA
.07	trace	NA	NA	NA	NA	0	2	0	NA	15	NA
.05	.2	.075	trace	NA	---	0	2	0	NA	15	NA
.02	.1	---	NA	NA	---	0	2	0	NA	10	.00305 Ohio
.03	.1	.075	NA	NA	.2125	0	3	0	NA	10	NA
.025	.5	---	---	NA	---	0	7.5	0	NA	22.5	NA
.008	.2	NA	NA	NA	NA	0	trace	0	NA	4	NA
.06	.9	.13986	.00259	NA	.23828	0	10	0	NA	28	NA
.04	.96	---	---	NA	---	0	9.6	0	NA	28.8	NA
.23	4.9	.2535	.0075	NA	1.1295	0	19	0	NA	100	NA
.13	2.8	---	---	NA	---	0	8	0	NA	63	NA
.013	.23	.0266	.0014	NA	.0912	0	3.3	0	NA	6	NA
.43	3.5	.1197	.0855	NA	3.0495	0	30	0	NA	22	NA
.61	4.9	2.769	.1362	NA	4.08	0	43	0	NA	30	NA
.24	2.8	---	---	NA	---	0	7	0	---	32	NA
.07	.8	.8925	.0175	.78	.455	0	12	0	.4	10	.0035 Amer.
.05	.5	---	---	NA	---	0	1.75	0	NA	55	NA
.05	.5	.06	.035	NA	.2	0	17.5	0	· NA	52.5	NA
.3	.25	.0375	.0105	NA	.180	0	15	0	NA	23	NA
.01	.2	---	---	NA	---	0	7	0	NA	12	NA
.01	.2	.0468	.00504	NA	.08	0	7	0	NA	11	NA
.048	.4	---	---	NA	---	0	5.6	0	NA	8	NA
.04	.3	.05	.006	NA	.117	0	10	0	NA	10.5	NA
.195	1.5	---	---	NA	---	0	19.5	0	NA	37.5	NA

Food and Amount	Iron mg.	Magnesium mg.	Phosphorus mg.	Potassium mg.	Sodium mg.
*Apple, raw, eaten w/o skin—1 apple, 2½" diam., 171 gm.	.48	8.5	16	176	1.6
Apple butter, canned—1 tablespoon, 20 gm.	.1	NA	4	50.4	.4
Apple cider—1 cup, 249 gm.	1.2	9.96	25	249	10
Apple jelly, sweetened—see Sweets, Sugars, Desserts, and Related Products					
Apple juice—1 cup, 248 gm.	1.5	10	22.5	252.5	2.5
Applesauce, canned, unsweetened—1 cup, 244 gm.	1.2	NA	12.5	195	5
Applesauce, canned, w/sugar added—1 cup, 255 gm.	1.3	12.5	12.5	162.5	5
Apricot nectar, canned—1 cup, 251 gm.	.5	...	30	377.5	trace
Apricots, candied—1 avg. (15 to a lb.), 30 gm.	.3	NA	6	...	...
Apricots, canned, halves, solids and liquid, heavy syrup—1 cup, 259 gm.	.8	18.13	38.8	606	2.59
Apricots, canned, halves, solids and liquid, water pack—1 cup, 240 gm.	.72	16.80	38.4	590.4	2.4
Apricots, dried, uncooked—1 cup (approx. 40 halves), 150 gm.	8.2	93	162	1,468.5	39
Apricots, dried, cooked, solids and liquid, unsweetened—1 cup, 285 gm.	5.1	57	99.75	906.3	22.8
Apricots, raw—1 apricot, 1½" diam., 38 gm.	.17	4.56	8.7	106.8	.38
*Avocado, raw, California variety—1 avocado, 3⅛" diam., 284 gm.	1.3	128.25	119.7	1,721	11.4
*Avocado, raw, Florida variety—1 avocado, 3½" diam., 454 gm.	1.8	204.30	189	2,718	18
Banana flakes—1 cup, 100 gm.	2.8	132	104	1,477	4
*Bananas, raw, common, 1 banana, medium size, 6½" x 1½", 175 gm.	.8	57.75	45.5	647.5	1.75
Blackberry jam, sweetened—see Sweets, Sugars, Desserts, and Related Products					
Blackberries, canned, solids and liquid, water pack—1 cup, 250 gm.	1.8	...	32.5	287.5	2.5
Blackberries, canned, solids and liquid, heavy syrup pack—1 cup, 250 gm.	1.5	...	30	272.5	2.5
Blackberries, raw (incl. boysenberries, dewberries, youngberries)—½ cup, 75 gm.	.65	22.5	14.25	127.5	.75
Blueberries, canned, solids and liquid, water pack—½ cup, 121 gm.	.8	4.84	11	73	1
Blueberries, canned, solids and liquid, heavy syrup pack—½ cup, 120 gm.	.7	4.80	10	66	1
Blueberries, frozen, not thawed, unsweetened—½ cup, 80 gm.	.64	4.8	1,014	64.8	.8
Blueberries, raw—½ cup, approx. 75 gm.	.7	4.5	9.75	60.75	.75
Boysenberries (also blackberries), frozen not thawed, unsweetened—1 cup, 150 gm.	2.4	27	36	229.5	1.5
Boysenberries, raw—see Blackberries, raw					

* Measure and weight apply to whole fruit, including parts not usually eaten; nutritive value given for edible portions only.

Food and Amount	Calories	Carbo-hydrate gm.	Protein gm.	Sat. Fatty Acids gm.	Unsat. Fatty Acids gm.	Vitamin A IU	Thiamin B₁ mg.
*Cantaloupe, raw—½ melon, 5″ diam., 1⅓ lb., 385 gm.	115.5	28.87	2.69	---	---	13,090	.15
Casaba melon, raw—¼ melon, 7″ diam., 390 gm.	105.3	25.35	4.68	NA	NA	117	.15
Cherries, canned, sour, red, solids and liquid, water pack—1 cup, 244 gm.	105	26	2	---	---	1,660	.07
Cherries, canned, sour, red, solids and liquid, heavy syrup pack—1 cup, 250 gm.	222.5	56.75	2	---	---	1,625	.075
Cherries, canned, sweet, solids and liquid, water pack—1 cup, 241 gm.	103.2	25.68	1.92	---	---	1,632	.072
Cherries, canned, sweet, solids and liquid, heavy syrup pack—1 cup, 250 gm.	222.5	56.75	2	---	---	1,625	.075
Cherries, frozen, not thawed, sour, red, unsweetened—½ cup, 125 gm.	68.75	16.75	1.25	---	---	1,250	.05
Cherries, maraschino, bottled, solids and liquid—1 large, 8.3 gm.	9.6	2.45	.016	---	---	---	---
Cherries, raw, sour, red—½ cup, 100 gm.	58	14.3	1.2	---	---	1,000	.05
Cherries, raw, sweet—1 cup, 190 gm.	133	33.06	2.47	---	---	209	.095
Crabapples, raw—1 crabapple, 1½″ diam., 15 gm.	10.2	2.67	.06	---	---	6	.004
Cranberry juice cocktail—1 cup, 250 gm.	165	42	trace	---	---	trace	.03
Cranberry sauce, sweetened, canned, strained—½ cup, 138 gm.	202.5	52	trace	---	---	30	.015
Cranberry sauce, sweetened, home prepared, unstrained—½ cup (scant), 100 gm.	178	45.5	.2	---	---	20	.01
Cranberry jelly—see Sweets, Sugars, Desserts, and Related Products							
Cranberry-orange relish, uncooked—1 tbsp., 12 gm.	21.36	5.44	.04	---	---	8.4	.003
Cranberries, raw—1 cup, 100 gm.	46	10.8	.4	---	---	40	.03
Currants, raw, black European—1 cup, 100 gm.	54	13.1	1.7	---	---	230	.05
Currants, raw, red and white—1 cup, 135 gm.	67.50	16.34	1.89	---	---	162	.054
Dates, dry, pitted, cut—1 cup, 178 gm.	490	130	4	---	---	90	.16
Dewberries—see Blackberries							
Figs, candied—1 piece (15 to a lb.), approx. 30 gm.	90	22.1	1.1	---	---	30	.02
Figs, canned, solids and liquid, water pack—1 cup, 240 gm.	115.2	29.76	1.2	---	---	72	.07
Figs, canned, solids and liquid, heavy syrup pack—½ cup, 125 gm.	105	27.25	.625	---	---	37.5	.0375
Figs, dried, uncooked—1 large, 2″ x 1″, or 3 small, 21 gm.	60	15	1	---	---	20	.02
Figs, raw—1 large, or 4 small (¾″), 50 gm.	40	10.15	.6	NA	NA	40	.03
Fruit cocktail, canned, solids and liquid, water pack—1 cup, 230 gm.	85.1	22.31	.92	---	---	345	.04

* Measure and weight apply to whole fruit, including parts not usually eaten; nutritive value given for edible portions only.

Food and Amount	Ribo-flavin B₂ mg.	Niacin mg.	B₆ mg.	Folic Acid mg.	PABA mg.	Panto-thenic Acid mg.	B₁₂ mcg.
*Cantaloupe, raw—½ melon, 5″ diam., 1⅓ lb., 385 gm.	.11	2.31	.331	.027	NA	.9625	0
Casaba melon, raw—¼ melon, 7″ diam., 390 gm.	.11	2.34	NA	NA	NA	NA	0
Cherries, canned, sour, red, solids and liquid, water pack—1 cup, 244 gm.	.05	.5	---	---	NA	---	0
Cherries, canned, sour, red, solids and liquid, heavy syrup pack—1 cup, 250 gm.	.05	.5	---	---	NA	•---	0
Cherries, canned, sweet, solids and liquid, water pack—1 cup, 241 gm.	.048	.48	---	---	NA	---	0
Cherries, canned, sweet, solids and liquid, heavy syrup pack—1 cup, 250 gm.	.05	.5	.075	.0075	NA	.3	0
Cherries, frozen, not thawed, sour, red, unsweetened—½ cup, 125 gm.	.0875	.375	---	---	NA	---	0
Cherries, maraschino, bottled, solids and liquid—1 large, 8.3 gm.	---	---	NA	NA	NA	NA	0
Cherries, raw, sour, red—½ cup, 100 gm.	.06	.4	.085	.006	NA	.07	0
Cherries, raw, sweet—1 cup, 190 gm.	.114	.76	.0608	.0114	NA	.4959	0
Crabapples, raw—1 crabapple, 1½″ diam., 15 gm.	.003	.015	NA	NA	NA	NA	0
Cranberry juice cocktail—1 cup, 250 gm.	.03	.1	NA	NA	NA	NA	0
Cranberry sauce, sweetened, canned, strained—½ cup, 138 gm.	.015	.05	.03	NA	NA	---	0
Cranberry sauce, sweetened, home prepared, unstrained—½ cup (scant), 100 gm.	.01	.1	.022	NA	NA	---	0
Cranberry jelly—see Sweets, Sugars, Desserts, and Related Products							
Cranberry-orange relish, uncooked—1 tbsp., 12 gm.	.002	.01	NA	NA	NA	NA	0
Cranberries, raw—1 cup, 100 gm.	.02	.1	NA	.002	NA	.2	0
Currants, raw, black European—1 cup, 100 gm.	.05	.3	NA	NA	NA	NA	0
Currants, raw, red and white—1 cup, 135 gm.	.0675	.135	NA	NA	NA	NA	0
Dates, dry, pitted, cut—1 cup, 178 gm.	.17	3.9	.2723	.0445	NA	1.3884	0
Dewberries—see Blackberries							
Figs, candied—1 piece (15 to a lb.), approx. 30 gm.	.02	.1	NA	NA	NA	NA	0
Figs, canned, solids and liquid, water pack—1 cup, 240 gm.	.07	.48	---	NA	NA	---	0
Figs, canned, solids and liquid, heavy syrup pack—½ cup, 125 gm.	.0375	.25	---	NA	NA	.08625	0
Figs, dried, uncooked—1 large, 2″ x 1″, or 3 small, 21 gm.	.02	.1	.03675	.00672	NA	.09135	0
Figs, raw—1 large, or 4 small (¾″), 50 gm.	.025	.2	.0555	.007	NA	.150	0
Fruit cocktail, canned, solids and liquid, water pack—1 cup, 230 gm.	.02	1.15	---	NA	NA	---	0

* Measure and weight apply to whole fruit, including parts not usually eaten; nutritive value given for edible portions only.

Vitamin C mg.	Vitamin D IU	Vitamin E IU	Calcium mg.	Iodine mg.	Iron mg.	Magnesium mg.	Phosphorus mg.	Potassium mg.	Sodium mg.
127.05	0	.539	54.5	.00089 Ohio	1.55	61.60	61.60	966.35	46.20
50.7	0	NA	54.6	NA	1.56	NA	62.4	978.9	46.8
12	0	NA	37	NA	.7	NA	32.5	325	5
12.5	0	NA	35	NA	.75	NA	30	310	2.5
12	0	NA	36	NA	.72	NA	31.2	312	4.8
12.5	0	NA	35	NA	.75	22.5	30	310	2.5
6.25	0	NA	16.25	NA	.875	12.5	27.50	235	2.5
...	0	NA	...	NA	...	NA	...	...	...
10	0	NA	22	NA	.4	14	19	191	2
19	0	NA	41.80	NA	.76	26.6	36.10	362.9	3.8
1.2	0	NA	.9	NA	.04	NA	1.95	16.5	.15
40	0	NA	13	NA	.8	...	7.5	25	2.5
3	0	NA	8.5	NA	.3	2.76	5.52	41.4	1.38
2	0	NA	7	NA	.2	2	5	38	1
2.16	NA	NA	2.28	.NA	.04	NA	.96	8.64	.12
11	0	NA	14	.029	.5	7	10	82	2
200	0	NA	60	NA	1.1	NA	40	372	3
55.35	0	NA	43.2	NA	1.35	20.25	31.05	347	2.7
0	0	NA	105	NA	5.3	103.24	112.14	1,153.4	1.78
trace	0	NA	20	NA	.2	NA	12	...	...
2.4	0	NA	33.6	NA	.96	NA	33.6	372	4.8
1.25	0	NA	16.25	NA	.5	...	16.25	186.25	2.5
0	0	NA	26	trace	.6	14.91	16.17	134.4	7.14
1	0	NA	17.5	.015	.3	10	11	97	1
4.6	0	NA	20.7	NA	.92	16.10	29.9	186.4	11.5

Food and Amount	Calories	Carbo-hydrate gm.	Protein gm.	Sat. Fatty Acids gm.	Unsat. Fatty Acids gm.	Vitamin A IU	Thiamin B₁ mg.
Fruit cocktail, canned, solids and liquid, heavy syrup pack—1 cup, 256 gm.	195	50	1	---	---	360	.05
Fruit salad, bottled "fresh," solids and liquid—1 cup, 280 gm.	98	25.48	1.12	---	---	1,316	.02
Fruit salad, canned, solids and liquid, water pack—1 cup, 270 gm.	94.5	24.57	1.08	---	---	1,269	.02
Fruit salad, canned, solids and liquid, heavy syrup pack—1 cup, 245 gm.	183.75	47.53	.735	---	---	1,102.5	.0245
Gooseberries, canned, solids and liquid, water pack—1 cup, 240 gm.	62.4	15.84	1.2	---	---	480	---
Gooseberries, canned, solids and liquid, heavy syrup pack—1 cup, 240 gm.	216	55.2	1.2	---	---	456	---
Gooseberries, raw—1 cup, 150 gm.	58.50	14.55	1.2	---	---	435	---
Grape juice, canned or bottled—1 cup, 253 gm.	165	42	1	---	---	---	.10
Grape juice, frozen concentrate, diluted w/3 pts. water—1 cup, 250 gm.	135	33	1	---	---	10	.05
Grape juice drink, canned—1 cup, 250 gm.	135	35	trace	---	---	---	.03
Grapefruit, canned, solids and liquid, water pack—½ cup, 100 gm.	30	7.6	.6	---	---	10	.03
Grapefruit, canned, solids and liquid, heavy syrup pack—1 cup, 254 gm.	180	45	2	---	---	30	.08
Grapefruit, raw, white—½ grapefruit, 3¾" diam., 241 gm.	45	12	1	---	---	10	.05
Grapefruit, raw, pink and red—½ grapefruit, 3¾" diam., 241 gm.	50	13	1	---	---	540	.05
Grapefruit juice, canned, white, sweetened—1 cup, 250 gm.	130	32	1	---	---	20	.07
Grapefruit juice, canned, white, unsweetened—1 cup, 247 gm.	100	24	1	---	---	20	.07
Grapefruit juice, fresh—1 cup, 246 gm.	95	23	1	---	---	20 white; 1,080 pink and red	.09
Grapefruit juice, frozen concentrate, diluted w/3 pts. water—1 cup, 247 gm.	100	24	1	---	---	20	.10
Grapefruit juice, dehydrated crystals, prepared w/water, 1 lb. = 1 gal.—1 cup, 247 gm.	100	24	1	---	---	20	.10
Grapes, canned, European green, water pack—½ cup, 100 gm.	51	13.6	.5	---	---	70	.04
Grapes, canned, European green, heavy syrup pack—½ cup, 100 gm.	77	20	.5	---	---	70	.04
Grapes, raw, American** type—1 cup, 153 gm.	65	15	1	---	---	100	.05
Grapes, raw, European† type—1 cup, 160 gm.	95	25	1	---	---	140	.07
Guavas, whole, raw, common—1 medium, 3½ oz., 100 gm.	62	15	.8	---	---	280	.05
Honeydew melon—¼ of small (5" diam.) melon, 100 gm.	33	7.7	.8	---	---	40	.04
Kumquats, raw—1 medium, 20 gm.	13	3.42	.18	---	---	120	.016
Lemon, raw—1 lemon, 2" diam., w/peel, 100 gm.	20	10.7	1.2	---	---	30	.05

** American type grapes are green Catawba, deep purple—Concord, and Delaware.

† European type grapes are green, Thompson seedless, Red Flame, Tokay and Cardinal, and deep red—Emperor.

Ribo-flavin B₂ mg.	Niacin mg.	B₆ mg.	Folic Acid mg.	PABA mg.	Panto-thenic Acid mg.	B₁₂ mcg.	Vitamin C mg.	Vitamin D IU	Vitamin E IU	Calcium mg.	Iodine mg.
.03	1.3	.08448	NA	NA	---	0	5	0	NA	23	NA
.08	1.68	NA	NA	NA	NA	0	8.4	0	NA	22.4	NA
.08	1.62	NA	NA	NA	.NA	0	8.1	0	NA	21.6	NA
.0735	1.47	NA	NA	NA	NA	0	4.9	0	NA	19.6	NA
---	---	NA	NA	NA	NA	0	26.4	0	NA	28.8	NA
---	---	NA	NA	NA	NA	0	24	0	NA	26.4	NA
---	---	NA	NA	NA	NA	0	49.5	0	NA	27	NA
.05	.5	---	---	NA	---	0	trace	0	NA	28	.0002 Ohio
.08	.5	.0525	.0075	NA	.1	0	0	0	NA	8	NA
.03	.3	NA	NA	NA	NA	0	0	0	NA	8	NA
.02	.2	---	---	NA	---	0	30	0	---	13	NA
.05	.5	.0508	---	NA	.3048	0	76	0	---	33	NA
.02	.2	.082	.00723	NA	.682	0	44	0	---	19	.003133
.02	.2	.082	.00723	NA	.682	0	44	0	---	20	NA
.04	.4	.0275	.005	NA	.325	0	78	0	.1	20	NA
.04	.4	.03211	.00469	NA	.41	0	84	0	.09	20	NA
.04	.4	.03458	.00321	NA	.39	0	92	0	---	22	NA
.04	.5	.03458	.0025	NA	.4	0	96	0	NA	25	NA
.05	.5	---	---	NA	---	0	91	0	NA	22	NA
.01	.2	NA	NA	NA	NA	0	2	0	NA	8	NA
.01	.2	NA	NA	NA	NA	0	2	0	NA	8	NA
.03	.2	.1224	.0076	NA	.11475	0	3	0	NA	15	NA
.04	.4	NA	NA	NA	NA	0	6	0	NA	17	NA
.05	1.2	NA	NA	NA	NA	0	242	0	NA	23	NA
.03	.6	.056	.005	NA	.207	0	23	0	NA	14	NA
.02	---	NA	NA	NA	NA	0	7.2	0	NA	12.6	NA
.04	.2	NA	NA	NA	NA	0	77	0	NA	61	NA

Food and Amount	Iron mg.	Magnesium mg.	Phosphorus mg.	Potassium mg.	Sodium mg.
Fruit cocktail, canned, solids and liquid, heavy syrup pack—1 cup, 256 gm.	1.0	17.92	30.72	412.16	12.8
Fruit salad, bottled "fresh," solids and liquid—1 cup, 280 gm.	.84	NA	30.8	389.2	2.8
Fruit salad, canned, solids and liquid, water pack—1 cup, 270 gm.	.81	NA	29.7	375.3	2.7
Fruit salad, canned, solids and liquid, heavy syrup pack—1 cup, 245 gm.	.735	NA	26.95	328.3	2.45
Gooseberries, canned, solids and liquid, water pack—1 cup, 240 gm.	.72	NA	24	252	2.4
Gooseberries, canned, solids and liquid, heavy syrup pack—1 cup, 240 gm.	.72	NA	21.6	235.2	2.4
Gooseberries, raw—1 cup, 150 gm.	.75	13.5	22.5	232.5	1.50
Grape juice, canned or bottled—1 cup, 253 gm.	.8	30.36	30.36	293.48	5.06
Grape juice, frozen concentrate, diluted w/3 pts. water—1 cup, 250 gm.	.3	10	10	85	2.5
Grape juice drink, canned—1 cup, 250 gm.	.3	NA	10	87.5	2.5
Grapefruit, canned, solids and liquid, water pack—½ cup, 100 gm.	.3	11.0	14	144	4
Grapefruit, canned, solids and liquid, heavy syrup pack—1 cup, 254 gm.	.8	27.94	35.56	342.9	2.54
Grapefruit, raw, white—½ grapefruit, 3¾" diam., 241 gm.	.05	28.92	38.56	325.35	2.41
Grapefruit, raw, pink and red—½ grapefruit, 3¾" diam., 241 gm.	.05	28.92	38.56	325.35	2.41
Grapefruit juice, canned, white, sweetened—1 cup, 250 gm.	1.0	---	35	405	2.5
Grapefruit juice, canned, white, unsweetened—1 cup, 247 gm.	1.0	NA	35	405	2.5
Grapefruit juice, fresh—1 cup, 246 gm.	.5	29.52	36.9	398.52	2.46
Grapefruit juice, frozen concentrate, diluted w/3 pts. water—1 cup, 247 gm.	.2	22.23	42	420	2.47
Grapefruit juice, dehydrated crystals, prepared w/water, 1 lb. = 1 gal.—1 cup, 247 gm.	.2	NA	39.5	412.5	2.47
Grapes, canned, European green, water pack—½ cup, 100 gm.	.3	NA	13	110	4
Grapes, canned, European green, heavy syrup pack—½ cup, 100 gm.	.3	NA	13	105	4
Grapes, raw, American** type—1 cup, 153 gm.	.4	19.89	18.36	241.7	4.6
Grapes, raw, European† type—1 cup, 160 gm.	.6	9.6	32	276.8	4.8
Guavas, whole, raw, common—1 medium, 3½ oz., 100 gm.	.9	13	42	289	4
Honeydew melon—⅛ of small (5" diam.) melon, 100 gm.	.4	---	16	251	12
Kumquats, raw—1 medium, 20 gm.	.08	NA	4.6	47.2	1.4
Lemon, raw—1 lemon, 2" diam., w/peel, 100 gm.	.7	NA	15	145	3

** American type grapes are green Catawba, deep purple—Concord, and Delaware. † European type grapes are green, Thompson seedless, Red Flame, Tokay and Cardinal, and deep red—Emperor.

Food and Amount	Calories	Carbo-hydrate gm.	Protein gm.	Sat. Fatty Acids gm.	Unsat. Fatty Acids gm.	Vitamin A IU	Thiamin B₁ mg.
Lemon, raw—1 lemon, 2½" diam., edible portion, peeled, 110 gm.	20	6	1	•••	•••	10	.03
Lemon juice, raw—1 tbsp., 15 gm.	3.75	1.25	.06	•••	•••	3.125	.00437
Lemon juice, canned or bottled, unsweetened—1 tbsp., 15 gm.	3.522	1.16375	.06	•••	•••	3.0625	.0046
Lemon juice, frozen, unsweetened, single strength juice—1 tbsp., 15 gm.	3.3	1.08	.06	•••	•••	3	.004
Lemon peel, candied—1 piece, ½" x ⅜", 1 gm.	3.16	.806	.004	NA	NA	•••	•••
Lemon peel, raw—1" x 1½", 2 gm.	NA	.32	.03	NA	NA	1	.001
Lemonade, frozen concentrate, diluted w/4½ pts. water—1 cup, 248 gm.	110	28	trace	•••	•••	trace	trace
Lime juice, fresh—1 tbsp., 15 gm.	4.06	1.375	.0625	•••	•••	1.25	.0031
Lime juice, canned, unsweetened—1 tbsp., 15 gm.	4.06	1.375	.0625	•••	•••	1.25	.0031
Lime juice, canned, sweetened—1 tbsp., 15 gm.	•••	•••	•••	NA	NA	•••	•••
Limeade, frozen concentrate, diluted w/4½ pts. water—1 cup, 247 gm.	100	27	trace	•••	•••	trace	trace
Limes, acid type, raw—1 lime, 1½" long, 40 gm.	11.2	3.8	.28	•••	•••	4	.01
Loganberries, canned, solids and liquid, water pack—½ cup, 100 gm.	40	9.4	.7	•••	•••	140	.01
Loganberries, canned, solids and liquid, heavy syrup pack—½ cup, 100 gm.	89	22.2	.6	•••	•••	130	.01
Loganberries, raw—1 cup, 150 gm.	93	22.35	1.5	•••	•••	300	.045
Mandarin oranges—see Tangerines							
Mangos, raw—1 medium, 198 gm.	130.68	33.264	1.386	•••	•••	9,504	.099
Melon balls, cantaloupe and honeydew, frozen, not thawed, heavy syrup pack—½ cup, 114 gm.	70.68	17.898	.684	•••	•••	1,756	.0342
Nectarines, raw—2" diam. 125 gm.	80	21.37	.75	•••	•••	2,062.5	•••
Oranges, fresh, peeled—1 section, 2¼" x ⁵⁄₁₆", 24 gm.	10.29	2.56	.21	•••	•••	42	.02
Orange juice, fresh—1 cup, 248 gm.	110	26	2	•••	•••	500	.22
Orange juice, canned, sweetened—1 cup, 250 gm.	130	30.5	1.75	•••	•••	500	.175
Orange juice, canned, concentrated, unsweetened, diluted w/5 pts. water—1 cup, 248 gm.	114.08	25.54	1.98	•••	•••	496	.19
Orange juice, canned, unsweetened—1 cup, 249 gm.	120	28	2	•••	•••	500	.17
Orange juice, frozen concentrate, unsweetened, diluted w/3 pts. water—1 cup, 249 gm.	120	29	2	•••	•••	550	.22
Orange juice, dehydrated crystals, prepared w/water, 1 lb. = 1 gal.—1 cup, 248 gm.	115	27	2	•••	•••	500	.20
Orange peel, candied—½" x 1", 1 gm.	3.16	.806	.004	NA	NA	•••	•••
Orange peel, raw—1" x 1½", 3 gm.	NA	.75	.045	NA	NA	12.6	.003
Orange-cranberry relish—see Cranberry-orange relish							

Food and Amount	Ribo-flavin B₂ mg.	Niacin mg.	B₆ mg.	Folic Acid mg.	PABA mg.	Panto-thenic Acid mg.	B₁₂ mcg.
Lemon, raw—1 lemon, 2½″ diam., edible portion, peeled, 110 gm.	.01	.1	NA	NA	NA	NA	0
Lemon juice, raw—1 tbsp., 15 gm.	.00125	.0125	.007	.00015	NA	.0157	0
Lemon juice, canned or bottled, unsweetened—1 tbsp., 15 gm.	.0015	.0153	.00765	.00003	NA	---	0
Lemon juice, frozen, unsweetened, single strength juice—1 tbsp., 15 gm.	.001	.015	.007	.00015	NA	.0157	0
Lemon peel, candied—1 piece, ½″ x ¾″, 1 gm.	---	---	NA	NA	NA	NA	0
Lemon peel, raw—1″ x 1½″, 2 gm.	.001	.008	NA	NA	NA	NA	0
Lemonade, frozen concentrate, diluted w/4⅓ pts. water—1 cup, 248 gm.	.02	.2	.0124	NA	NA	.02728	0
Lime juice, fresh—1 tbsp., 15 gm.	.00125	.0125	---	NA	NA	---	0
Lime juice, canned, unsweetened—1 tbsp., 15 gm.	.00125	.0125	---	NA	NA	---	0
Lime juice, canned, sweetened—1 tbsp., 15 gm.	---	---	---	NA	NA	.0471	0
Limeade, frozen concentrate, diluted w/4⅓ pts. water—1 cup, 247 gm.	trace	trace	NA	NA	NA	NA	0
Limes, acid type, raw—1 lime, 1½″ long, 40 gm.	.008	.08	NA	NA	NA	NA	0
Loganberries, canned, solids and liquid, water pack—½ cup, 100 gm.	.02	.2	NA	NA	NA	NA	0
Loganberries, canned, solids and liquid, heavy syrup pack—½ cup, 100 gm.	.02	.2	NA	NA	NA	NA	0
Loganberries, raw—1 cup, 150 gm.	.06	.6	NA	NA	NA	NA	0
Mandarin oranges—see Tangerines							
Mangos, raw—1 medium, 198 gm.	.099	2.178	NA	NA	NA	NA	0
Melon balls, cantaloupe and honeydew, frozen, not thawed, heavy syrup pack—½ cup, 114 gm.	.0228	.57	NA	NA	NA	NA	0
Nectarines, raw—2″ diam. 125 gm.	---	---	.02125	.025	NA	---	0
Oranges, fresh, peeled—1 section, 2¼″ x ⅝″, 24 gm.	.0084	.08	.0144	.0012	NA	.06	0
Orange juice, fresh—1 cup, 248 gm.	.07	1.0	.0992	.00496	NA	.4712	0
Orange juice, canned, sweetened—1 cup, 250 gm.	.05	.75	---	---	NA	---	0
Orange juice, canned, concentrated, unsweetened, diluted w/5 pts. water—1 cup, 248 gm.	.04	.74	---	---	NA	---	0
Orange juice, canned, unsweetened—1 cup, 249 gm.	.05	.7	.08715	.005	NA	.3735	0
Orange juice, frozen concentrate, unsweetened, diluted w/3 pts. water—1 cup, 249 gm.	.02	1.0	.06972	.00498	NA	.40836	0
Orange juice, dehydrated crystals, prepared w/water, 1 lb. = 1 gal.—1 cup, 248 gm.	.07	1.0	---	---	NA	---	0
Orange peel, candied—½″ x ½″, 1 gm.	---	---	NA	NA	NA	NA	0
Orange peel, raw—1″ x 1½″, 3 gm.	.002	.027	NA	NA	NA	NA	0
Orange-cranberry relish—see Cranberry-orange relish							

Vitamin C mg.	Vitamin D IU	Vitamin E IU	Calcium mg.	Iodine mg.	Iron mg.	Magnesium mg.	Phosphorus mg.	Potassium mg.	Sodium mg.
39	0	NA	19	NA	.4	NA	17.6	151.8	2.2
7	0	NA	1.06	.0008	.0312	1.22	1.525	21.5025	.1525
6.43125	0	NA	1.0719	NA	.0306	NA	1.53125	21.5906	.1531
6.6	0	NA	1.05	NA	.04	1.05	1.35	21.15	.15
...	0	NA	...	NA	...	NA	...	...	...
2.58	0	NA	2.68	NA	.016	...	.24	3.2	.12
17	0	NA	2	.0017 Ohio	trace	2.48	2.48	39.68	trace
4.9375	0	NA	1.375	NA	.03125	...	1.69125	15.9875	.15375
1.25	0	NA	1.375	NA	.03125	...	1.69125	15.9875	.15375
...	0	NA	...	NA	...	...	...	...	...
5	0	NA	2	NA	trace	...	2.47	32.11	trace
14.8	0	NA	13.2	NA	.24	NA	7.2	40.8	.8
8	0	NA	24	NA	.8	NA	11	115	1
8	0	NA	22	NA	.8	NA	11	109	1
36	0	NA	52.5	NA	1.8	37.5	25.5	255	1.5
69.3	0	NA	19.8	NA	.792	NA	25.74	374.2	13.86
18.24	0	NA	11.4	NA	3.42	NA	13.68	214.32	10.26
16.25	0	NA	5	NA	.62	16.25	30	367.5	7.5
10.5	0	...	8.61	...	.08	2.64	4.2	42	.21
124	0	.0992	27	.00372	.5	27.28	42.16	496	2.48
100	0	NA	25	NA	1	NA	45	497.5	2.5
116.56	0	NA	24.8	NA	.74	29.76	44.64	476.16	2.48
100	0	NA	25	NA	1.0	...	44.82	495.51	2.49
120	0	NA	25	NA	.2	24.9	39.84	463.14	2.49
109	0	NA	25	NA	.5	NA	39.68	518.32	2.48
...	0	NA	...	NA	...	NA	...	...	...
4.08	0	NA	4.83	NA	.024	...	.63	6.36	.09

Food and Amount	Calories	Carbo-hydrate gm.	Protein gm.	Sat. Fatty Acids gm.	Unsat. Fatty Acids gm.	Vitamin A IU	Thiamin B₁ mg.
Oranges, fresh, peeled—1 orange, 2⅝″ diam., 180 gm.	65	16	1	---	---	260	.13
Papaya, raw—1 whole papaya—300 gm.	117	30	1.8	---	---	5 250	.12
Papaya, raw, ½″ cubes—1 cup, 182 gm.	70	18	1	---	---	3,190	.07
Peaches, yellow flesh, canned, solids and liquid, halves or slices, heavy syrup pack—1 cup, 257 gm.	200	52	1	---	---	1,100	.02
Peaches, yellow flesh, canned, solids and liquid, water pack—1 cup, 245 gm.	75	20	1	---	---	1,100	.02
Peaches, dried, uncooked—1 cup, 160 gm.	420	109	5	---	---	6,240	.02
Peaches, dried, cooked, w/o added sugar—1 cup, 270 gm.	220	58	3	---	---	3,290	.01
Peaches, sliced, frozen, not thawed, sweetened—1 cup, 250 gm.	220	56.5	1	---	---	1,625	.025
*Peaches, raw—1 whole peach, 2″ diam., 114 gm.	35	10	1	---	---	1,320 yel. flesh	.02
Peaches, raw, slices—1 cup, 168 gm.	65	16	1	---	---	2,230 yel. flesh	.03
Pear nectar, canned—1 cup, 250 gm.	130	33	.75	---	---	trace	trace
*Pears, raw—1 pear, 3″ x 2½″ diam., 182 gm.	100	25	1	---	---	30	.04
Pears, candied—1 piece, 2″ x 1 x ½″, 75 gm.	227.25	56.92	.97	NA	NA	---	---
Pears, canned, solids and liquid, heavy syrup pack—1 cup, 255 gm.	195	50	1	---	---	trace	.03
Pears, canned, solids and liquid, water pack—1 cup, 250 gm.	80	20.75	.5	---	---	trace	.025
Pears, dried, uncooked—4 halves, 75 gm.	201	50.47	2.32	---	---	52.5	.007
Pears, dried, cooked, unsweetened— 1 cup, 304 gm.	383.04	96.36	4.56	---	---	91.2	trace
Persimmons, raw, Japanese or Kaki— 1 med., 2½″ diam., 125 gm.	96.25	24.62	.875	---	---	3,387.5	.0375
Persimmons, raw, native—1 med., 1¼″ diam., 75 gm.	95.25	25.12	.60	NA	NA	---	---
Pineapple, candied—1 slice, 50 gm.	158	40	.4	---	---	---	---
Pineapple, canned, heavy syrup pack, crushed—1 cup, 260 gm.	195	50	1	---	---	120	.20
Pineapple, canned, slices and juice, heavy syrup pack—2 slices w/juice, 122 gm.	90	24	trace	---	---	50	.09
Pineapple, canned, all styles except crushed, water pack—½ cup, 125 gm.	48.75	12.75	.375	---	---	62.50	10.00
Pineapple, frozen chunks, sweetened, not thawed—½ cup, 130 gm.	110.5	28.86	.52	---	---	39	.130
Pineapple, raw—1 slice, 4½″ x ⅜″, 72 gm.	37.44	9.86	.28	---	---	50.4	.06
Pineapple, raw, diced—1 cup, 140 gm.	75	19	1	---	---	100	.12
Pineapple juice, canned, unsweetened— 1 cup, 249 gm.	135	34	1	---	---	120	.12

* Measure and weight apply to whole fruit, including parts not usually eaten; nutritive value given for edible portions only.

Riboflavin B$_2$ mg.	Niacin mg.	B$_6$ mg.	Folic Acid mg.	PABA mg.	Pantothenic Acid mg.	B$_{12}$ mcg.	Vitamin C mg.	Vitamin D IU	Vitamin E IU	Calcium mg.	Iodine mg.
.05	.5	.108	.009	NA	.45	0	66	0	---	54	.0288
.12	.9	NA	NA	NA	NA	0	168	0	NA	60	NA
.08	.5	NA	NA	NA	NA	0	102	0	NA	36	NA
.06	1.4	.04883	.00257	NA	.1285	0	7	0	NA	10	NA
.06	1.4	.04655	.00245	NA	.1225	0	7	0	NA	10	.004 Ohio
.31	8.5	.160	.008	NA	---	0	28	0	NA	77	.0026 S. Car.
.15	4.2	---	---	NA	---	0	6	0	NA	41	NA
.1	1.75	.045	.010	NA	.330	0	27.5	0	NA	10	NA
.05	1.0	.02736	.00456	NA	.1938	0	7	0	NA	9	NA
.08	1.6	.04032	.00672	NA	.2856	0	12	0	NA	15	NA
.05	trace	NA	NA	NA	NA	0	trace	0	NA	7.5	NA
.07	.2	.03094	.00364	NA	.1274	0	7	0	NA	13	NA
---	---	NA	NA	NA	NA	0	---	0	NA	---	NA
.05	.3	.0357	NA	NA	.0561	0	4	0	NA	13	NA
.05	.3	---	NA	NA	---	0	2.5	0	NA	12.5	.00055 Ohio
.13	.45	NA	NA	NA	NA	0	5.25	0	NA	26.25	NA
.24	.91	NA	NA	NA	NA	0	6.08	0	NA	48.64	NA
.0250	.125	NA	NA	NA	NA	0	13.75	0	NA	7.5	NA
---	---	NA	NA	NA	NA	0	49.5	0	NA	20.25	NA
---	---	NA	NA	NA	NA	0	---	0	NA	---	NA
.06	.5	.1924	.0026	---	.260	0	17	0	NA	29	NA
.03	.2	.09028	.00122	---	.122	0	8	0	NA	13	NA
.025	.25	---	---	---	---	0	8.75	0	NA	15	.00275
.039	.39	---	---	---	---	0	10.4	0	NA	11.7	NA
.02	.14	.06336	.00432	---	.1152	0	12.24	0	NA	12.24	NA
.04	.3	.1232	.0084	---	.224	0	24	0	NA	24	NA
.04	.5	.23904	.00249	.44	.249	0	22	0	NA	37	NA

Food and Amount	Iron mg.	Mag-nesium mg.	Phos-phorus mg.	Potas-sium mg.	Sodium mg.
Oranges, fresh, peeled—1 orange, 2⅝″ diam., 180 gm.	.5	19.8	36	360	1.8
Papaya, raw—1 whole papaya—300 gm.	.9	- - -	48	702	9
Papaya, raw, ½″ cubes—1 cup, 182 gm.	.5	- - -	29.12	425.88	5.46
Peaches, yellow flesh, canned, solids and liquid, halves or slices, heavy syrup pack—1 cup, 257 gm.	.8	15.42	30.84	334.1	5.14
Peaches, yellow flesh, canned, solids and liquid, water pack—1 cup, 245 gm.	.7	14.7	31.85	335.65	4.9
Peaches, dried, uncooked—1 cup, 160 gm.	9.6	76.80	187.2	1,520	25.6
Peaches, dried, cooked, w/o added sugar—1 cup, 270 gm.	5.1	40.50	99.9	801.9	13.5
Peaches, sliced, frozen, not thawed, sweetened—1 cup, 250 gm.	1.25	15	32.5	310	5
*Peaches, raw—1 whole peach, 2″ diam., 114 gm.	.5	11.4	21.66	230.28	1.14
Peaches, raw, slices—1 cup, 168 gm.	.8	16.8	31.92	339.36	1.68
Pear nectar, canned—1 cup, 250 gm.	.25	- - -	12.5	97.5	2.5
*Pears, raw—1 pear, 3″ x 2½″ diam., 182 gm.	.5	12.74	20.02	236.6	3.64
Pears, candied—1 piece, 2″ x 1 x ½″, 75 gm.	- - -	- - -	- - -	- - -	- - -
Pears, canned, solids and liquid, heavy syrup pack—1 cup, 255 gm.	.5	12.75	17.5	210	2.55
Pears, canned, solids and liquid, water pack—1 cup, 250 gm.	.5	12.50	17.5	220	2.5
Pears, dried, uncooked—4 halves, 75 gm.	.97	23.25	36	430	5.25
Pears, dried, cooked, unsweetened—1 cup, 304 gm.	1.82	45.6	69.92	817.76	9.12
Persimmons, raw, Japanese or Kaki—1 med., 2½″ diam., 125 gm.	.375	10	32.50	217.5	7.5
Persimmons, raw, native—1 med., 1¾″ diam., 75 gm.	1.87	NA	19.5	232.5	.75
Pineapple, candied—1 slice, 50 gm.	- - -	NA	- - -	- - -	- - -
Pineapple, canned, heavy syrup pack, crushed—1 cup, 260 gm.	.8	20.8	13	249.6	2.6
Pineapple, canned, slices and juice, heavy syrup pack—2 slices w/juice, 122 gm.	.4	9.76	6.1	117.12	1.22
Pineapple, canned, all styles except crushed, water pack—½ cup, 125 gm.	.375	NA	6.25	123.75	1.25
Pineapple, frozen chunks, sweetened, not thawed—½ cup, 130 gm.	.52	NA	5.2	130	2.6
Pineapple, raw—1 slice, 4½″ x ¾″, 72 gm.	.36	9.36	5.76	105.12	.72
Pineapple, raw, diced—1 cup, 140 gm.	.7	18.2	11.2	204.4	1.4
Pineapple juice, canned, unsweetened—1 cup, 249 gm.	.7	29.88	22.41	371.01	2.49

* Measure and weight apply to whole fruit, including parts not usually eaten; nutritive value given for edible portions only.

Food and Amount	Calories	Carbo-hydrate gm.	Protein gm.	Sat. Fatty Acids gm.	Unsat. Fatty Acids gm.	Vitamin A IU	Thiamin B₁ mg.
Pineapple juice, frozen concentrate, diluted w/3 pts. water, unsweetened—1 cup, 250 gm.	130	32	1	•••	•••	25	.17
Plantain (baking banana), raw—1 small (5″ long), 100 gm.	119	31.2	1.1	•••	•••	10—white 1,200—yellow	.06
Plums, canned (Italian prunes), solids and liquid, heavy syrup pack—1 cup, 256 gm.	205	53	1	•••	•••	2,970	.05
Plums, canned (Italian prunes), solids and liquid, water pack—½ cup, 125 gm.	57.5	14.875	.5	•••	•••	1,562.5	.025
Plums, raw, all types except prune—1 plum, 2″ diam., 60 gm.	25	7	trace	•••	•••	140	.02
Pomegranate pulp, raw—1 tbsp., 14 gm.	8.82	2.29	.07	•••	•••	trace	.004
Prune juice, canned or bottled—1 cup, 256 gm.	200	49	1	•••	•••	•••	.03
Prunes, dehydrated, uncooked—1 large, 12 gm.	41.28	10.95	.396	•••	•••	260.4	.0144
Prunes, dried, "softenized," uncooked—1 medium prune, 8 gm.	17.5	4.5	.25	•••	•••	110	.005
Prunes, dried, "softenized," cooked (solids and liquid), unsweetened—1 cup, 270 gm.	295	78	2	•••	•••	1,860	.08
Prickly pear, fresh and raw—1 piece, 2″ x 1″ x 1″, 80 gm.	33.6	8.72	.4	•••	•••	48	.009
Quinces, raw—1 quince, 3″ x 2½″, 240 gm.	136.8	36.72	.96	•••	•••	96	.04
Raisins, seedless, raw—1 package, ½ oz. or 1½ tbsp., 14 gm.	40	11	trace	•••	•••	trace	.02
Raisins, seedless, raw—1 cup (pressed down), 165 gm.	480	128	4	•••	•••	30	.18
Raspberries, canned, red, solids and liquid, water pack—1 cup, 200 gm.	70	17.6	1.4	•••	•••	180	.02
Raspberries, canned, black, solids and liquid, water pack—1 cup, 200 gm.	102	21.4	2.2	•••	•••	trace	.02
Raspberries, red, frozen, sweetened, not thawed—½ cup, 123 gm.	121	30.3	.8	•••	•••	86	.02
Raspberries, raw, black—1 cup, 150 gm.	109.5	23.5	2.25	•••	•••	trace	.045
Raspberries, raw, red—1 cup, 123 gm.	70	17	1	•••	•••	160	.04
Rhubarb, raw, cubed—1 cup, 125 gm.	20	4.625	.75	•••	•••	125	.0375
Rhubarb, cooked, sugar added—1 cup, 150 gm.	211	54	.75	•••	•••	120	.03
Rhubarb, frozen, sweetened, not thawed—1 cup, 264 gm.	377.5	95.56	1.32	•••	•••	184.8	.0528
Strawberries, canned, solids and liquid, water pack—1 cup, 260 gm.	57.2	14.56	1.04	•••	•••	104	.026
Strawberries, frozen, sweetened, not thawed, whole—½ cup, 122 gm.	112	28.7	.5	•••	•••	37	.02
Strawberries, raw—1 cup, 149 gm.	55	13	1	•••	•••	90	.04
Tangerine juice, raw—1 cup, 250 gm.	107.5	25.25	1.25	•••	•••	1,050	.15
Tangerine juice, canned, unsweetened—1 cup, 250 gm.	107.5	25.5	1.25	•••	•••	1,050	.15

Food and Amount	Riboflavin B_2 mg.	Niacin mg.	B_6 mg.	Folic Acid mg.	PABA mg.	Pantothenic Acid mg.	B_{12} mcg.
Pineapple juice, frozen concentrate, diluted w/3 pts. water, unsweetened—1 cup, 250 gm.	.05	.50	---	---	NA	---	0
Plantain (baking banana), raw—1 small (5" long), 100 gm.	.04	.6	NA	NA	NA	NA	0
Plums, canned (Italian prunes), solids and liquid, heavy syrup pack—1 cup, 256 gm.	.05	.9	.06912	.00256	NA	.18432	0
Plums, canned (Italian prunes), solids and liquid, water pack—½ cup, 125 gm.	.025	.5	---	---	NA	---	0
Plums, raw, all types except prune—1 plum, 2" diam., 60 gm.	.02	.3	.0312	NA	NA	.1116	0
Pomegranate pulp, raw—1 tbsp., 14 gm.	.004	.04	NA	NA	NA	NA	0
Prune juice, canned or bottled—1 cup, 256 gm.	.03	1.0	NA	NA	NA	NA	0
Prunes, dehydrated, uncooked—1 large, 12 gm.	.0264	.252	---	---	NA	---	0
Prunes, dried, "softenized," uncooked—1 medium prune, 8 gm.	.01	.1	.0192	.0004	NA	.0368	0
Prunes, dried, "softenized," cooked (solids and liquid), unsweetened—1 cup, 270 gm.	.18	1.7	---	---	NA	---	0
Prickly pear, fresh and raw—1 piece, 2" x 1" x 1", 80 gm.	.02	.32	NA	NA	NA	NA	0
Quinces, raw—1 quince, 3" x 2½", 240 gm.	.07	.48	NA	NA	NA	NA	0
Raisins, seedless, raw—1 package, ½ oz. or 1½ tbsp., 14 gm.	.01	.1	.03316	.0014	NA	.0063	0
Raisins, seedless, raw—1 cup (pressed down), 165 gm.	.13	.8	.396	.0165	NA	.07425	0
Raspberries, canned, red, solids and liquid, water pack—1 cup, 200 gm.	.08	1	---	---	NA	---	0
Raspberries, canned, black, solids and liquid, water pack—1 cup, 200 gm.	.08	1	NA	NA	NA	NA	0
Raspberries, red, frozen, sweetened, not thawed—½ cup, 123 gm.	.07	.7	.04674	.00615	NA	.3321	0
Raspberries, raw, black—1 cup, 150 gm.	.135	1.35	NA	NA	NA	NA	0
Raspberries, raw, red—1 cup, 123 gm.	.11	1.1	.0738	.00615	NA	.2952	0
Rhubarb, raw, cubed—1 cup, 125 gm.	.0875	.375	---	---	NA	---	0
Rhubarb, cooked, sugar added—1 cup, 150 gm.	.07	.45	.0435	.006	NA	.1	0
Rhubarb, frozen, sweetened, not thawed—1 cup, 264 gm.	.1056	.528	---	---	NA	---	0
Strawberries, canned, solids and liquid, water pack—1 cup, 260 gm.	.078	1.04	---	---	NA	---	0
Strawberries, frozen, sweetened, not thawed, whole—½ cup, 122 gm.	.07	.6	.05246	.01098	NA	.1647	0
Strawberries, raw—1 cup, 149 gm.	.10	1.0	.08195	.01341	NA	.5066	0
Tangerine juice, raw—1 cup, 250 gm.	.05	.25	---	NA	NA	---	0
Tangerine juice, canned, unsweetened—1 cup, 250 gm.	.05	.25	.08	NA	NA	---	0

Vitamin C mg.	Vitamin D IU	Vitamin E IU	Calcium mg.	Iodine mg.	Iron mg.	Magnesium mg.	Phosphorus mg.	Potassium mg.	Sodium mg.
30	0	NA	27.5	NA	.75	22.50	20	340	2.5
14	0	NA	7	NA	.7	NA	30	385	5
4	0	NA	22	NA	2.2	12.8	25.6	363.52	2.56
2.5	0	NA	11.25	NA	1.25	NA	12.5	185	2.50
3	0	NA	7	.0003 Ohio	.3	5.4	9	141	.9
.56	0	NA	.42	NA	.04	NA	1.12	36.26	.42
5	0	NA	36	NA	10.5	25.6	51.2	601.6	5.12
.48	0	NA	10.8	NA	.528	NA	12.84	112.8	1.32
.25	0	NA	3.5	trace Ore.	.275	3.2	6.32	55.52	.64
2	0	NA	60	.00135 Ohio	4.5	54	99.9	882.9	10.8
17.6	0	NA	16	NA	.24	NA	22.4	132.8	1.6
36	0	NA	26.4	NA	1.68	NA	40.8	473	9.6
trace	0	NA	9	trace Eur.	.5	4.9	14.14	106.82	3.78
2	0	NA	102	.00053 Eur.	5.8	57.75	166.65	1,258.95	44.55
18	0	NA	30	NA	1.2	26	30	228	2
12	0	NA	40	NA	1.2	NA	30	270	2
26	0	NA	16	NA	.7	13.53	21	123	1
27	0	NA	.45	NA	1.35	45	33	298.5	1.5
31	0	NA	27	NA	1.1	24.6	27.06	206.64	1.23
11.25	0	NA	120	NA	1	20	22.5	313.75	2.5
9	0	NA	117	NA	.9	19.5	22.5	304	3
15.84	0	NA	205.9	NA	1.848	11.68	31.68	464.64	7.92
52	0	---	36.4	NA	1.82	NA	36.4	288.6	2.6
67	0	.2562	16	NA	.7	10.98	20	127	1
88	0	.1937	31	NA	1.5	17.88	31.29	244.36	1.49
77.5	0	NA	45	NA	.5	---	35	445	2.5
77.5	0	NA	45	NA	.5	---	35	445	2.5

Food and Amount	Calories	Carbo-hydrate gm.	Protein gm.	Sat. Fatty Acids gm.	Unsat. Fatty Acids gm.	Vitamin A IU	Thiamin B₁ mg.
Tangerine juice, canned, sweetened—1 cup, 249 gm.	125	30	1	---	---	1,050	.15
Tangerine juice, frozen concentrate, unsweetened, diluted, 3 pts. water—1 cup, 250 gm.	115	27	1.25	---	---	1,025	.15
*Tangerines, raw, medium size—1 tangerine, 2½" diam., 116 gm.	40	10	1	---	---	360	.05
Watermelon, raw—1 wedge, 4" x 8", 925 gm.	115	27	2	---	---	2,510	.13
Watermelon, raw, diced—1 cup,158 gm.	41.08	10.112	.79	---	---	932.2	.0474
Youngberries—see Blackberries							

* Measure and weight apply to whole fruit, including parts not usually eaten; nutritive value given for edible portions only.

GRAINS, CEREALS, AND RELATED PRODUCTS

Food and Amount	Calories	Carbo-hydrate gm.	Protein gm.	Sat. Fatty Acids gm.	Unsat. Fatty Acids gm.	Vitamin A IU	Thiamin B₁ mg.
Alimentary pastes—see Macaroni, Noodles, Spaghetti							
Bagels, egg—1 bagel, 3" diam., 55 gm.	165	28	6	---	---	30	.14
Bagels, water—1 bagel, 3" diam., 55 gm.	165	30	6	---	---	0	.15
Barley, pearled, light, uncooked—1 cup, 200 gm.	700	158	16	trace	2	0	.24
Barley, pearled, Pot or Scotch, uncooked—1 tbsp., 14 gm.	49	11	1.3	trace	NA	0	.02
Biscuit dough, commercial, w/enriched flour, chilled in cans—1 piece, 2" x ½", 40 gm.	110.8	18.56	2.92	---	---	trace	.1
Biscuit dough, commercial, w/enriched flour, frozen—1 piece, 2" diam. x ⅓", 38 gm.	124.26	18.58	2.16	---	---	trace	.08
Biscuits, baking powder, from home recipe, made w/enriched flour—1 biscuit, 2" diam., 35 gm.	129	16	2.6	1.4	4.2	trace	.07
Biscuits, baking powder, from home recipe, made w/unenriched flour—1 biscuit, 2" diam., 35 gm.	129	16	2.6	1.4	4.2	trace	.014
Biscuits, baking powder, from home recipe, made w/self-rising flour, enriched—one 2" biscuit, 35 gm.	130	16.1	2.5	1.4	4.2	trace	.08
Biscuits, baking powder, made from mix, with enriched flour, made with milk—1 biscuit, 2" diam., 28 gm.	90	15	2	1	2	trace	.08
Boston Brown Bread—1 slice, 3" x ¾", 48 gm.	100	22	3	NA	NA	0	.05
Bran, plain, prepared—1 cup, 60 gm.	144	44.6	7.6	NA	NA	0	.06
Bran, added sugar and malt extract—1 tbsp., 3 gm.	7.2	2.22	.37	NA	NA	0	.003
Bran, added sugar and defatted wheat germ—1 tbsp., 3 gm.	7.14	2.36	.32	NA	NA	0	.008
Branflakes (40% bran), added thiamin and iron—1 cup, 35 gm.	105	28	4	---	---	0	.14

Ribo-flavin B_2 mg.	Niacin mg.	B_6 mg.	Folic Acid mg.	PABA mg.	Panto-thenic Acid mg.	B_{12} mcg.	Vitamin C mg.	Vitamin D IU	Vitamin E IU	Calcium mg.	Iodine mg.
.05	.2	---	NA	NA	---	0	55	0	NA	45	NA
.05	.25	---	NA	NA	---	0	67.5	0	NA	45	NA
.02	.1	.07772	.00812	NA	.232	0	27	0	NA	34	NA
.13	.7	.629	.00925	NA	2.775	0	30	0	NA	30	NA
.0474	.316	.10744	.00158	NA	.474	0	11.06	0	NA	11.06	NA

GRAINS, CEREALS, AND RELATED PRODUCTS

Ribo-flavin B_2 mg.	Niacin mg.	B_6 mg.	Folic Acid mg.	PABA mg.	Panto-thenic Acid mg.	B_{12} mcg.	Vitamin C mg.	Vitamin D IU	Vitamin E IU	Calcium mg.	Iodine mg.
.10	1.2	NA	NA	NA	NA	NA	0	NA	NA	9	NA
.11	1.4	NA	NA	NA	NA	0	0	NA	NA	8	NA
.10	6.2	.448	---	NA	1.0	0	0	NA	7.6	32	.0146
.009	.51	NA	NA	NA	NA	0	0	NA	NA	5	NA
.06	.84	NA	NA	NA	NA	NA	0	NA	NA	21.2	NA
.06	.64	NA	NA	NA	NA	NA	trace	NA	NA	26.98	NA
.07	.6	NA	NA	NA	NA	NA	trace	NA	NA	42	NA
.04	.2	NA	NA	NA	NA	NA	trace	NA	NA	42	NA
.08	.7	NA	NA	NA	NA	NA	trace	NA	NA	73	NA
.07	.6	NA	NA	NA	NA	NA	trace	NA	NA	19	NA
.03	.6	NA	NA	NA	NA	NA	0	NA	NA	43	NA
.174	10.7	.828	.117	NA	1.8	0	trace	0	NA	42	NA
.008	.53	NA	NA	NA	NA	0	trace	0	NA	2.10	NA
.006	.42	NA	NA	NA	NA	0	0	0	NA	2.19	NA
.06	2.2	.134	NA	NA	.306	0	0	0	NA	25	NA

Food and Amount	Iron mg.	Mag-nesium mg.	Phos-phorus mg.	Potas-sium mg.	Sodium mg.
Tangerine juice, canned, sweetened—1 cup, 249 gm.	.5	---	34.86	443.22	2.49
Tangerine juice, frozen concentrate, unsweetened, diluted, 3 pts. water—1 cup, 250 gm.	.5	---	35	435	250
*Tangerines, raw, medium size—1 tangerine, 2¾" diam., 116 gm.	.3	---	20.88	146.16	2.32
Watermelon, raw—1 wedge, 4"x 8", 925 gm.	2.1	74	92.5	925	9.25
Watermelon, raw, diced—1 cup,158 gm.	.79	12.64	15.8	158	1.58
Youngberries—see Blackberries					

* Measure and weight apply to whole fruit, including parts not usually eaten; nutritive value given for edible portions only.

GRAINS, CEREALS, AND RELATED PRODUCTS

Food and Amount	Iron mg	Mag-nesium mg.	Phos-phorus mg.	Potas-sium mg.	Sodium mg.
Alimentary pastes—see Macaroni, Noodles, Spaghetti					
Bagels, egg—1 bagel, 3" diam., 55 gm.	1.2	NA	NA	NA	NA
Bagels, water—1 bagel, 3" diam., 55 gm.	1.2	NA	NA	NA	NA
Barley, pearled, light, uncooked—1 cup, 200 gm.	4.0	74	378	320	6
Barley, pearled, Pot or Scotch, uncooked—1 tbsp., 14 gm.	.37	NA	40	41	---
Biscuit dough, commercial, w/enriched flour, chilled in cans—1 piece, 2"x ½", 40 gm.	.68	NA	198.8	26	347.2
Biscuit dough, commercial, w/enriched flour, frozen—1 piece, 2" diam. x ⅜", 38 gm.	.53	NA	152	32.68	345.8
Biscuits, baking powder, from home recipe, made w/enriched flour—1 biscuit, 2" diam., 35 gm.	.6	---	61	41	219
Biscuits, baking powder, from home recipe, made w/unenriched flour—1 biscuit, 2" diam., 35 gm.	.2	NA	61	41	219
Biscuits, baking powder, from home recipe, made w/self-rising flour, enriched—one 2" biscuit, 35 gm.	.6	---	111	22	231
Biscuits, baking powder, made from mix, with enriched flour, made with milk—1 biscuit, 2" diam., 28 gm.	.6	NA	65	32	272
Boston Brown Bread—1 slice, 3"x ¾", 48 gm.	.9	NA	77	140	120
Bran, plain, prepared—1 cup, 60 gm.	NA	NA	706	639	636
Bran, added sugar and malt extract—1 tbsp., 3 gm.	.24	12.6	35.28	32.10	31.80
Bran, added sugar and defatted wheat germ—1 tbsp., 3 gm.	.26	---	29.31	---	14.70
Branflakes (40% bran), added thiamin and iron—1 cup, 35 gm.	12.3	---	173	---	324

Food and Amount	Calories	Carbo-hydrate gm.	Protein gm.	Sat. Fatty Acids gm.	Unsat. Fatty Acids gm.	Vitamin A IU	Thiamin B₁ mg.
Branflakes w/raisins, added thiamin and iron—1 cup, 50 gm.	145	40	4	---	---	trace	.16
Bread, cracked wheat—1 slice, ½″, 25 gm.	65	13	2	---	---	trace	.03
Bread, French or Vienna, enriched—1 slice, ¾″, 28 gm.	81	15	2.5	.28	.56	trace	.07
Bread, French or Vienna, unenriched—1 slice, ¾″, 28 gm.	81	15	2.5	.28	.56	trace	.02
Bread, Italian, enriched—1 slice, ¾″, 28 gm.	77	16	2.5	NA	NA	0	.08
Bread, Italian, unenriched—1 slice, ¾″, 28 gm.	77	16	2.5	NA	NA	0	.02
Bread Raisin—1 slice, ½″, 25 gm.	65	13	2	---	---	trace	.01
Bread, Rye, American (⅓ rye, ⅔ clear flour)—1 slice, ½″, 25 gm.	60	13	2	---	---	0	.05
Bread, Rye, Pumpernickel—1 slice, ⅜″, 32 gm.	79	17	2.9	---	---	0	.07
Bread, Salt-rising—1 slice, ½″, 26 gm.	69	13	2.05	.26	.52	2.6	.01
Bread, White, enriched, made w/1–2% nonfat dry milk—1 slice, ½″, 23 gm.	62	11.6	2	---	---	trace	.06
Bread, White, enriched, made w/3–4% nonfat dry milk—1 slice, ½″, 23 gm.	62	11.6	2	.23	.46	trace	.06
Bread, White, enriched, made w/5–6% nonfat dry milk—1 slice, ½″, 23 gm.	63	11.5	2.1	.23	.46	trace	.06
Bread, White, enriched, diet slice—1 slice, ¼″, 12.5 gm.	31	5.8	1	---	---	trace	.03
Bread, White, unenriched, made w/1–2% nonfat dry milk—1 slice, ½″, 23 gm.	62	11.5	2	.23	.46	trace	.02
Bread, White, unenriched, made w/3–4% nonfat dry milk—1 slice, ½″, 23 gm.	62	11.6	2	.23	.46	trace	.01
Bread, White, unenriched, made w/5–6% nonfat dry milk—1 slice, ½″, 23 gm.	63	11.5	2.07	.23	.46	trace	.01
Bread, Whole Wheat, made w/2% nonfat dry milk—1 slice, ½″, 23 gm.	56	11	2.4	.23	.46	trace	.06
Breadcrumbs, dry, grated—1 cup, 100 gm.	390	73	13	1	6	trace	.22
Breadcrumbs, dry, grated—1 tbsp., 6 gm.	23	4.4	.75	.06	.24	trace	.01
Breadsticks—see Saltsticks							
Breadstuffing, prepared from mix, dry, crumbly, w/water and table fat—½ cup, 95 gm.	352	68.7	12.2	10.45	8.55	trace	.32
Breadstuffing, prepared from mix, moist: prepared w/water, egg, table fat—1 cup, 205 gm.	426	40	9	14.35	12.30	861	.10
Breakfast cereals—see Corn, Oats, Rice, Wheat, Bran, Farina							
Brownies—see Cookies							
Buckwheat, whole-grain—1 cup, 208 gm.	696.8	151.63	24.33	---	---	0	1.24
Buckwheat flour, dark—1 cup sifted, 100 gm.	333	72	11.7	---	---	0	.58
Buckwheat flour, light—1 cup, 98 gm.	340	78	6	---	---	0	.08

Food and Amount	Ribo-flavin B₂ mg.	Niacin mg.	B₆ mg.	Folic Acid mg	PABA mg.	Panto-thenic Acid mg.	B₁₂ mcg.
Branflakes w/raisins, added thiamin and iron—1 cup, 50 gm.	.07	2.7	---	NA	NA	---	0
Bread, cracked wheat—1 slice, ½", 25 gm.	.02	.3	.023	.006	NA	.151	NA
Bread, French or Vienna, enriched—1 slice, ¾", 28 gm.	.06	.7	.013	.002	NA	.094	NA
Bread, French or Vienna, unenriched—1 slice, ¾", 28 gm.	.02	.22	NA	NA	NA	NA	NA
Bread, Italian, enriched—1 slice, ¾", 28 gm.	.05	.72	NA	---	NA	NA	NA
Bread, Italian, unenriched—1 slice, ¾", 28 gm.	.01	.22	NA	NA	NA	NA	NA
Bread Raisin—1 slice, ½", 25 gm.	.02	.2	NA	NA	NA	NA	NA
Bread, Rye, American (⅓ rye, ⅔ clear flour)—1 slice, ½", 25 gm.	.02	.4	.025	.004	NA	.112	NA
Bread, Rye, Pumpernickel—1 slice, ⅜", 32 gm.	.04	.4	.051	NA	NA	.160	NA
Bread, Salt-rising—1 slice, ½", 26 gm.	.01	.15	NA	NA	NA	NA	NA
Bread, White, enriched, made w/1-2% nonfat dry milk—1 slice, ½", 23 gm.	.04	.5	---	---	NA	---	---
Bread, White, enriched, made w/3-4% nonfat dry milk—1 slice, ½", 23 gm.	.05	.6	.009	.003	NA	.098	trace
Bread, White, enriched made w/5-6% nonfat dry milk—1 slice, ½", 23 gm.	.04	.6	---	---	NA	---	---
Bread, White, enriched, diet slice—1 slice, ¼", 12.5 gm.	.02	.25	---	---	NA	---	---
Bread, White, unenriched, made w/1-2% nonfat dry milk—1 slice, ½", 23 gm.	.01	.27	NA	NA	NA	NA	NA
Bread, White, unenriched, made w/3-4% nonfat dry milk—1 slice, ½", 23 gm.	.02	.25	NA	NA	NA	NA	NA
Bread, White, unenriched, made w/5-6% nonfat dry milk—1 slice, ½", 23 gm.	.02	.20	NA	.003	NA	NA	NA
Bread, Whole Wheat, made w/2% nonfat dry milk—1 slice, ½", 23 gm.	.02	.6	.0966	.006	NA	.174	0
Breadcrumbs, dry, grated—1 cup, 100 gm.	.30	3.5	NA	NA	NA	NA	NA
Breadcrumbs, dry, grated—1 tbsp., 6 gm.	.01	.21	NA	NA	NA	NA	NA
Breadsticks—see Saltsticks							
Breadstuffing, prepared from mix, dry, crumbly, w/water and table fat—½ cup, 95 gm.	.25	3	NA	NA	NA	NA	NA
Breadstuffing, prepared from mix, moist; prepared w/water, egg, table fat—1 cup, 205 gm.	.18	1.64	NA	NA	NA	NA	NA
Breakfast cereals—see Corn, Oats, Rice, Wheat, Bran, Farina							
Brownies—see Cookies							
Buckwheat, whole-grain—1 cup, 208 gm.	---	9.15	NA	NA	NA	NA	0
Buckwheat flour, dark—1 cup sifted, 100 gm.	.15	2.9	NA	NA	NA	NA	0
Buckwheat flour, light—1 cup, 98 gm.	.04	.4	NA	NA	NA	NA	0

Vitamin C mg.	Vitamin D IU	Vitamin E IU	Calcium mg.	Iodine mg.	Iron mg.	Mag-nesium mg.	Phos-phorus mg.	Potas-sium mg.	Sodium mg.
0	0	NA	28	NA	13.5	---	198	---	400
trace	NA	NA	22	NA	.3	9	32	33	132
trace	NA	NA	12	NA	.61	6.16	24	25	162
trace	NA	NA	12	NA	.19	6.16	24	25	162
0	NA	NA	5	NA	.61	---	21	21	164
0	NA	NA	5	NA	.19	NA	21	21	164
trace	NA	NA	18	NA	.3	6	22	58	91
0	NA	NA	19	NA	.4	10.5	37	36	139
0	NA	NA	27	NA	.8	23	73	145	182
trace	NA	NA	6	NA	.15	NA	18	17	69
trace	---	---	16	.00304 Ohio	.6	4	20	20	117
trace	---	.02	19	.00304 Ohio	.6	5	22	24	117
trace	---	---	22	.00304 Ohio	.6	6	24	28	114
trace	---	---	8	.00152 Ohio	.3	2	10	10	58.5
trace	NA	---	16	.00304 Ohio	.16	NA	20	19	116
trace	NA	---	19	.00304 Ohio	.16	5	22	24	116
trace	NA	---	22	.00304 Ohio	.16	NA	23	28	114
trace	NA	.10	23	.00248 Ohio	.5	18	52	63	121
trace	NA	NA	122	NA	3.6	NA	141	152	736
trace	NA	NA	7.3	NA	.21	NA	8	9.1	44
trace	NA	NA	118	NA	3.0	NA	180	163	1,264
trace	NA	NA	82	NA	2.05	NA	135	119	1,033
0	NA	NA	237.12	NA	6.44	476.32	586.56	931.84	---
0	NA	NA	33	NA	2.8	---	347	---	---
0	NA	NA	11	NA	1.0	47.04	86	313	---

Food and Amount	Calories	Carbohydrate gm.	Protein gm.	Sat. Fatty Acids gm.	Unsat. Fatty Acids gm.	Vitamin A IU	Thiamin B₁ mg.
Buckwheat pancake mix—see Pancake mix							
Bulgur (parboiled wheat) (Pilaf), dry, commerical, made from club wheat—1 tbsp., 14 gm.	50.26	11.13	1.21	---	---	0	.04
Bulgur (parboiled wheat), dry, commercial, made from hard, red, winter wheat—1 tbsp., 14 gm.	49.56	10.59	1.56	---	---	0	.008
Bulgur (parboiled wheat), dry, commercial, made from white wheat—1 tbsp., 14 gm.	49.98	10.93	1.44	---	---	0	.04
Bulgur, canned, made from hard, red, winter wheat, unseasoned—1 cup, 135 gm.	226.8	47.25	8.37	---	---	0	.06
Bulgur, canned, made from hard, red, winter wheat, seasoned—1 cup, 135 gm.	245	44	8	---	---	0	.08
Cake, from home recipe, Angelfood—1 piece, 1/12 of 8" cake, 40 gm.	107.6	24.08	2.84	NA	NA	0	.004
Cake, from home recipe, Boston cream pie—1 piece, 1/12 of 8" diam., 69 gm.	210	34	4	2	4	140	.02
Cake, from home recipe, Caramel, w/o icing—1 piece, 1/12 of 8" cake, 56 gm.	215.6	30.07	2.52	NA	NA	100.8	.01
Cake, from home recipe, Chocolate (devil's food), w/o icing—1 piece, 1/12 of 8" cake, 56 gm.	205	29.12	2.68	NA	NA	84	.01
Cake, from home recipe, Fruitcake, made with enriched flour, dark—1 slice, 1/30 of 8" loaf, 15 gm.	55	9	1	trace	1	20	.02
Cake, from home recipe, Fruitcake, made with enriched flour, light—1 piece, 2" x 2" x 1/2", 30 gm.	116.7	17.2	1.8	1.8	2.7	21	.03
Cake, from home recipe, Gingerbread, made with enriched flour—1 piece, 2" x 2" x 2", 54 gm.	171.1	28.08	2.05	2	4	48.6	.06
Cake, from home recipe, Plain cake or cupcake, w/o icing—1 piece, 1/6 of 9" square, 86 gm.	315	48	4	3	8	150	.02
Cake, from home recipe, Old-fashioned Pound cake (equal wts. flour, sugar, table fat, eggs)—1/2" slice, 30 gm.	140	14	2	2	5	80	.01
Cake, from home recipe, Sponge—1 piece, 1/12 of 10" diam. cake, 66 gm.	195	36	5	1	2	300	.03
Cake, from home recipe, White, w/o icing—1 piece, 3" x 2" x 1 1/2", 54 gm.	203	29	2.48	2	4.8	16.2	.005
Cake, from home recipe, Yellow, w/o icing—2 layer, 1 piece, 1/16 of 9" diam., 54 gm.	200	32	2	2	4	80	.01
Cakes made from mixes—see Sweets, Sugars, Desserts, and Related Products							
Cake icings—see Sweets, Sugars, Desserts, and Related Products							
Carob flour (St. Johnsbread)—1 piece, 4", 10 gm.	18	NA	.45	NA	NA	---	---
Cereals, breakfast—see Corn, Oats, Rice, Wheat, Bran, Farina							
Cookies, Assorted, packaged, commercial—1 cookie, 10 gm.	48	7.1	.51	---	---	8.0	.003

Ribo-flavin B_2 mg.	Niacin mg.	B_6 mg.	Folic Acid mg.	PABA mg.	Panto-thenic Acid mg.	B_{12} mcg.	Vitamin C mg.	Vitamin D IU	Vitamin E IU	Calcium mg.	Iodine mg.
.01	.58	NA	NA	NA	NA	0	0	NA	NA	4.2	NA
.004	.13	NA	NA	NA	NA	0	0	NA	NA	4.06	NA
.01	.58	NA	NA	NA	NA	0	0	NA	NA	5.04	NA
.04	3.24	NA	NA	NA	NA	0	0	NA	NA	27	NA
.05	4.1	NA	NA	NA	NA	0	0	NA	NA	27	NA
.056	.08	NA	NA	NA	NA	NA	0	NA	NA	3.6	NA
.08	.1	NA	NA	NA	NA	NA	trace	NA	NA	46	NA
.04	.11	NA	NA	NA	NA	NA	trace	NA	NA	43.68	NA
.05	.11	---	NA	NA	NA	---	trace	NA	.12 (chocolate)	41.44	NA
.02	.1	NA	NA	NA	NA	NA	trace	NA	NA	11	NA
.03	.21	NA	NA	NA	NA	NA	trace	NA	NA	20.4	NA
.05	.48	NA	NA	NA	NA	NA	0	NA	NA	36.7	NA
.08	.2	.0344	NA	NA	---	---	trace	NA	NA	55	NA
.03	.1	NA	NA	NA	NA	NA	0	NA	.33	6	NA
.09	.1	NA	NA	NA	NA	NA	trace	NA	NA	20	NA
.04	.1	NA	NA	NA	NA	NA	trace	NA	NA	34	NA
.04	.1	NA	NA	NA	NA	NA	trace	NA	NA	39	NA
---	---	NA	NA	NA	NA	NA	---	NA	NA	35	NA
.005	.04	NA	NA	NA	NA	NA	trace	NA	---	3.7	NA

Food and Amount	Iron mg.	Mag- nesium mg.	Phos- phorus mg.	Potas- sium mg.	Sodium mg.
Buckwheat pancake mix—see Pancake mix					
Bulgur (parboiled wheat) (Pilaf), dry, commerical, made from club wheat— 1 tbsp., 14 gm.	.65	NA	44.66	36.68	---
Bulgur (parboiled wheat), dry, com- mercial, made from hard, red, winter wheat—1 tbsp., 14 gm.	.51	NA	47.32	32.06	---
Bulgur (parboiled wheat), dry, com- mercial, made from white wheat— 1 tbsp., 14 gm.	.65	NA	42	43.4	---
Bulgur, canned, made from hard, red, winter wheat, unseasoned—1 cup, 135 gm.	1.75	NA	270	117.45	808.65
Bulgur, canned, made from hard, red, winter wheat, seasoned—1 cup, 135 gm.	1.9	NA	263.25	151.2	621
Cake, from home recipe, Angelfood— 1 piece, ½₂ of 8″ cake, 40 gm.	.08	---	8.8	35.2	113.2
Cake, from home recipe, Boston cream pie—1 piece, ½₂ of 8″ diam., 69 gm.	.3	NA	69.69	61.41	128.3
Cake, from home recipe, Caramel, w/o icing—1 piece, ½₂ of 8″ cake, 56 gm.	.72	NA	59.36	38.08	170.8
Cake, from home recipe, Chocolate (devil's food), w/o icing—1 piece, ½₂ of 8″ cake, 56 gm.	.50	---	76.72	78.4	164.6
Cake, from home recipe, Fruitcake, made with enriched flour, dark— 1 slice, ½₀ of 8″ loaf, 15 gm.	.4	---	16.95	74.4	23.7
Cake, from home recipe, Fruitcake, made with enriched flour, light— 1 piece, 2″ x 2″ x ½″, 30 gm.	.48	NA	34.5	70	57.9
Cake, from home recipe, Gingerbread, made with enriched flour—1 piece, 2″ x 2″ x 2″, 54 gm.	1.24	---	35.1	245	128
Cake, from home recipe, Plain cake or cupcake, w/o icing—1 piece, ⅑ of 9″ square, 86 gm.	.3	---	87.72	68	258
Cake, from home recipe, Old-fashioned Pound cake (equal wts. flour, sugar, table fat, eggs)—½″ slice, 30 gm.	.2	---	23.7	18	33
Cake, from home recipe, Sponge— 1 piece, ½₂ of 10″ diam. cake, 66 gm.	.8	---	73.92	57.4	110
Cake, from home recipe, White, w/o icing—1 piece, 3″ x 2″ x 1½″, 54 gm.	.10	NA	49.14	41	174
Cake, from home recipe, Yellow, w/o icing—2 layer, 1 piece, ½₆ of 9″ diam., 54 gm.	.2	NA	60.4	42	139
Cakes made from mixes—see Sweets, Sugars, Desserts, and Related Products					
Cake icings—see Sweets, Sugars, Desserts, and Related Products					
Carob flour (St. Johnsbread)—1 piece, 4″, 10 gm.	---	NA	8.1	---	---
Cereals, breakfast—see Corn, Oats, Rice, Wheat, Bran, Farina					
Cookies, Assorted, packaged, com- mercial—1 cookie, 10 gm.	.07	1.5	16.3	6.7	36.5

Food and Amount	Calories	Carbo-hydrate gm.	Protein gm.	Sat. Fatty Acids gm.	Unsat. Fatty Acids gm.	Vitamin A IU	Thiamin B₁ mg.
Cookies, Brownies w/nuts, from home recipe, with enriched flour—1 brownie, 2″, 20 gm.	95	10	1	1	4	40	.04
Cookies, Brownies w/nuts, from mix—1 brownie, 2″, 20 gm.	85	13	1	1	3	20	.03
Cookies, Butter, thin, rich—1 cookie, 8 gm.	36	5.67	.48	NA	NA	52	.006
Cookies, Chocolate—1 cookie, 4 gm.	18	2.85	.28	.04	.12	6.4	.001
Cookies, Chocolate Chip, from home recipe, with enriched flour—1 cookie, 1½″, 10 gm.	50	6	1	1	2	10	.01
Cookies, Chocolate Chip, commercial type—1 cookie, 1½″, 10 gm.	50	7	1	1	1	10	trace
Cookies, Coconut bars—1 bar, 14 gm.	69	9	.86	NA	NA	22	.005
Cookies, Fig bars, commercial—1 fig bar, 14 gm.	50	11	1	----	----	20	trace
Cookies, Gingersnaps—1 piece, 1½″ diam., 6 gm.	25	4.8	.33	.06	.18	4.2	.002
Cookies, Ladyfingers—1 piece, 3″, 12 gm.	43	7.7	.93	----	----	78	.007
Cookies, Macaroons—1 cookie, 2″ diam., 22 gm.	105	14.5	1.16	3.52	1.32	0	.008
Cookies, Marshmallow—1 cookie, 2″ diam., 14 gm.	57	10.12	.56	1.12	.84	36.4	.002
Cookies, Molasses—1 cookie, 2½″ diam., 10 gm.	42	7.6	.64	.10	.30	8	.004
Cookies, Oatmeal with raisins—1 piece, 3″ diam., 11 gm.	49	8.08	.63	.44	1.21	5.5	.01
Cookies, Peanut—1 piece, 2″ diam., 6 gm.	28	4.02	.60	.24	.66	12	004
Cookies, Raisin—1 cookie, 2″ diam., 9 gm.	34	7.27	.39	----	----	19	.003
Cookies, Sandwich type—1 cookie, 1½″ diam., 10 gm.	50	7	1	1	1	0	trace
Cookies, Shortbread—2″ sq., 8 gm.	40	5	.57	.32	.88	6.4	.003
Cookies, Sugar, soft, thick, with enriched flour, from home recipe—1 piece, 3″ diam., 14 gm.	62	9.5	.84	.56	1.54	15.4	.02
Cookies, Sugar wafers—1 cookie, 3″ long, 3 gm.	14	2.2	.14	.12	.33	4.2	.0003
Cookies, Vanilla wafers—1 cookie, 2″ diam., 3 gm.	14	2.2	.16	.12	.33	3.9	.0006
Cornflakes, added nutrients, plain—1 cup, 25 gm.	100	21	2	----	----	0	.11
Cornflakes, added nutrients, sugar-covered—1 cup, 40 gm.	155	36	2	----	----	0	.16
Cornflour—1 cup sifted, 110 gm.	405	84.5	8.6	trace	2.20	374*	.22
Corn fritters—2¾″ diam. x ½″, 43 gm.	162.11	17.07	3.35	----	----	172	.06
Corn (Hominy) grits, degermed, enriched, cooked—1 cup, 245 gm.	125	27	3	----	----	150*	.10
Corn (Hominy) grits, degermed, unenriched, cooked—1 cup, 245 gm.	125	27	3	----	----	150*	.05
Corn Muffins—see Muffins, corn							

* Based on yellow varieties of corn; white varieties contain only a trace.

Food and Amount	Ribo-flavin B₂ mg.	Niacin mg.	B₆ mg.	Folic Acid mg.	PABA mg.	Panto-thenic Acid mg.	B₁₂ mcg.
Cookies, Brownies w/nuts, from home recipe, with enriched flour— 1 brownie, 2″, 20 gm.	.02	.1	NA	NA	NA	NA	NA
Cookies, Brownies w/nuts, from mix— 1 brownie, 2″, 20 gm.	.02	.1	NA	NA	NA	NA	NA
Cookies, Butter, thin, rich—1 cookie, 8 gm.	.01	.08	NA	NA	NA	NA	NA
Cookies, Chocolate—1 cookie, 4 gm.	.003	.02	NA	NA	NA	NA	NA
Cookies, Chocolate Chip, from home recipe, with enriched flour—1 cookie, 1½″, 10 gm.	.01	.1	NA	NA	NA	NA	NA
Cookies, Chocolate Chip, commercial type—1 cookie, 1½″, 10 gm.	trace	trace	NA	NA	NA	NA	NA
Cookies, Coconut bars—1 bar, 14 gm.	.008	.056	NA	NA	NA	NA	NA
Cookies, Fig bars, commercial— 1 fig bar, 14 gm.	.01	.1	NA	NA	NA	NA	NA
Cookies, Gingersnaps—1 piece, 1½″ diam., 6 gm.	.00:	.024	NA	NA	NA	NA	NA
Cookies, Ladyfingers—1 piece, 3″, 12 gm.	.01	.02	NA	NA	NA	NA	NA
Cookies, Macaroons—1 cookie, 2″ diam., 22 gm.	.03	.13	NA	NA	NA	NA	NA
Cookies, Marshmallow—1 cookie, 2″ diam., 14 gm.	.008	.02	NA	NA	·NA	NA	NA
Cookies, Molasses—1 cookie, 2½″ diam., 10 gm.	.006	.07	NA	NA	NA	NA	NA
Cookies, Oatmeal with raisins—1 piece, ·3″ diam., 11 gm.	.008	.05	NA	NA	NA	NA	NA
Cookies, Peanut—1 piece, 2″ diam., 6 gm.	.004	.16	NA	NA	NA	NA	NA
Cookies, Raisin—1 cookie, 2″ diam., 9 gm.	.007	.05	NA	NA	NA	NA	NA
Cookies, Sandwich type—1 cookie, 1½″ diam., 10 gm.	trace	.1	NA	NA	NA	NA	NA
Cookies, Shortbread—2″ sq., 8 gm.	.004	.04	NA	NA	NA	NA	NA
Cookies, Sugar, soft, thick, with enriched flour, from home recipe— 1 piece, 3″ diam., 14 gm.	.02	.18	NA	NA	NA	NA	NA
Cookies, Sugar wafers—1 cookie, 3″ long, 3 gm.	.0012	.015	NA	NA	NA	NA	NA
Cookies, Vanilla wafers—1 cookie, 2″ diam., 3 gm.	.002	.009	NA	NA	NA	NA	NA
Cornflakes ,added nutrients, plain— 1 cup, 25 gm.	.02	.5	.01625	.0015	NA	.04625	0
Cornflakes, added nutrients, sugar-covered—1 cup, 40 gm.	.02	.8	---	---	NA	---	0
Cornflour—1 cup sifted, 110 gm.	.06	1.5	NA	NA	NA	NA	0
Corn fritters—2¾″ diam. x ½″, 43 gm.	.08	.68	NA	NA	NA	NA	NA
Corn (Hominy) grits, degermed, enriched, cooked—1 cup. 245 gm.	.07	1.0	.0147	.01102	NA.	.83	0
Corn (Ho.niny) grits, degermed, unenriched, cooked—1 cup, 245 gm.	.02	.5	---	---	NA	---	0
Corn Muffins—see Muffins, corn							

* Based on yellow varieties of corn; white varieties contain only a trace.

Vitamin C mg.	Vitamin D IU	Vitamin E IU	Calcium mg.	Iodine mg.	Iron mg.	Magnesium mg.	Phosphorus mg.	Potassium mg.	Sodium mg.
trace	NA	NA	8	NA	.4	---	29.6	38	50.2
trace	NA	NA	9	NA	.4	NA	25	35.8	40
0	NA	NA	10	NA	.04	NA	7.5	4.8	33
trace	NA	NA	2.08	NA	.04	NA	5.08	5.12	5.5
trace	NA	NA	4	NA	.2	NA	10	11.7	35
trace	NA	NA	4	NA	.2	NA	11.4	13.4	40
0	NA	NA	10	NA	.19	NA	17	32	20.7
trace	NA	NA	11	NA	.2	---	8.4	28	35
trace	NA	NA	4.3	NA	.13	NA	2.8	28	34
0	NA	NA	4.9	NA	.18	NA	19.6	8.5	8.52
0	NA	NA	5.9	NA	.19	NA	18	102	7.5
trace	NA	NA	2.9	NA	.07	NA	8	12.7	29
0	NA	NA	5.1	NA	.21	NA	8.3	13.8	38
trace	NA	---	2.3	NA	.31	NA	11	40.7	18
trace	NA	---	2.5	NA	.05	NA	6.9	10	10
trace	NA	NA	6.39	NA	.18	NA	14.13	24.48	4.68
0	NA	.12	2	NA	.1	NA	24	3.8	48
0	NA	.03	5.6	NA	.04	2.8	12	5.2	4.8
trace	NA	NA	11	NA	.19	NA	14	10.6	44
0	NA	.01	1.08	NA	.009	NA	2.4	1.8	5.67
0	NA	.01	1.23	NA	.01	1.05	1.9	2.2	7.56
0	0	.03	4	NA	.4	4	11.25	30	251.25
0	0	---	5	NA	.4	6.4	11	---	120
0	NA	NA	7	NA	2	NA	180	---	1
.86	NA	NA	27.52	NA	.73	---	66.65	57.19	205.11
0	NA	.75	2	NA	.7	7.35	25	27	---
0	NA	.75	2	NA	.2	7.35	25	27	---

Food and Amount	Calories	Carbo-hydrate gm.	Protein gm.	Sat. Fatty Acids gm.	Unsat. Fatty Acids gm.	Vitamin A IU	Thiamin B₁ mg.
Corn, puffed, added nutrients—1 cup, 28 gm.	111.72	22.62	2.26	---	---	0	.24
Corn, puffed, pre-sweetened, added nutrients—1 cup, 30 gm.	115	27	1	---	---	0	.13
Corn, puffed, pre-sweetened, cocoa-flavored, added nutrients—1 cup, 30 gm.	117	26.01	1.86	---	---	0	.23
Corn, puffed, pre-sweetened, fruit-flavored, added nutrients—1 cup, 30 gm.	118.5	26.22	1.68	---	---	0	.29
Corn, rice and wheat flakes, mixed, added nutrients—1 cup, 32 gm.	124.48	27.55	2.36	---	---	0	.12
Corn bread, Southern style, home recipe, made w/whole-ground cornmeal—1 piece, 2″ sq., 45 gm.	93	13.1	3.3	.90	1.80	68	.06
Corn bread, Northern style (Johnny-cake), home recipe, made w/enriched, yellow, degermed cornmeal—1 piece, 2″ sq., 40 gm.	107	18.2	3.5	.80	1.60	136	.08
Corn bread–Spoonbread, made w/white whole-ground cornmeal—1 piece, 2″ sq., 50 gm.	97.5	8.45	3.35	---	---	145	.045
Corn bread, from mix, w/egg and milk—1 piece, 2″ sq., 42 gm.	97.86	13.81	2.56	1.26	2.1	113.4	.06
Corn pone, made w/white whole-ground cornmeal—1 piece, 5″ long, 40 gm.	81.6	14.48	1.8	---	---	trace	.06
Corn meal, white or yellow, whole-ground, unbolted—1 cup, 122 gm.	435	90	11	1	4	620*	.46
Corn meal, white or yellow, whole-ground, bolted (nearly whole-grain)—1 cup, 122 gm.	440	91	11	trace	.3	590*	.37
Corn meal, white or yellow, degermed, enriched, cooked—1 cup, 240 gm.	120	26	3	---	---	140*	.14
Corn meal, white or yellow, degermed, unenriched, cooked—1 cup, 240 gm.	120	26	3	---	---	140*	.05
Cottonseed flour—1 cup, 108 gm.	384	35.6	51.9	2.16	7.56	64.8	1.3
Crackers, Animal—1 cracker, 1¼″ x ¾″, 2 gm.	9	1.6	.13	.06	.16	2.6	.0008
Crackers, Butter—1 cracker, 1¾″ diam., 3.9 gm.	1.8	2.6	.027	.117	.312	8.5	.0003
Crackers, Cheese—1 cracker, 1¼″ diam., 3.5 gm.	17	2.11	.39	.280	.385	13	.0003
Crackers, Graham, plain—2½″ square, 1 cracker, 7 gm.	27	5.13	.56	.49	1.12	0	.002
Crackers, Graham, chocolate-covered—2½″ square, 1 cracker, 8 gm.	38	5.43	.40	.56	1.28	4.8	.005
Crackers, Graham, sugar-honey coated—2½″ sq., 1 cracker, 7 gm.	29	5.34	.46	.21	.56	---	.002
Cracker: meal—1 cup, 128 gm.	538	93.1	12.3	---	---	0	.077
Crackers, Saltines—4 crackers, 11 gm.	50	8	1	---	1	0	trace
Crackers, Sandwich-type, Peanut cheese—1 piece, 1¾″ diam., 7 gm.	34	4	1	.42	1.19	2.8	.002
Crackers, Soda—2½″ diam., 7 gm.	31	5	.64	.21	.56	0	.007

* Based on yellow varieties of corn; white varieties contain only a trace.

Ribo-flavin B₂ mg.	Niacin mg.	B₆ mg.	Folic Acid mg.	PABA mg.	Panto-thenic Acid mg.	B₁₂ mcg.	Vitamin C mg.	Vitamin D IU	Vitamin E IU	Calcium mg.	Iodine mg.
.05	.75	---	NA	NA	.08064	0	0	0	---	5.6	NA
.05	.6	---	NA	NA	---	0	0	0	---	3	NA
.05	.75	---	NA	NA	---	0	0	0	---	6	NA
.05	.75	---	NA	NA	---	0	31.8	0	---	9	NA
---	1.02	NA	NA	NA	NA	0	0	0	---	12.48	NA
.09	.3	NA	NA	NA	NA	NA	trace	NA	NA	54	NA
.12	.6	NA	NA	NA	NA	NA	trace	NA	NA	44	NA
.09	.2	NA	NA	NA	NA	NA	trace	NA	NA	48	NA
.08	.5	NA	NA	NA	NA	NA	trace	NA	NA	37.38	NA
.02	.36	NA	NA	NA	NA	NA	0	NA	NA	24.8	NA
.13	2.4	.305	---	.36	.7076	0	0	NA	.78	24	NA
.10	2.3	---	---	.36	---	0	0	NA	.78	21	NA
.10	1.2	---	.0216	---	---	0	0	NA	1.53	2	NA
.02	.2	---	---	---	---	0	0	NA	---	2	NA
.90	7.02	NA	NA	NA	NA	0	---	NA	NA	305.6	NA
.002	.006	NA	NA	NA	NA	NA	trace	NN	NA	1	NA
.0015	.039	NA	NA	NA	NA	NA	0	NA	NA	5.7	NA
.0035	.028	NA	NA	NA	NA	NA	0	NA	NA	12	NA
.014	.105	NA	NA	NA	NA	NA	0	NA	NA	2.8	NA
.022	.096	NA	NA	NA	NA	NA	0	NA	NA	9.04	NA
.001	.07	NA	NA	NA	NA	NA	0	NA	NA	6.2	NA
.064	1.4	NA	NA	NA	NA	NA	0	0	NA	26	NA
trace	.1	.007	NA	NA	---	0	0	NA	NA	2	NA
.005	.24	NA	NA	NA	NA	NA	0	NA	NA	4	NA
.003	.07	NA	NA	NA	NA	NA	0	NA	.05	1.5	NA

Food and Amount	Iron mg.	Mag-nesium mg.	Phos-phorus mg.	Potas-sium mg.	Sodium mg.
Corn, puffed, added nutrients—1 cup, 28 gm.	1.62	---	25.2	---	296.8
Corn, puffed, pre-sweetened, added nutrients—1 cup, 30 gm.	.5	---	8.4	---	90
Corn, puffed, pre-sweetened, cocoa-flavored, added nutrients—1 cup, 30 gm.	1.8	---	27	---	255
Corn, puffed, pre-sweetened, fruit-flavored, added nutrients—1 cup, 30 gm.	1.5	---	21	---	180
Corn, rice and wheat flakes, mixed, added nutrients—1 cup, 32 gm.	.57	---	38.4	---	304
Corn bread, Southern style, home recipe, made w/whole-ground cornmeal—1 piece, 2'' sq., 45 gm.	.5	---	95	71	283
Corn bread, Northern style (Johnny-cake), home recipe, made w/enriched, yellow, degermed cornmeal—1 piece, 2'' sq., 40 gm.	.7	---	62	75	276
Corn bread-Spoonbread, made w/white whole-ground cornmeal—1 piece, 2'' sq., 50 gm.	.5	---	82	66	241
Corn bread, from mix, w/egg and milk—1 piece, 2'' sq., 42 gm.	.5	NA	112.56	53.34	312.48
Corn pone, made w/white whole-ground cornmeal—1 piece, 5'' long, 40 gm.	.48	---	65.2	24.4	158.4
Corn meal, white or yellow, whole-ground, unbolted—1 cup, 122 gm.	2.9	129.32	312	346	1.2
Corn meal, white or yellow, whole-ground, bolted (nearly whole-grain)—1 cup, 122 gm.	2.2	129.32	272	303	1.2
Corn meal, white or yellow, degermed, enriched, cooked—1 cup, 240 gm.	1.0	16.8	33	38	---
Corn meal, white or yellow, degermed, unenriched, cooked—1 cup, 240 gm.	.5	16.8	33	38	---
Cottonseed flour—1 cup, 108 gm.	13.6	702	1,201	---	---
Crackers, Animal—1 cracker, 1¼'' x ¾'', 2 gm.	.01	NA	2.3	1.9	6.06
Crackers, Butter—1 cracker, 1¾'' diam., 3.9 gm.	.02	NA	10	4.4	42
Crackers, Cheese—1 cracker, 1¾'' diam., 3.5 gm.	.031	NA	11	4	36
Crackers, Graham, plain—2½'' square, 1 cracker, 7 gm.	.10	3.7	10	27	47
Crackers, Graham, chocolate-covered—2½'' square, 1 cracker, 8 gm.	.20	NA	16	26	13
Crackers, Graham, sugar-honey coated—2½'' sq., 1 cracker, 7 gm.	.11	NA	23	19	35
Cracker: meal—1 cup, 128 gm.	1.4	NA	123	---	---
Crackers, Saltines—4 crackers, 11 gm.	.1	---	10	13	121
Crackers, Sandwich-type, Peanut cheese—1 piece, 1¾'' diam., 7 gm.	.04	NA	12	16	69
Crackers, Soda—2½'' diam., 7 gm.	.10	2	6	8	77

* Based on yellow varieties of corn; white varieties contain only a trace.

Food and Amount	Calories	Carbo-hydrate gm.	Protein gm.	Sat. Fatty Acids gm.	Unsat. Fatty Acids gm.	Vitamin A IU	Thiamin B₁ mg.
Crackers, Wholewheat—1¾″ diam., 1 cracker, 2 gm.	8	1.3	.16	.06	.16	0	.001
Danish pastry—see Rolls and Buns							
Doughnuts, cake type—1 doughnut, 32 gm.	125	16	1	1	4	30	.05
Doughnuts, glazed—1 doughnut, 37 gm.	151	21.7	2.1	---	---	41	.07
Farina, enriched, regular, cooked—1 cup, 238 gm.	100	20.7	.09	---	---	0	.09
Farina, enriched, quick-cooking, cooked—1 cup, 245 gm.	105	22	3	---	---	0	.12
Farina, enriched, instant-cooking, cooked—1 cup, 242 gm.	133	27	4	---	---	0	.16
Farina, unenriched, regular, cooked—1 cup, 240 gm.	101	21	1.12	---	---	0	.02
Gluten flour—see Wheat flours							
Griddlecakes—see Pancakes							
Grits—see Corn Grits							
Macaroni, enriched, cooked, firm stage—1 cup, 130 gm.	190	39	6	---	---	0	.23
Macaroni, enriched, cooked, tender stage—1 cup, 140 gm.	155	32	5	---	---	0	.20
Macaroni, unenriched, cooked, firm stage—1 cup, 130 gm.	190	39	6	---	---	0	.03
Macaroni, unenriched, cooked, tender stage—1 cup, 140 gm.	155	32	5	---	---	0	.01
Macaroni (enriched) and cheese, baked, home recipe—1 cup, 200 gm.	430	40	17	10	11	860	.20
Macaroni and cheese, baked, canned—1 cup, 240 gm.	230	26	9	4	4	260	.12
Malt—1 tbsp., 10 gm.	36.8	7.74	1.31	NA	NA	---	.049
Millet, proso (broomcorn, hogmillet), whole-grain—1 cup, 200 gm.	654	145.8	19.8	2	4	0	1.46
Muffin, Plain, from home recipe, made w/enriched flour—1 muffin, 3″ diam., 40 gm.	120	17	3	1	3	40	.07
Muffin, Blueberry, from home recipe, made w/enriched flour—1 muffin, 3″ diam., 40 gm.	112	16.8	2.9	1.2	2.4	88	.06
Muffin, Bran, from home recipe, made w/enriched flour—1 muffin, 2¾″ diam., 45 gm.	117	19	3	2.25	1.8	103	.06
Muffin, Corn, from home recipe, made w/enriched, degermed cornmeal—1 muffin, 2⅜″ diam., 40 gm.	125	19	3	2	2	120*	.08
Muffin, Corn, from home recipe, made w/whole-ground cornmeal—1 muffin, 2½″ diam., 45 gm.	130	19.1	3.2	1.8	2.25	140	.08
Muffin, Corn, from mix with enriched flour, made w/egg and milk—1 muffin, 2⅜″ diam., 40 gm.	130	20	3	1	3	100	.07
Muffin, Corn, from mix with cake flour, nonfat dry milk, made with egg, water—1 muffin, 2¾″ diam., 45 gm.	184	32	2.8	1.8	2.25	45	.05

* Based on yellow varieties of corn; white varieties contain only a trace.

Food and Amount	Ribo-flavin B₂ mg.	Niacin mg.	B₆ mg.	Folic Acid mg.	PABA mg.	Panto-thenic Acid mg.	B₁₂ mcg.
Crackers, Wholewheat—1¾″ diam., 1 cracker, 2 gm.	.008	.02	NA	NA	NA	NA	NA
Danish pastry—see Rolls and Buns							
Doughnuts, cake type—1 doughnut, 32 gm.	.05	.4	---	NA	NA	.123	---
Doughnuts, glazed—1 doughnut, 37 gm.	.06	.5	---	NA	NA	---	---
Farina, enriched, regular, cooked—1 cup, 238 gm.	.07	.95	NA	NA	NA	NA	NA
Farina, enriched, quick-cooking, cooked—1 cup, 245 gm.	.07	1.0	NA	NA	NA	NA	NA
Farina, enriched, instant-cooking, cooked—1 cup, 242 gm.	.09	1.2	NA	NA	NA	NA	NA
Farina, unenriched, regular, cooked—1 cup, 240 gm.	.02	.24	NA	NA	NA	NA	NA
Gluten flour—see Wheat flours							
Griddlecakes—see Pancakes							
Grits—see Corn Grits							
Macaroni, enriched, cooked, firm stage—1 cup, 130 gm.	.14	1.8	NA	NA	NA	NA	0
Macaroni, enriched, cooked, tender stage—1 cup, 140 gm.	.11	1.5	NA	NA	NA	NA	0
Macaroni, unenriched, cooked, firm stage—1 cup, 130 gm.	.03	.5	NA	NA	NA	NA	0
Macaroni, unenriched, cooked, tender stage—1 cup, 140 gm.	.01	.4	NA	NA	NA	NA	0
Macaroni (enriched) and cheese, baked, home recipe—1 cup, 200 gm.	.40	1.8	NA	NA	NA	NA	NA
Macaroni and cheese, baked, canned—1 cup, 240 gm.	.24	1.0	NA	NA	NA	NA	NA
Malt—1 tbsp., 10 gm.	.031	.9	NA	NA	---	NA	NA
Millet, proso (broomcorn, hogmillet), whole-grain—1 cup, 200 gm.	.76	4.6	NA	NA	NA	NA	0
Muffin, Plain, from home recipe, made w/enriched flour—1 muffin, 3″ diam., 40 gm.	.09	.6	NA	NA	NA	NA	NA
Muffin, Blueberry, from home recipe, made w/enriched flour—1 muffin, 3″ diam., 40 gm.	.08	.5	NA	NA	NA	NA	NA
Muffin, Bran, from home recipe, made w/enriched flour—1 muffin, 2¾″ diam., 45 gm.	.10	.18	NA	NA	NA	NA	NA
Muffin, Corn, from home recipe, made w/enriched, degermed cornmeal—1 muffin, 2⅜″ diam., 40 gm.	.09	.6	NA	NA	NA	NA	NA
Muffin, Corn, from home recipe, made w/whole-ground cornmeal—1 muffin, 2½″ diam., 45 gm.	.08	.5	NA	NA	NA	NA	NA
Muffin, Corn, from mix with enriched flour, made w/egg and milk—1 muffin, 2⅜″ diam., 40 gm.	.08	.6	NA	NA	NA	NA	NA
Muffin, Corn, from mix with cake flour, nonfat dry milk, made with egg, water—1 muffin, 2¾″ diam., 45 gm.	.06	.5	NA	NA	NA	NA	NA

* Based on yellow varieties of corn; white varieties contain only a trace.

Vitamin C mg.	Vitamin D IU	Vitamin E IU	Calcium mg.	Iodine mg.	Iron mg.	Magnesium mg.	Phosphorus mg.	Potassium mg.	Sodium mg.
0	NA	NA	.46	NA	.006	NA	3.8	---	11
trace	NA	NA	13	NA	.4	---	61	29	160
trace	NA	NA	12	NA	.6	8	26	---	---
0	NA	NA	10	NA	.7	7	29	21	343
0	NA	NA	147	NA	.7	7.35	162	24	404
0	NA	NA	186	NA	.7	9.7	145	31	455
0	NA	NA	9.6	NA	.5	7.2	29	22	345
0	NA	NA	14	NA	1.4	26	84	103	1.3
0	NA	NA	8	NA	1.3	25.2	70	85	1.4
0	NA	NA	14	NA	.7	26	84	103	1.3
0	NA	NA	11	NA	.6	25	70	85	1.4
trace	NA	NA	362	NA	1.8	---	322	240	1,086
trace	NA	NA	199	NA	1.0	---	182	139	729
---	NA	NA	---	NA	.4	NA	---	---	---
0	NA	NA	40	NA	13.6	324	622	860	---
trace	NA	NA	42	NA	.6	11	60	50	176
.4	NA	NA	34	NA	.6	10	53	46	253
trace	NA	NA	64	NA	1.6	NA	182	194	201
trace	NA	NA	42	NA	.7	---	67	54	192
trace	NA	NA	50	NA	.6	48	97	59	223
trace	NA	NA	96	NA	.6	---	152	44	191
trace	NA	NA	100	NA	.4	NA	147	60	365

Food and Amount	Calories	Carbo-hydrate gm.	Protein gm.	Sat. Fatty Acids gm.	Unsat. Fatty Acids gm.	Vitamin A IU	Thiamin B₁ mg.
Noodles, chow mein, canned—1 cup, 72 gm.	352.08	41.76	9.5	---	---	---	---
Noodles, egg, enriched, cooked—1 cup, 160 gm.	200	37	7	1	1	110	.22
Noodles, egg, unenriched, cooked—1 cup, 160 gm.	200	37	7	1	1	110	.05
Oat cereal w/toasted wheat germ and soygrits, cooked—1 cup, 220 gm.	136.4	20.90	7.26	---	---	0	.35
Oatflakes, maple flavored, instant cooking, cooked—1 cup, 230 gm.	158.7	29.90	5.98	---	---	0	.13
Oat granules, maple flavored, quick-cooking, cooked—1 cup, 230 gm.	138	26	5.29	---	---	0	.13
Oat and wheat cereal, cooked—1 cup, 220 gm.	143	26	5.7	---	---	0	.19
Oatmeal or rolled oats, cooked—1 cup, 240 gm.	130	23	5	---	1	0	.19
Oats (with or without corn), puffed, added nutrients—1 cup, 25 gm.	100	19	3	---	---	0	.24
Oats (w/ or w/o corn, wheat), puffed, added nutrients, sugar-covered—1 cup, 28 gm.	110	23.9	1.87	---	---	0	.28
Oats (with soy flour and rice), flaked, added nutrients—1 cup, 30 gm.	119	21.2	4.47	---	---	0	.21
Pancakes, Buckwheat and other cereal flours, made from mix, prepared w/egg, milk—one 4" cake, 27 gm.	55	6	2	1	1	60	.03
Pancakes, from home recipe, made w/enriched flour—4" diam., 1 cake, 27 gm.	60	9	2	trace	1	30	.05
Pancakes, from home recipe, made w/unenriched flour—4" diam., 1 cake, 27 gm.	62	9	2	.54	1.35	32	.04
Pancakes, Plain and Buttermilk, from pancake and waffle mix w/enriched flour, made with milk—4" cake, 27 gm.	54.54	8.61	1.64	1	.8	32.4	.03
Pancakes, Plain and Buttermilk, from pancake and waffle mix w/enriched flour, made with egg, milk—one 4" cake, 27 gm.	60	9	2	1	1	70	.04
Pancakes, Plain and Buttermilk, from mix w/unenriched flour, made with milk—4" pancake, 28 gm.	56	9	1.7	.56	.84	33	.01
Pancakes, Plain and Buttermilk, from mix w/unenriched flour, made with egg, milk—4" cake, 28 gm.	63	9	2	.84	1.4	70	.01
Pastry shell, plain—see Piecrust							
Pie—see Sweets, Sugars, Desserts, and Related Products							
Piecrust, from mix, prepared w/water, baked—one 9" shell, 160 gm.	742	70	10	11.2	38.4	0	.04
Piecrust or plain pastry, baked, w/enriched flour—one 9" shell, 180 gm.	900	79	11	16	40	0	.36
Piecrust or plain pastry, baked, w/unenriched flour—one 9" shell, 180 gm.	900	79	11	16	40	0	.05
Popcorn, popped, plain—1 cup, 6 gm.	25	5	1	---	---	---	---

Ribo-flavin B_2 mg.	Niacin mg.	B_6 mg.	Folic Acid mcg.	PABA mg.	Panto-thenic Acid mg.	B_{12} mcg.	Vitamin C mg.	Vitamin D IU	Vitamin E IU	Calcium mg.	Iodine mg.
---	---	NA	NA	NA	NA	NA	---	NA	NA	---	NA
.13	1.9	---	NA	NA	---	NA	0	NA	NA	16	NA
.03	.6	---	NA	NA	---	NA	0	NA	NA	16	NA
.06	.44	NA	---	---	NA	0	0	0	---	28.6	NA
---	---	NA	---	---	NA	0	0	0	---	23	NA
---	---	NA	---	---	NA	0	0	0	---	23	NA
.06	1.10	NA	---	---	NA	0	0	0	---	24	NA
.05	.2	NA	.079	.79	NA	0	0	0	4.8	22	.03768 Ohio
.04	.5	NA	NA	NA	NA	0	0	0	.15	44	NA
.03	.47	NA	NA	NA	NA	0	0	0	---	20	NA
.09	2.55	NA	NA	NA	NA	0	0	0	---	45	NA
.04	.2	NA	NA	NA	NA	NA	trace	NA	NA	59	NA
.06	.4	NA	NA	NA	NA	NA	trace	NA	NA	27	NA
.05	.35	NA	NA	NA	NA	NA	trace	NA	NA	27	NA
.06	.21	NA	NA	NA	NA	NA	trace	NA	NA	59.67	NA
.06	.2	NA	NA	NA	NA	NA	trace	NA	NA	58	NA
.04	.11	NA	NA	NA	NA	NA	trace	NA	NA	62	NA
.04	.11	NA	NA	NA	NA	NA	trace	NA	NA	60	NA
.04	.8	NA	NA	NA	NA	NA	0	NA	NA	65	NA
.25	3.2	NA	NA	NA	NA	NA	0	NA	NA	25	NA
.05	.9	NA	NA	NA	NA	NA	0	NA	NA	25	NA
.01	.1	---	NA	NA	---	0	0	NA	NA	1	NA

Food and Amount	Iron mg.	Mag- nesium mg.	Phos- phorus mg.	Potas- sium mg.	Sodium mg.
Noodles, chow mein, canned—1 cup, 72 gm.	...	NA	...	...	...
Noodles, egg, enriched, cooked—1 cup, 160 gm.	1.4	---	94	70	3
Noodles, egg, unenriched, cooked— 1 cup, 160 gm.	1.0	NA	94	70	3
Oat cereal w/toasted wheat germ and soygrits, cooked—1 cup, 220 gm.	2.42	---	211.2	trace	642
Oatflakes, maple flavored, instant cooking, cooked—1 cup, 230 gm.	1.38	---	149.5	---	246
Oat granules, maple flavored, quick-cooking, cooked—1 cup, 230 gm.	1.38	---	145	---	165
Oat and wheat cereal, cooked—1 cup, 220 gm.	1.54	---	165	---	369
Oatmeal or rolled oats, cooked—1 cup, 240 gm.	1.4	50	136	146	523
Oats (with or without corn), puffed, added nutrients—1 cup, 25 gm.	1.2	28	102	---	316
Oats (w/ or w/o corn, wheat), puffed, added nutrients, sugar-covered— 1 cup, 28 gm.	1.23	31.36	56	---	164
Oats (with soy flour and rice), flaked, added nutrients—1 cup, 30 gm.	2.55	---	105	---	360
Pancakes, Buckwheat and other cereal flours, made from mix, prepared w/egg, milk—one 4" cake, 27 gm.	.4	---	91	66	125
Pancakes, from home recipe, made w/enriched flour—4" diam., 1 cake, 27 gm.	.4	---	37	33	114
Pancakes, from home recipe, made w/unenriched flour—4" diam., 1 cake, 27 gm.	.35	---	37	33	114
Pancakes, Plain and Buttermilk, from pancake and waffle mix w/enriched flour, made with milk—4" cake, 27 gm.	.24	NA	65.34	42.12	121.77
Pancakes, Plain and Buttermilk, from pancake and waffle mix w/enriched flour, made with egg, milk—one 4" cake, 27 gm.	.3	NA	70	41	152
Pancakes, Plain and Buttermilk, from mix w/unenriched flour, made with milk—4" pancake, 28 gm.	.11	NA	67	43	126
Pancakes, Plain and Buttermilk, from mix w/unenriched flour, made with egg, milk—4" cake, 28 gm.	.19	NA	72	43	158
Pastry shell, plain—see Piecrust					
Pie—see Sweets, Sugars, Desserts, and Related Products					
Piecrust, from mix, prepared w/water, baked—one 9" shell, 160 gm.	.64	---	136	90	1,300
Piecrust or plain pastry, baked, w/enriched flour—one 9" shell, 180 gm.	3.1	---	90	90	1,100
Piecrust or plain pastry, baked, w/unenriched flour—one 9" shell, 180 gm.	.9	---	90	90	1,100
Popcorn, popped, plain—1 cup, 6 gm.	.2	---	17	---	.18

Food and Amount	Calories	Carbo-hydrate gm.	Protein gm.	Sat. Fatty Acids gm.	Unsat. Fatty Acids gm.	Vitamin A IU	Thiamin B₁ mg.
Popcorn, popped, w/oil (butter) and salt—1 cup, 9 gm.	40	5	1	1	trace	---	---
Popcorn, popped, sugar-coated—1 cup, 35 gm.	135	30	2	---	---	---	---
Popovers, baked, from home recipe with enriched flour—3½″, 50 gm.	112	12.9	4.4	1.5	2.5	165	.07
Potato flour—1 cup, 150 gm.	526	120	12	---	---	trace	.63
Pretzels, Dutch, twisted—1 pretzel, 16 gm.	60	12	2	---	---	0	trace
Pretzels, Stick, small, 2¼″—10 sticks, 3 gm.	10	2	trace	---	---	0	trace
Pretzels, Stick, regular, 3⅛″—5 sticks, 3 gm.	10	2	trace	---	---	0	trace
Pretzels, Thin, twisted—1 pretzel, 6 gm.	25	5	1	---	---	0	trace
Rice, Brown, cooked—1 cup, 150 gm.	178	38.2	3.8	---	---	0	.14
Rice, White (fully milled or polished), enriched, all common commercial varieties, cooked—1 cup, 205 gm.	225	50	4	---	---	0	.23
Rice, White (polished), enriched, long grain, parboiled, cooked—1 cup, 175 gm.	185	41	4	---	---	0	.19
Rice, White (polished), enriched, instant, cooked—1 cup, 165 gm.	180	40	4	---	---	0	.21
Rice, White (polished), unenriched, all common commercial varieties, cooked—1 cup, 205 gm.	225	50	4	---	---	0	.04
Rice (hot cereal), granulated, added nutrients, cooked—1 cup, 220 gm.	110	24.64	1.76	---	---	0	.13
Rice flakes, added nutrients—1 cup, 32 gm.	125	28	1.88	---	---	0	.11
Rice, puffed, added nutrients, w/o salt —1 cup, 15 gm.	60	13	1	---	---	0	.07
Rice, puffed or oven-popped, pre-sweetened, honey, and added nutrients—1 cup, 17 gm.	65.9	15.4	.71	---	---	0	.05
Rice, puffed or oven-popped, pre-sweetened, honey or cocoa, and added nutrients, incl. fat—1 cup, 17 gm.	68.17	14.73	.76	---	---	0	.07
Rice, shredded, added nutrients— 1 cup, 30 gm.	117.6	26.64	1.56	NA	NA	0	.11
Rice, w/protein concentrate (cereal), mainly casein, other added nutrients —1 cup, 28 gm.	106.9	15.3	11.2	---	---	0	.47
Rice, w/protein concentrate (cereal), mainly wheat gluten, other added nutrients—1 cup, 30 gm.	115.8	22.3	6	---	---	0	.42
Rolls, baked from packaged dough, enriched—3″ diam., 35 gm.	108	19.6	2.97	---	---	trace	.09
Rolls, baked from packaged dough, unenriched—3″ diam., 38 gm.	118	21.2	3.23	---	---	trace	.03
Rolls, baked from mix, made w/water —3″ diam., 38 gm.	113	20.7	3.42	---	---	trace	.01
Rolls and buns, baked, from home recipe, with milk and enriched flour —3″ diam., 40 gm.	135.6	22.4	3.28	.8	2.4	32	.10

Food and Amount	Riboflavin B₂ mg.	Niacin mg.	B₆ mg.	Folic Acid mg.	PABA mg.	Pantothenic Acid mg.	B₁₂ mcg.
Popcorn, popped, w/oil (butter) and salt—1 cup, 9 gm.	.01	.2	.01836	NA	NA	---	0
Popcorn, popped, sugar-coated—1 cup, 35 gm.	.02	.4	---	NA	NA	---	NA
Popovers, baked, from home recipe with enriched flour—3½", 50 gm.	.12	.5	NA	NA	NA	NA	NA
Potato flour—1 cup, 150 gm.	.21	5.1	NA	NA	NA	NA	0
Pretzels, Dutch, twisted—1 pretzel, 16 gm.	trace	.1	.00304	NA	NA	.0864	trace
Pretzels, Stick, small, 2¼"—10 sticks, 3 gm.	trace	trace	.00057	NA	NA	.0162	trace
Pretzels, Stick, regular, 3⅛"—5 sticks, 3 gm.	trace	trace	.00057	NA	NA	.0162	trace
Pretzels, Thin, twisted—1 pretzel, 6 gm.	trace	trace	.00114	NA	NA	.0324	trace
Rice, Brown, cooked—1 cup, 150 gm.	.03	2.1	.93	.03	NA	2.28	0
Rice, White (fully milled or polished), enriched, all common commercial varieties, cooked—1 cup, 205 gm.	.02	2.1	.07585	.0328	---	1.53	0
Rice, White (polished), enriched, long grain, parboiled, cooked—1 cup, 175 gm.	---	2.1	.175	.03325	---	2.39	0
Rice, White (polished), enriched, instant, cooked—1 cup, 165 gm.	---	1.7	---	---	---	---	0
Rice, White (polished), unenriched, all common commercial varieties, cooked—1 cup, 205 gm.	.02	.8	---	---	---	---	0
Rice (hot cereal), granulated, added nutrients, cooked—1 cup, 220 gm.	.02	1.76	NA	NA	---	NA	0
Rice flakes, added nutrients—1 cup, 32 gm.	.01	1.7	.04	.00256	NA	.1088	0
Rice, puffed, added nutrients, w/o salt—1 cup, 15 gm.	.01	.7	.024	---	NA	.12096	0
Rice, puffed or oven-popped, pre-sweetened, honey, and added nutrients—1 cup, 17 gm.	---	.78	---	---	NA	---	0
Rice, puffed or oven-popped, pre-sweetened, honey or cocoa, and added nutrients, incl. fat—1 cup, 17 gm.	.01	1.07	---	---	NA	---	0
Rice, shredded, added nutrients—1 cup, 30 gm.	---	2.1	NA	NA	NA	NA	0
Rice, w/protein concentrate (cereal), mainly casein, other added nutrients—1 cup, 28 gm.	.58	4.92	NA	NA	NA	NA	0
Rice, w/protein concentrate (cereal), mainly wheat gluten, other added nutrients—1 cup, 30 gm.	.51	.51	NA	NA	NA	NA	0
Rolls, baked from packaged dough, enriched—3" diam., 35 gm.	.07	.80	---	NA	NA	---	---
Rolls, baked from packaged dough, unenriched—3" diam., 38 gm.	.03	.38	---	NA	NA	---	---
Rolls, baked from mix, made w/water—3" diam., 38 gm.	.04	.26	---	NA	NA	---	---
Rolls and buns, baked, from home recipe, with milk and enriched flour—3" diam., 40 gm.	.10	.92	.014	NA	NA	.124	---

Vitamin C mg.	Vitamin D IU	Vitamin E IU	Calcium mg.	Iodine mg.	Iron mg.	Magnesium mg.	Phosphorus mg.	Potassium mg.	Sodium mg.
0	NA	NA	1	NA	.2	---	19	---	175
0	NA	NA	2	NA	.5	NA	47	---	.35
trace	NA	NA	48	NA	.8	12	70	75	110
28.5	NA	NA	50	NA	25.8	NA	267	2,382	51
0	NA	.02	4	NA	.2	NA	---	---	---
0	NA	trace	1	NA	trace	NA	---	---	---
0	NA	trace	1	NA	trace	NA	---	---	---
0	NA	trace	1	NA	.1	NA	---	---	---
0	0	NA	18	NA	.8	45	110	105	423
0	0	.82	21	.00615	1.8	16	57	57	766
0	0	---	33	NA	1.4	---	1.4	0	75
0	0	---	5	NA	1.3	---	31	trace	450
0	0	---	21	NA	.4	---	57	57	766
0	0	NA	4.4	NA	1.54	---	28.6	trace	387.2
0	0	.01	9	NA	.51	---	42	57	315
0	0	---	3	.00227	.3	---	14	15	.30
0	0	---	7.8	NA	.15	---	12.58	---	120
0	0	NA	8.67	NA	.56	---	13.94	10	60.8
0	0	---	4.2	NA	.54	---	28.5	---	253.8
14.84	NA	---	44.5	NA	4.92	---	89	---	168
10.5	NA	---	15.9	NA	3.72	---	56	---	240
trace	NA	NA	13.6	NA	.70	---	30.8	33.6	196
trace	NA	NA	14.8	NA	.38	---	33.4	36.4	212
trace	NA	NA	21.2	NA	.22	---	36.8	46.7	119
trace	NA	NA	18.8	NA	.84	---	40.8	46.8	111

Food and Amount	Calories	Carbo-hydrate gm.	Protein gm.	Sat. Fatty Acids gm.	Unsat. Fatty Acids gm.	Vitamin A IU	Thiamin B₁ mg.
Rolls and buns, baked, commercial, Danish pastry—1 piece, 4¼" x 1", 65 gm.	275	30	5	5	10	200	.05
Rolls and buns, baked commercially, Hard rolls, enriched—3½" diam., 35 gm.	109	21	3.4	.35	1.4	trace	.09
Rolls and buns, baked commercially, Hard rolls, unenriched—3½" diam., 35 gm.	109	21	3.4	.35	1.4	trace	.01
Rolls and buns, baked commercially, Plain (pan rolls), enriched—3½" diam., 38 gm.	113	20.1	3.1	.38	1.52	trace	.11
Rolls and buns, baked commercially, Plain (pan rolls), unenriched—3" diam., 38 gm.	113	20.1	3.1	.38	1.52	trace	.02
Rolls and buns, baked commercially, Raisin rolls or buns—1 piece, 2½" diam., 43 gm.	118	24	2.96	.43	1.72	trace	.02
Rolls and buns, baked commercially, Sweet rolls—1 piece, 4" x 1", 55 gm.	178	29.6	4.7	---	---	0	.03
Rolls and buns, baked commercially, Whole-wheat rolls—1 piece, 3" diam., 35 gm.	90	18.3	3.5	.35	1.4	trace	.12
Rye, whole-grain—1 cup, 120 gm.	400	88	14.5	---	---	0	.51
Rye flour, light—1 cup sifted, 80 gm.	285	62	7.5	---	---	0	.12
Rye flour, medium—1 cup sifted, 102 gm.	357	76	11.6	---	---	0	.30
Rye flour, dark—1 cup sifted, 125 gm.	409	85	20	NA	NA	0	.76
Rye wafers, whole-grain—1⅞" x 3½", 2 wafers, 13 gm.	45	10	2	---	---	0	.04
St. Johnsbread—see Carob flour							
Salt sticks, regular type—1 stick, 3" long, 14 gm.	53	10.5	1.68	NA	NA	trace	.008
Salt sticks, Vienna bread type—1 stick, 3" long, 14 gm.	42	8.12	1.33	NA	NA	trace	.007
Shortbread—see Cookies							
Spaghetti, enriched, cooked, firm stage —1 cup, 146 gm.	216	44	7.3	---	---	0	.26
Spaghetti, enriched, cooked, tender stage—1 cup, 140 gm.	155	32	5	---	---	0	.20
Spaghetti, unenriched, cooked, firm stage—1 cup, 146 gm.	216	44	7.3	---	---	0	.03
Spaghetti, unenriched, cooked, tender stage—1 cup, 150 gm.	166	34.5	5.1	---	---	0	.015
Spaghetti in tomato sauce w/cheese, cooked, home recipe—1 cup, 250 gm.	260	37	9	2	6	1,080	.25
Spaghetti in tomato sauce w/cheese, canned—1 cup, 250 gm.	190	38	6	1	2	930	.35
Spaghetti w/meat balls in tomato sauce, cooked, home recipe—1 cup, 248 gm.	330	39	19	4	7	1,590	.25
Spaghetti w/meat balls in tomato sauce, canned—1 cup, 250 gm.	260	28	12	2	7	1,000	.15
Spanish rice, cooked from home recipe—1 cup, 150 gm.	130	24.9	2.7	NA	NA	990	.06

Riboflavin B2 mg.	Niacin mg.	B6 mg.	Folic Acid mg.	PABA mg	Pantothenic Acid mg.	B12 mcg.	Vitamin C mg.	Vitamin D IU	Vitamin E IU	Calcium mg.	Iodine mg.
.10	.5	NA	NA	NA	NA	NA	trace	NA	NA	33	NA
.08	.94	---	NA	NA	---	---	trace	NA	NA	16	NA
.03	.28	NA	NA	NA	NA	NA	trace	NA	NA	16	NA
.07	.8	.0133	NA	NA	.1178	---	trace	NA	NA	28	NA
.03	.3	.0133	NA	NA	.1178	---	trace	NA	NA	28	NA
.04	.3	NA	NA	NA	NA	NA	trace	NA	NA	32	NA
.07	.6	NA	NA	NA	NA	NA	0	NA	NA	35	NA
.05	1.1	NA	NA	NA	NA	NA	trace	NA	NA	37	NA
.26	1.9	NA	NA	NA	NA	0	0	NA	3.63	45	.00036
.05	.48	.072	.128	NA	.576	0	0	NA	---	17	NA
.12	2.55	NA	NA	NA	NA	0	0	NA	---	27	NA
.27	3.37	NA	NA	NA	NA	0	NA	NA	---	67	NA
.03	.2	NA	NA	NA	NA	NA	0	NA	---	7	NA
.009	.14	NA	NA	NA	NA	NA	trace	NA	NA	3.92	NA
.01	.11	NA	NA	NA	NA	NA	trace	NA	NA	6.30	NA
.15	2	NA	NA	NA	NA	NA	0	NA	NA	16	NA
.11	1.5	NA	NA	NA	NA	NA	0	NA	NA	11	NA
.03	.6	NA	NA	NA	NA	NA	0	NA	NA	16	NA
.015	.4	NA	NA	NA	NA	NA	0	NA	NA	12	NA
.18	2.3	NA	NA	NA	NA	NA	13	NA	NA	80	NA
.28	4.5	NA	NA	NA	NA	NA	10	NA	NA	40	NA
.30	4.0	NA	NA	NA	NA	NA	22	NA	NA	124	NA
.18	2.3	NA	NA	NA	NA	NA	5	NA	NA	53	NA
.04	1.1	NA	NA	NA	NA	NA	22	NA	NA	21	NA

Food and Amount	Iron mg.	Magnesium mg.	Phosphorus mg.	Potassium mg.	Sodium mg.
Rolls and buns, baked, commercial, Danish pastry—1 piece, 4¼″ x 1″, 65 gm.	.6	---	70	72	238
Rolls and buns, baked commercially, Hard rolls, enriched—3½″ diam., 35 gm.	.8	---	32	34	219
Rolls and buns, baked commercially, Hard rolls, unenriched—3½″ diam., 35 gm.	.28	---	32	34	219
Rolls and buns, baked commercially, Plain (pan rolls), enriched—3½″ diam., 38 gm.	.7	14	32	36	192
Rolls and buns, baked commercially, Plain (pan rolls), unenriched—3″ diam., 38 gm.	.3	14	32	36	192
Rolls and buns, baked commercially, Raisin rolls or buns—1 piece, 2½″ diam., 43 gm.	.6	---	39	105	165
Rolls and buns, baked commercially, Sweet rolls—1 piece, 4″ x 1″, 55 gm.	.3	18	57	68	214
Rolls and buns, baked commercially, Whole-wheat rolls—1 piece, 3″ diam., 35 gm.	.8	40	98	102	197
Rye, whole-grain—1 cup, 120 gm.	4.44	138	451	560	1.2
Rye flour, light—1 cup sifted, 80 gm.	.88	58	148	125	.80
Rye flour, medium—1 cup sifted, 102 gm.	2.65	NA	267	207	1.0
Rye flour, dark—1 cup sifted, 125 gm.	5.6	NA	670	1,075	1.25
Rye wafers, whole-grain—1⅞″ x 3½″, 2 wafers, 13 gm.	.5	---	50	78	115
St. Johnsbread—see Carob flour					
Salt sticks, regular type—1 stick, 3″ long, 14 gm.	.12	NA	13.8	13	234
Salt sticks, Vienna bread type—1 stick, 3″ long, 14 gm.	.11	NA	12.4	13	219
Shortbread—see Cookies					
Spaghetti, enriched, cooked, firm stage—1 cup, 146 gm.	1.6	29	95	115	1
Spaghetti, enriched, cooked, tender stage—1 cup, 140 gm.	1.3	---	70	85	1
Spaghetti, unenriched, cooked, firm stage—1 cup, 146 gm.	.7	29	95	115	1
Spaghetti, unenriched, cooked, tender stage—1 cup, 150 gm.	.6	27	75	92	2
Spaghetti in tomato sauce w/cheese, cooked, home recipe—1 cup, 250 gm.	2.3	---	135	407	955
Spaghetti in tomato sauce w/cheese, canned—1 cup, 250 gm.	2.8	---	87	302	955
Spaghetti w/meat balls in tomato sauce, cooked, home recipe—1 cup, 248 gm.	3.7	---	235	664	1,009
Spaghetti w/meat balls in tomato sauce, canned—1 cup, 250 gm.	3.3	---	112	245	1,220
Spanish rice, cooked from home recipe—1 cup, 150 gm.	.9	NA	58	347	475

Food and Amount	Calories	Carbohydrate gm.	Protein gm.	Sat. Fatty Acids gm.	Unsat. Fatty Acids gm.	Vitamin A IU	Thiamin B₁ mg.
Waffles, from home recipe, made w/enriched flour—1 waffle, 6″ diam., 75 gm.	210	28	7	2	5	250	.13
Waffles, from home recipe, made w/unenriched flour—1 waffle, 6″ diam., 75 gm.	209	28.1	7	2	5	248	.04
Waffles, frozen, made w/enriched flour—6″ diam., 75 gm.	189.75	31.5	5.32	1.5	3.75	97.5	.12
Waffles, made from mix w/enriched flour, prepared with water—6″ diam., 74 gm.	225.7	29.74	3.55	2.22	7.4	59.2	.08
Waffles, made from mix w/unenriched flour, prepared with water—6″ diam., 74 gm.	225.7	29.74	3.55	2.22	7.4	59.2	.01
Waffles, made from mix w/enriched flour, made w/egg, milk—1 waffle, 7″ diam., 75 gm.	205	27	7	3	4	170	.11
Waffles, made with egg, milk, made from mix w/unenriched flour—6½″ diam., 77 gm.	211.75	27.87	6.77	3.08	4.62	177.1	.06
Wheat bran, crude, commercially milled—1 tbsp., 10 gm.	36.3	4.67	2.66	---	---	0	.201
Wheat flour, whole (from hard wheats) —1 cup, 120 gm.	400	85	16	trace	2	0	.66
Wheat flour, 80% extraction (from hard wheats)—1 cup sifted, 110 gm.	401	81	13	NA	NA	0	.28
Wheat flour, straight, hard wheat— 1 cup, 115 gm.	419	85	13	---	---	0	.13
Wheat flour, straight, soft wheat— 1 cup, 113 gm.	411	86	10.9	---	---	0	.09
Wheat flour, all-purpose, enriched— 1 cup sifted, 115 gm.	420	88	12	---	---	0	.51
Wheat flour, all-purpose, unenriched— 1 cup sifted, 110 gm.	400	83.7	11.6	---	---	0	.07
Wheat flour, bread flour, enriched— 1 cup sifted, 112 gm.	409	83.7	13.2	---	---	0	.49
Wheat flour, bread flour, unenriched— 1 cup sifted, 112 gm.	409	83.7	13.2	---	---	0	.09
Wheat flour, cake or pastry flour— 1 cup, 96 gm.	350	76	7	---	---	0	.03
Wheat flour, Gluten flour—1 cup, 140 gm.	529	66.1	58	---	---	0	---
Wheat flour, self-rising, enriched— 1 cup, 125 gm.	440	93	12	---	---	0	.55
Wheat germ, crude, commercially milled—1 tbsp., 10 gm.	36	4.7	2.7	.20	.80	0	.2
Wheat, par boiled—see Bulgur							
Wheat, puffed, added nutrients, w/o salt—1 cup, 15 gm.	55	12	2	---	---	0	.08
Wheat, puffed, added nutrients w/sugar and honey—1 cup, 15 gm.	56	13	.90	---	---	0	.07
Wheat, rolled (hot cereal), cooked— 1 cup, 220 gm.	165	37	4.84	---	---	0	.15
Wheat, shredded, no additives—1 two inch biscuit, 25 gm.	90	20	2	---	---	0	.06

Food and Amount	Ribo-flavin B₂ mg.	Niacin mg.	B₆ mg.	Folic Acid mg.	PABA mg.	Panto-thenic Acid mg.	B₁₂ mcg.
Waffles, from home recipe, made w/enriched flour—1 waffle, 6" diam., 75 gm.	.19	1.0	---	NA	NA	.487	---
Waffles, from home recipe, made w/unenriched flour—1 waffle, 6" diam., 75 gm.	.14	.3	---	NA	NA	.487	NA
Waffles, frozen, made w/enriched flour—6" diam., 75 gm.	.12	.9	---	NA	NA	---	NA
Waffles, made from mix w/enriched flour, prepared with water—6" diam., 74 gm.	.08	.74	---	NA	NA	---	NA
Waffles, made from mix w/unenriched flour, prepared with water—6" diam., 74 gm.	.03	.22	---	NA	NA	---	NA
Waffles, made from mix w/enriched flour, made w/egg, milk—1 waffle, 7" diam., 75 gm.	.17	.7	---	NA	NA	---	NA
Waffles, made with egg, milk, made from mix w/unenriched flour— 6½" diam., 77 gm.	.14	.3	---	NA	NA	---	NA
Wheat bran, crude, commercially milled—1 tbsp., 10 gm.	.068	.42	---	---	NA	---	0
Wheat flour, whole (from hard wheats) —1 cup, 120 gm.	.14	5.2	.396	.0456	---	1.29	0
Wheat flour, 80% extraction (from hard wheats)—1 cup sifted, 110 gm.	.07	2.2	---	---	NA	---	0
Wheat flour, straight, hard wheat— 1 cup, 115 gm.	.08	1.61	---	---	NA	---	0
Wheat flour, straight, soft wheat— 1 cup, 113 gm.	.05	1.35	---	---	NA	---	0
Wheat flour, all-purpose, enriched— 1 cup sifted, 115 gm.	.30	4.0	.069	.009	NA	.534	0
Wheat flour, all-purpose, unenriched— 1 cup sifted, 110 gm.	.06	1	.066	.008	NA	.511	0
Wheat flour, bread flour, enriched— 1 cup sifted, 112 gm.	.29	3.9	---	---	NA	---	0
Wheat flour, bread flour, unenriched— 1 cup sifted, 112 gm.	.07	1.1	---	---	NA	---	0
Wheat flour, cake or pastry flour— 1 cup, 96 gm.	.03	.7	.043	.004	NA	.211	0
Wheat flour, Gluten flour—1 cup, 140 gm.	---	---	---	---	NA	---	0
Wheat flour, self-rising, enriched— 1 cup, 125 gm.	.33	4.4	---	---	NA	---	0
Wheat germ, crude, commercially milled—1 tbsp., 10 gm.	.07	.4	.115	.030	.17	.12	0
Wheat, par boiled—see Bulgur							
Wheat, puffed, added nutrients, w/o salt—1 cup, 15 gm.	.03	1.2	.025	NA	NA	---	0
Wheat, puffed, added nutrients w/sugar and honey—1 cup, 15 gm.	.02	.96	---	NA	NA	---	0
Wheat, rolled (hot cereal), cooked— 1 cup, 220 gm.	.06	1.98	NA	.1078	---	NA	0
Wheat, shredded, no additives—1 two inch biscuit, 25 gm.	.03	1.1	.061	.013	NA	.176	0

Vitamin C mg.	Vitamin D IU	Vitamin E IU	Calcium mg.	Iodine mg.	Iron mg.	Magnesium mg.	Phosphorus mg.	Potassium mg.	Sodium mg.
trace	NA	NA	85	NA	1.3	19	130	109	356
trace	NA	NA	85	NA	.7	19	130	109	356
trace	NA	NA	91.5	NA	1.35	NA	156	118.5	483
trace	NA	NA	56.24	NA	.74	NA	93.98	40.7	414.4
trace	NA	NA	56.24	NA	.29	NA	93.98	40.7	414.4
trace	NA	NA	179	NA	1.0	NA	257	146	514
trace	NA	NA	184.03	NA	.69	NA	264.11	150.15	528.22
0	NA	NA	7.2	NA	.94	---	111.8	82.7	.3
0	NA	3.12	49	0 Neb.	4.0	135.6	446	444	3.6
0	NA	2.97	26	0 Neb.	1.4	---	210	104	2.2
0	NA	NA	23	0 Neb.	1.61	---	111	109	2.3
0	NA	NA	22	0 Neb.	1.24	---	109	107	2.26
0	NA	NA	18	0 Neb.	3.3	28	100	109	2.3
0	NA	NA	18	0 Neb.	.9	28	96	105	2
0	NA	NA	18	0 Neb.	3.2	28	106	106	2
0	NA	NA	18	0 Neb.	1	28	106	106	2
0	NA	NA	16	0 Neb.	.5	---	70	91	2
0	NA	NA	56	0 Neb.	---	---	196	84	3
0	NA	NA	331	0 Neb.	3.6	---	582	---	1,348
0	NA	2.7	7	NA	.9	34	112	83	trace
0	0	NA	4	NA	.6	---	48	51	.60
0	0	NA	4	NA	.5	---	22	15	24
0	0	NA	17.6	NA	1.54	---	167	184	trace
0	0	NA	11	NA	.9	33	97	87	.75

Food and Amount	Calories	Carbo-hydrate gm.	Protein gm.	Sat. Fatty Acids gm.	Unsat. Fatty Acids gm.	Vitamin A IU	Thiamin B₁ mg.
Wheat, shredded, w/malt, salt and sugar added—1 two inch biscuit, 25 gm.	91	20	2.27	---	---	0	.02
Wheat, whole-meal, cooked—1 cup, 230 gm.	103	21.6	4.14	---	---	0	.13
Wheat, whole-grain, hard red winter—1 cup, 210 gm.	693	150	25.8	NA	NA	0	1.09
Wheat bran cereal—see Bran							
Wheat flakes, added nutrients—1 cup, 68 gm.	241	54	6.9	---	---	0	.43
Wheat germ cereal, added nutrients, toasted—1 cup, 113 gm.	442	55.9	33.9	---	---	124	1.86
Wheat and malted barley flakes, nutrients added—1 cup, 25 gm.	98	21	2.2	---	---	0	.11
Wheat and malted barley granules, nutrients added—1 cup, 26 gm.	101	22	2.6	---	---	0	.11
Wheat and malted barley cereal, toasted, quick-cooking, cooked—1 cup, 220 gm.	143	29.04	4.40	---	---	0	.11
Wheat and malted barley cereal, toasted, instant-cooking, cooked—1 cup, 220 gm.	176	35.42	6.60	---	---	0	.15
Wild rice, cooked—1 cup, 190 gm.	670	143	26.7	---	---	0	.85
Zwieback—1 piece, 7 gm.	30	5	.74	.14	.42	3	.003

MEAT, POULTRY, GAME, ETC.

Food and Amount	Calories	Carbo-hydrate gm.	Protein gm.	Sat. Fatty Acids gm.	Unsat. Fatty Acids gm.	Vitamin A IU	Thiamin B₁ mg.
Bacon, cured, cooked, broiled or fried, drained—one 7″ slice, 5 gm.	30.5	.16	1.52	.85	1.5	0	.02
Bacon, Canadian, cooked, broiled or fried, drained—2¼″ x ³⁄₁₆″, 30 gm.	83.1	.09	8.28	1.5	2.1	0	.27
Beans and frankfurters, canned—1 cup, 245 gm.	352.8	30.87	18.62	---	---	318.5	.17
BEEF, RETAIL CUTS, CHOICE GRADE, LEAN ONLY, SEPARABLE FAT REMOVED							
Beef, Brisket cut, Corned Beef—see Beef, Corned							
Beef, Brisket cut, Beef Brisket—moist*, cooked, 1 sl., 5″ x 1″ x ¾″, 95 gm.	411	0	17.3	5.03	4.94	---	.048
Beef, Chuck cut, Arm Pot Roast—moist* cooked, 1 sl., 4¼″ x 1¼″ x 1″, 83 gm.	218	0	27.4	4.15	3.73	---	.083
Beef, Chuck cut, Rolled Neck—moist* cooked, 1 sl., 4″ x 2″ x 1″, 132 gm.	325	0	40.3	6.6	5.94	---	.066
Beef, Chuck cut, Boneless Neck—moist* cooked, 1 sl., 4″ x 2″ x 1″, 132 gm.	325	0	40.3	6.6	5.94	---	.066
Beef, Chuck cut, Triangle Pot Roast—moist* cooked, 1 sl., 4″ x 1¼″ x ½″, 48 gm.	102.7	0	14.4	2.4	2.16	9.6	.02
Beef, Chuck cut, Boneless Chuck Pot Roast—moist* cooked, 1 sl., 4″ x 1¼″ x ½″, 46 gm.	98.4	0	13.8	2.3	2.07	9.2	.02

* Dry cooking; broiling, roasting—Moist cooking: stewing, braising.

Riboflavin B_2 mg.	Niacin mg.	B_6 mg.	Folic Acid mg.	PABA mg.	Pantothenic Acid mg.	B_{12} mcg.	Vitamin C mg.	Vitamin D IU	Vitamin E IU	Calcium mg.	Iodine mg.
.03	1.2	---	---	NA	---	0	0	0	NA	9.7	NA
.04	1.38	NA	---	NA	NA	0	0	0	NA	16.1	NA
.25	9.03	.714	.0798	1.17	2.31	0	0	NA	NA	96.6	0 Neb.
.09	3.3	.198	.031	NA	.318	0	0	0	NA	28	NA
1.10	5.98	---	---	---	---	0	11	0	NA	53	NA
.02	.97	NA	NA	NA	NA	0	0	0	NA	12.25	NA
.01	1.37	NA	NA	NA	NA	0	0	0	NA	13.78	NA
.02	---	NA	NA	NA	NA	0	0	0	1.34	19.8	NA
.04	---	NA	NA	NA	NA	0	0	0	1.34	19.8	NA
1.19	11.78	NA	NA	NA	NA	NA	0	NA	NA	36.1	NA
.004	.063	NA	NA	NA	NA	NA	0	NA	NA	.91	NA

MEAT, POULTRY, GAME, ETC.

Riboflavin B_2 mg.	Niacin mg.	B_6 mg.	Folic Acid mg.	PABA mg.	Pantothenic Acid mg	B_{12} mcg.	Vitamin C mg.	Vitamin D IU	Vitamin E IU	Calcium mg.	Iodine mg.
.01	.26	.00625 (raw)	---	NA	.0165 (raw)	.03 (raw)	---	0	.02	.70	.00081 (raw) Ohio
.05	1.5	---	---	NA	---	---	---	0	---	5.7	NA
.14	3.18	NA	NA	NA	NA	NA	trace	NA	NA	90.65	NA
.219	3.7	---	---	.28 (raw)	---	---	0	0	---	11	NA
.191	3.6	---	---	.24 (raw)	---	---	0	0	---	7	NA
.03	5.1	---	---	.39 (raw)	---	---	0	0	---	15	NA
.03	5.1	---	---	.39 (raw)	---	---	0	0	---	15	NA
.11	2.20	---	---	.14 (raw)	---	---	0	0	---	6.24	NA
.10	2.11	---	---	.13 (raw)	---	---	0	0	---	5.98	NA

Food and Amount	Iron mg.	Magnesium mg.	Phosphorus mg.	Potassium mg.	Sodium mg.
Wheat, shredded, w/malt, salt and sugar added—1 two inch biscuit, 25 gm.	.85	---	92	---	174
Wheat, whole-meal, cooked—1 cup, 230 gm.	1.15	---	119	110	487
Wheat, whole-grain, hard red winter—1 cup, 210 gm.	7.14	336	743	777	6.3
Wheat bran cereal—see Bran					
Wheat flakes, added nutrients—1 cup, 68 gm.	3	---	210	---	701
Wheat germ cereal, added nutrients, toasted—1 cup, 113 gm.	10.05	---	1,225	1,070	2.2
Wheat and malted barley flakes, nutrients added—1 cup, 25 gm.	.65	---	62	---	195
Wheat and malted barley granules, nutrients added—1 cup, 26 gm.	.72	---	45	59	184
Wheat and malted barley cereal, toasted, quick-cooking, cooked—1 cup, 220 gm.	.88	---	129	trace	158
Wheat and malted barley cereal, toasted, instant-cooking, cooked—1 cup, 220 gm.	1.98	68.2	180	trace	224
Wild rice, cooked—1 cup, 190 gm.	7.98	212.8	644	418	13
Zwieback—1 piece, 7 gm.	.04	NA	5	10	17

MEAT, POULTRY, GAME, ETC.

Food and Amount	Iron mg.	Magnesium mg.	Phosphorus mg.	Potassium mg.	Sodium mg.
Bacon, cured, cooked, broiled or fried, drained—one 7" slice, 5 gm.	.16	1.25	11.2	11.8	51
Bacon, Canadian, cooked, broiled or fried, drained—2¼" x ⁷⁄₁₆", 30 gm.	1.23	7.2	65.4	129.6	766.5
Beans and frankfurters, canned—1 cup, 245 gm.	4.65	NA	291.55	641.9	1,320.55
BEEF, RETAIL CUTS, CHOICE GRADE, LEAN ONLY, SEPARABLE FAT REMOVED					
Beef, Brisket cut, Corned Beef—see Beef, Corned					
Beef, Brisket cut, Beef Brisket—moist*, cooked, 1 sl., 5" x 1" x ¾", 95 gm.	---	12.7	123	285	52
Beef, Chuck cut, Arm Pot Roast—moist* cooked, 1 sl., 4" x 1¼" x 1", 83 gm.	---	16.4	158	320	45
Beef, Chuck cut, Rolled Neck—moist* cooked, 1 sl., 4" x 2" x 1", 132 gm.	---	27	230	396	72
Beef, Chuck cut, Boneless Neck—moist* cooked, 1 sl., 4" x 2" x 1", 132 gm.	---	27	230	396	72
Beef, Chuck cut, Triangle Pot Roast—moist* cooked, 1 sl., 4" x 1¼" x ½", 48 gm.	1.82	7.2	76.8	---	---
Beef, Chuck cut, Boneless Chuck Pot Roast—moist* cooked, 1 sl., 4" x 1¼" x ½", 46 gm.	1.74	6.9	73.6	---	---

*Dry cooking; broiling, roasting—Moist cooking: stewing, braising.

Food and Amount	Calories	Carbo-hydrate gm.	Protein gm.	Sat. Fatty Acids gm.	Unsat. Fatty Acids gm.	Vitamin A IU	Thiamin B1 mg.
Beef, Chuck cut, Blade Steak—dry* cooked, 1 sl., 3″ x 2″ x ½″, 90 gm.	384.3	0	20.16	4.5	4.05	63	.03
Beef, Chuck cut, Blade Pot Roast—moist* cooked, 1 sl., 4″ x 1¼″ x 1″, 83 gm.	218	0	27.4	4.15	3.73	---	.083
Beef, Chuck cut, Ground Chuck—dry* cooked, 2½″ diam., ¾″ thick, ¼ lb. raw, 85 gm.	363	0	19.04	4.25	3.82	39.2	.03
Beef, Shank cut, Knuckle Soup Bone—moist* cooked, 1–3″ bone, 19 gm., (meat only)	34.96	0	5.83	---	---	1.9	.01
Beef, Plate cut, Short Ribs—moist* cooked, 1 piece, 2″ x 1″, 14 gm.	31.08	0	4.15	---	---	2.8	.008
Beef, Plate cut, Plate Boiling Beef—moist* cooked, 2″ x 2″ x ¾″, 48 gm.	106.56	0	14.25	---	---	9.6	.02
Beef, Flank, Flank Steak—moist* cooked, 4″ x 2″ x ⅝″, 141 gm.	331	0	47.1	5.64	4.23	---	.07
Beef, Fat—1 cubic inch, 38 gm. (1.35 oz.)	277.02	0	2.166	14.06	14.93	---	---
Beef, Flank, Flank Stew Meat—moist* cooked, 1 piece, 1¼′ x 1¼″ x 1″, 35 gm.	68.6	0	10.67	1.4	1.05	---	.02
Beef, Flank, Rolled Flank—moist* cooked, 4″ x 2″ x ⅝″, 141 gm.	331	0	47.1	5.64	4.23	---	.07
Beef, Rib cut, Standing Rib Roast—dry* cooked, 1 sl., 4″ x 2½″ x 1″, 106 gm.	302	0	28.4	7.1	7.1	---	.064
Beef, Rib cut, Rolled Rib Roast—dry* cooked, 1 sl., 4″ x 2½″ x 1″, 106 gm.	302	0	28.4	7.1	7.1	---	.064
Beef, Rib cut, Rib Steak—dry* cooked, 1 piece, 4″ x 3″ x ½″, 94 gm.	246	0	24	6.29	6.29	---	.056
Beef, Short Loin cut, Porterhouse Steak—dry* cooked, 4″ x 3″ x ½″, 100 gm.	242	0	25.4	5.3	5.3	---	.1
Beef, Short Loin cut, T-Bone Steak—dry* cooked, 3¼″ x 3⅛″ x ½″, 95 gm.	235	0	24	5.03	5.03	---	.095
Beef, Short Loin cut, Club Steak—dry* cooked, 3¼″ x 3⅛″ x ½″, 93 gm.	260	0	23.9	4.92	4.92	---	.093
Beef, Short Loin cut, Filet Mignon—dry* cooked, 2″ diam. x 1½″ thick, 180 gm.	395	0	52.1	9.09	9.09	---	.14
Beef, Short Loin cut, N.Y. Strip or Shell Steak—dry* cooked, 5″ x 2¾″ x ¾″ (widest point), 170 gm.	380	0	51.3	9.01	9.01	34	.13
Beef, Short Loin cut, Tenderloin Steak—dry* cooked, 4″ x 3″ x ¼″, 66 gm.	148	0	17.2	3.49	3.49	---	.066
Beef, Loin End cut, Sirloin Steak—dry* cooked, 1 sl., 3″ x 2½″ x 1″, 125 gm.	260	0	31.9	4.75	4.5	---	.125
Beef, Loin End Cut, Pin Bone Sirloin Steak—dry* cooked, 1 sl., 3″ x 2½″ x 1″, 125 gm.	260	0	31.9	4.75	4.5	---	.125
Beef, Loin End cut, Ground Sirloin Beef—dry* cooked, 2½″ diam., ¾″ thick, ¼ lb. raw, 85 gm.	346.8	0	18.87	3.23	3.06	51	.05
Beef, Rump cut, Rump Roast—moist* cooked, 1 sl., 4″ x 1¼″ x 1″, 80 gm.	188	0	25.6	3.76	3.68	---	.08
Beef, Rump cut, Rolled Rump—dry* cooked, 4″ x 1½″ x ¾″, 95 gm.	197.6	0	27.64	4.46	4.37	19	.06
Beef, Round cut, Round Steak—dry* cooked, 1 piece, 4″ x 3″ x 1″, 112 gm.	292.32	0	32.03	3.47	3.36	33.6	.08

* Dry cooking: broiling, roasting—Moist cooking: stewing, braising.

Food and Amount	Riboflavin B_2 mg.	Niacin mg.	B_6 mg.	Folic Acid mg.	PABA mg.	Pantothenic Acid mg.	B_{12} mcg.
Beef, Chuck cut, Blade Steak—dry* cooked, 1 sl., 3″ x 2″ x ½″, 90 gm.	.15	3.15	---	---	.27 (raw)	---	---
Beef, Chuck cut, Blade Pot Roast—moist* cooked, 1 sl., 4″ x 1¼″ x 1″, 83 gm.	.191	3.6	---	---	.24 (raw)	---	---
Beef, Chuck cut, Ground Chuck—dry* cooked, 2½″ diam., ¾″ thick, ¼ lb. raw, 85 gm.	.14	2.97	.36975 (raw)	.00935	.25 (raw)	.527 (raw)	1.53 (raw)
Beef, Shank cut, Knuckle Soup Bone—moist* cooked, 1–3″ bone, 19 gm., (meat only)	.04	.89	NA	NA	.05 (raw)	NA	NA
Beef, Plate cut, Short Ribs—moist* cooked, 1 piece, 2″ x 1″, 14 gm.	.03	.63	---	---	.04 (raw)	---	---
Beef, Plate cut, Plate Boiling Beef—moist* cooked, 2″ x 2″ x ¾″, 48 gm.	.1	2.16	---	---	.14 (raw)	---	---
Beef, Flank, Flank Steak—moist* cooked, 4″ x 2″ x ⅝″, 141 gm.	.226	3.9	---	---	.42 (raw)	---	---
Beef, Fat—1 cubic inch, 38 gm. (1.35 oz.)	---	---	NA	NA	NA	NA	NA
Beef, Flank, Flank Stew Meat—moist* cooked, 1 piece, 1¼′ x 1¼″ x 1″, 35 gm.	.08	1.61	---	---	.1 (raw)	---	---
Beef, Flank, Rolled Flank—moist* cooked, 4″ x 2″ x ⅝″, 141 gm.	.226	3.9	---	---	.42 (raw)	---	---
Beef, Rib cut, Standing Rib Roast— dry* cooked, 1 sl., 4″ x 2½″ x 1″, 106 gm.	.223	4.2	.4611 (raw)	.01166	.31 (raw)	.6572 (raw)	1.9 (raw)
Beef, Rib cut, Rolled Rib Roast—dry* cooked, 1 sl., 4″ x 2½″ x 1″, 106 gm.	.223	4.2	.4611 (raw)	.01166	.31 (raw)	.6572 (raw)	1.9 (raw)
Beef, Rib cut, Rib Steak—dry* cooked, 1 piece, 4″ x 3″ x ½″, 94 gm.	.197	3.8	.4089 (raw)	.01034	.28 (raw)	.5828 (raw)	1.69 (raw)
Beef, Short Loin cut, Porterhouse Steak —dry* cooked, 4″ x 3″ x ½″, 100 gm.	.12	6.1	.435 (raw)	.011	.3 (raw)	.62 (raw)	1.8 (raw)
Beef, Short Loin cut, T-Bone Steak—dry* cooked, 3¼″ x 3⅛″ x ½″, 95 gm.	.114	5.8	.41325 (raw)	.01045	.28 (raw)	.589 (raw)	1.71 (raw)
Beef, Short Loin cut, Club Steak—dry* cooked, 3¼″ x 3⅛″ x ½″, 93 gm.	.112	5.7	.40455 (raw)	.01023	.27 (raw)	.5766 (raw)	1.67 (raw)
Beef, Short Loin cut, Filet Mignon—dry* cooked, 2″ diam. x 1½″ thick, 180 gm.	.41	10.07	.7402 (raw)	.0189	.54 (raw)	1.055 (raw)	3.07 (raw)
Beef, Short Loin cut, N.Y. Strip or Shell Steak—dry* cooked, 5″ x 2¾″ x ¾″ (widest point), 170 gm.	.39	10.03	.7395 (raw)	.0187	.51 (raw)	1.054 (raw)	3.06 (raw)
Beef, Short Loin cut, Tenderloin Steak—dry* cooked, 4″ x 3″ x ¼″, 66 gm.	.304	2.2	.2871 (raw)	.00726	.19 (raw)	.4092 (raw)	1.18 (raw)
Beef, Loin End cut, Sirloin Steak—dry* cooked, 1 sl., 3″ x 2½″ x 1″, 125 gm.	.575	4.1	.54375 (raw)	.01375	.37 (raw)	.775 (raw)	2.25 (raw)
Beef, Loin End Cut, Pin Bone Sirloin Steak—dry* cooked, 1 sl., 3″ x 2½″ x 1″, 125 gm.	.575	4.1	.54375 (raw)	.01375	.37 (raw)	.775 (raw)	2.25 (raw)
Beef, Loin End cut, Ground Sirloin Beef —dry* cooked, 2½″ diam., ¾″ thick, ¼ lb. raw, 85 gm.	.15	3.91	(raw)	.00935	.25 (raw)	.527 (raw)	1.53 (raw)
Beef, Rump cut, Rump Roast—moist* cooked, 1 sl., 4″ x 1¼″ x 1″, 80 gm.	.184	.34	---	---	.24 (raw)	---	---
Beef, Rump cut, Rolled Rump—dry* cooked, 4″ x 1½″ x ¾″, 95 gm.	.2	4.94	.41325 (raw)	.01045	.28 (raw)	.589 (raw)	1.71 (raw)
Beef, Round cut, Round Steak—dry* cooked, 1 piece, 4″ x 3″ x 1″, 112 gm.	.24	6.27	.4872 (raw)	.01232	.33 (raw)	.6944 (raw)	2.01 (raw)

*** Dry cooking: broiling, roasting—Moist cooking: stewing, braising.**

Vitamin C mg.	Vitamin D IU	Vitamin E IU	Calcium mg.	Iodine mg.	Iron mg.	Mag-nesium mg.	Phos-phorus mg.	Potas-sium mg.	Sodium mg.
0	0	---	9	.00828 Ohio	2.61	26.1	99	333	54
0	0	---	7	NA	---	16.4	158	320	45
0	0	.11	8.5	.00782 Ohio	---	17.85	93.5	314.5	51
0	0	---	2.66	NA	.74	2.85	28.69	70.3	11.4
0	0	---	1.82	NA	.53	2.1	20.44	51.8	8.4
0	0	---	6.24	NA	1.82	7.2	70.08	177.6	28.8
0	0	---	20	NA	---	30	299	344	67
0	0	NA	---	NA	---	---	---	140.6	22.8
0	0	---	4.9	NA	1.33	5.25	52.5	129.5	21
0	0	---	20	NA	---	30	299	344	67
0	0	.13	8	.00975 Ohio	3.5	24	217	438	57
0	0	.13	8	.00975 Ohio	3.5	24	217	438	57
0	0	.12	7	.00865 Ohio	3.6	22	159	388	50
0	0	.13	11	.0092 Ohio	---	20	183	398	52
0	0	.12	10	.00874 Ohio	3.6	19	172	378	49
0	0	.12	10	.00856 Ohio	---	17.9	151	370	48
0	0	.23	20.7	.01656 Ohio	6.31	50.2	412	632	104
0	0	.22	20.4	.01564 Ohio	6.29	49.3	411	629	102
0	0	.08	10	.00607 Ohio	2.6	15	137	288	30
0	0	.16	18	.0115 Ohio	4.8	26	282	545	57
0	0	.16	18	.0115 Ohio	4.8	26	282	545	57
0	0	.11	8.5	.00782 Ohio	2.46	21.25	158	314.5	51
0	0	---	7	.00736 Ohio	3.8	16	158	309	43
0	0	.12	11.4	.00874 Ohio	3.51	27.55	230.85	351.5	57
0	0	.14	13.44	.01030 Ohio	3.92	32.48	280	414.4	67.2

Food and Amount	Calories	Carbo-hydrate gm.	Protein gm.	Sat. Fatty Acids gm.	Unsat. Fatty Acids gm.	Vitamin A IU	Thiamin B₁ mg.
Beef, Round cut, Top Round Steak—dry* cooked, 1 piece, 4″ x 3″ x 1″, 111 gm.	254	0	43.1	3.44	3.33	---	.111
Beef, Round cut, Bottom Round Steak (Swiss Steak)—dry* cooked, 4″ x 3″ x 1″, 114 gm.	271	0	40.5	3.53	3.42	---	.148
Beef, Round cut, Eye Round Roast—dry* cooked, 3″ x 2″ x 1¼″, 130 gm.	339.3	0	37.18	4.03	3.9	39	.1
Beef, Round cut, Heel of Round—moist* cooked, 1 sl., 3½″ x 2″ x 1″, 118 gm.	261	0	36.8	3.65	3.54	---	.118
Beef, Round cut, Ground Round Beef—dry* cooked, 3″ diam. x 1″ thick, ½ lb. raw, 172 gm.	448.92	0	49.18	5.32	5.16	51.6	.12
Beef and Vegetable Stew, home recipe, w/lean beef chuck—1 cup, 280 gm.	249.2	17.36	17.92	5.6	5.6	2,744	.16
Beef and Vegetable Stew, canned— 1 cup, 280 gm.	221.2	19.88	16.24	---	---	2,716	.08
Beef, Corned, boneless, medium-fat, cooked—1 sl., 7″ x 2″ x ¼″, 60 gm.	223.2	0	13.74	9	8.4	---	.01
Beef, Corned, boneless, canned, lean— 1 sl., 3″ x 2″ x ¼″, 28 gm.	60	0	7.1	1.68	1.68	---	.006
Beef, Corned, boneless, canned corned beef hash, w/potato—½ cup, 115 gm.	229	9.3	10.2	5.75	5.75	trace	.034
Beef, dried, chipped, uncooked—1 thin slice, 4″ x 5″, 14 gm.	28.42	0	4.8	.42	.42	---	.009
Beef, dried, chipped, cooked, creamed— ½ cup, 120 gm.	209	6.1	16.1	7.2	3.6	437	.068
Beef potpie, home prepared, baked— 1 pie, 4¼″ diam., 8 oz. raw, 227 gm.	443	37	16.6	9.08	22.7	1,401	.2
Beef, potted—see Sausage, Cold Cuts, and Luncheon Meats							
Bockwurst—see Sausage, Cold Cuts, and Luncheon Meats							
Bologna—see Sausage, Cold Cuts, and Luncheon Meats							
Brains, all kinds, raw—2½″ x 1½″ x 1″, 48 gm.	60	.38	4.99	---	---	0	.11
Capicola—see Sausage, Cold Cuts, and Luncheon Meats							
Chicken, broiled—½ chicken, 7½″ x 4″, 207 gm.	281.52	0	49.25	2.07	4.14	186.3	.08
Chicken, light meat, w/o skin, roasted— 1 sl., 3½″ x 2½″ x ¼″, 35 gm.	63.7	0	11.3	.7	1.05	38.5	.02
Chicken, dark meat, w/o skin, roasted— 1 sl., 3½″ x 2½″ x ¼″, 36 gm.	66.24	0	10.54	.72	1.98	57.6	.04
Chicken breast (½), edible portion, broiled—4″ x 4½″, 78 gm.	106.08	0	18.56	.78	1.56	70.2	.03
Chicken breast (½), edible portion, fried**—4″ x 3″, 48 gm.	116	1.6	13.4	1.92	3.84	230	.039
Chicken, drumstick, edible portion, broiled—5″ x 1½″ diam., 46 gm.	62.56	0	10.94	.46	.92	41.4	.02
Chicken, drumstick, edible portion, fried**—4¼″ x 1½″ diam., 40 gm.	64	1.5	10.5	1.6	3.2	161	.043
Chicken, wing, edible portion, broiled— 3″ x 1½″, 25 gm.	34	0	5.95	.25	.5	22.5	.01
Chicken, wing, edible portion, fried**— 3″ x 1½″, 23 gm.	61.64	.62	6.67	.92	1.84	57.5	.01

* Dry cooking: broiling, roasting—Moist cooking: stewing, braising.
** Pan fried—chicken fried in deep fat has vitamin values of 0.

Riboflavin B2 mg.	Niacin mg.	B6 mg.	Folic Acid mg.	PABA mg.	Pantothenic Acid mg.	B12 mcg.	Vitamin C mg.	Vitamin D IU	Vitamin E IU	Calcium mg.	Iodine mg.
.344	6.3	.48287 (raw)	.01221 (raw)	.33 (raw)	.6882 (raw)	1.99 (raw)	0	0	.14	9	.01021 Ohio
.376	6.5	.4959 (raw)	.01254 (raw)	.34 (raw)	.7068 (raw)	2.05 (raw)	0	0	.14	14	.01049 Ohio
.28	7.28	.5655 (raw)	.0143 (raw)	.34 (raw)	.806 (raw)	2.34 (raw)	0	0	.16	15.6	.01196 Ohio
.271	5.1	---	---	.35 (raw)	---	---	0	0	---	10	NA
.36	9.62	.7482 (raw)	.01892 (raw)	.5 (raw)	1.0664 (raw)	3.08 (raw)	0	0	.22	20.64	.01582 Ohio
.19	5.32	NA	NA	NA	NA	NA	19.6	0	NA	33.6	NA
.14	2.8	---	NA	NA	---	1.82	8.4	0	NA	33.6	NA
.1	.9	---	---	NA	---	---	0	0	---	5.4	NA
.067	1	---	---	NA	-.-	.51	0	0	---	6	NA
.161	3.3	---	---	NA	.08625	---	0	0	---	30	NA
.044	.532	---	---	NA	---	---	0	0	---	2.8	NA
.268	1.6	---	---	NA	---	---	0	2	---	106	NA
.27	4.7	---	---	NA	---	---	6.81	0	---	14	NA
.12	2.11	NA	NA	NA	NA	NA	8.64	0	NA	4.8	NA
.37	18.2	---	---	NA	---	---	---	NA	---	18.63	NA
.03	4.13	---	---	NA	---	---	---	NA	---	3.85	NA
.06	1.9	---	---	NA	---	---	---	NA	---	5.04	NA
.14	6.86	.53274	.00234	NA	.624	.35	---	NA	.28	7.02	NA
.052	5.1	---	---	NA	---	---	0	NA	---	10	NA
.08	4.04	.1495	.00138	NA	.46	.18	---	NA	---	4.14	NA
.113	2.4	---	---	NA	---	---	0	NA	---	9	NA
.04	2.2	---	-.--	NA	---	---	---	NA	---	2.25	NA
.05	1.56	---	---	NA	---	---	---	NA	---	2.3	NA

Food and Amount	Iron mg.	Mag-nesium mg.	Phos-phorus mg.	Potas-sium mg.	Sodium mg.
Beef, Round cut, Top Round Steak—dry* cooked, 1 piece, 4″ x 3″ x 1″, 111 gm.	6.5	28	268	547	46
Beef, Round cut, Bottom Round Steak (Swiss Steak)—dry* cooked, 4″ x 3″ x 1″, 114 gm.	6.1	28	260	552	51
Beef, Round cut, Eye Round Roast—dry* cooked, 3″ x 2″ x 1¼″, 130 gm.	4.55	37.7	325	481	78
Beef, Round cut, Heel of Round—moist* cooked, 1 sl., 3½″ x 2″ x 1″, 118 gm.	5.5	28	204	455	64
Beef, Round cut, Ground Round Beef— dry* cooked, 3″ diam. x 1″ thick, ½ lb. raw, 172 gm.	6.02	43	430	636.4	103.2
Beef and Vegetable Stew, home recipe, w/lean beef chuck—1 cup, 280 gm.	3.36	---	210	700	103.6
Beef and Vegetable Stew, canned— 1 cup, 280 gm.	2.52	---	126	487.2	1,150.8
Beef, Corned, boneless, medium-fat, cooked—1 sl., 7″ x 2″ x ¼″, 60 gm.	1.74	---	55.8	90	1,044
Beef, Corned, boneless, canned, lean— 1 sl., 3″ x 2″ x ¼″, 28 gm.	1.2	---	30	17	268
Beef, Corned, boneless, canned corned beef hash, w/potato—½ cup, 115 gm.	1.4	---	80	230	997
Beef, dried, chipped, uncooked—1 thin slice, 4″ x 5″, 14 gm.	.71	---	56.56	28	602
Beef, dried, chipped, cooked, creamed— ½ cup, 120 gm.	2.1	---	232	183.6	1,161
Beef potpie, home prepared, baked— 1 pie, 4¼″ diam., 8 oz. raw, 227 gm.	3.4	---	117	160.93	1,008
Beef, potted—see Sausage, Cold Cuts, and Luncheon Meats					
Bockwurst—see Sausage, Cold Cuts, and Luncheon Meats					
Bologna—see Sausage, Cold Cuts, and Luncheon Meats					
Brains, all kinds, raw—2½″ x 1½″ x 1″, 48 gm.	1.15	---	149.76	105.12	60
Capicola—see Sausage, Cold Cuts, and Luncheon Meats					
Chicken, broiled—½ chicken, 7½″ x 4″, 207 gm.	3.5	---	416.07	567.18	136.62
Chicken, light meat, w/o skin, roasted— 1 sl., 3½″ x 2½″ x ¼″, 35 gm.	.45	8.05 (raw)	95.2	147.7	23.1
Chicken, dark meat, w/o skin, roasted— 1 sl., 3½″ x 2½″ x ¼″, 36 gm.	.64	---	84.6	118.8	31.68
Chicken breast (½), edible portion, broiled—4″ x 4½″, 78 gm.	1.32	14.82	156.78	213.72	51.48
Chicken breast (½), edible portion, fried**—4″ x 3″, 48 gm.	.7	11.04 (raw)	123	---	---
Chicken, drumstick, edible portion, broiled—5″ x 1½″ diam., 46 gm.	.78	---	92.46	126.04	30.36
Chicken, drumstick, edible portion, fried**—4¼″ x 1½″ diam., 40 gm.	1	---	97	---	---
Chicken, wing, edible portion, broiled— 3″ x 1½″, 25 gm.	.42	---	50.25	68.5	16.5
Chicken, wing, edible portion, fried**— 3″ x 1½″, 23 gm.	.46	---	54.28	---	---

* Dry cooking: broiling, roasting—Moist cooking: stewing, braising.
** Pan fried—chicken fried in deep fat has vitamin values of 0.

Food and Amount	Calories	Carbo-hydrate gm.	Protein gm.	Sat. Fatty Acids gm.	Unsat. Fatty Acids gm.	Vitamin A IU	Thiamin B₁ mg.
Chicken, thigh, edible portion, broiled—3¼" x 2½", 58 gm.	78.88	0	13.8	.58	1.16	52.2	.02
Chicken, thigh, edible portion, fried**—3" x 2½", 42 gm.	99.54	1.05	12.22	1.68	3.36	84	.02
Chicken, canned, meat only, boned—1 tbsp., 15 gm.	27	05	3.05	.6	.9	---	trace
Chicken, potted—see Sausage, Cold Cuts, and Luncheon Meats							
Chicken potpie, home-prepared, baked—½ pie, 2" sq. serving, 116 gm.	230	20.2	9.6	5.8	9.28	143	.087
Chickens, Capon, flesh and skin, roasted—1 sl., 3" x 3" x ¼", 32 gm.	90.56	0	6.84	---	---	---	---
Chickens, Hens and cocks, flesh and skin, cooked, stewed—1 sl., 3" x 3" x ¼", 45 gm.	142.65	0	11.74	3.15	6.3	301.5	.01
Chickens, Hens and cocks, flesh only, cooked, stewed—1 sl., 3" x 3" x ¼", 40 gm.	83	0	10.6	---	---	100	.021
Chickens, Hens and cocks, flesh only, dark meat, stewed—1 sl., 3" x 3" x ¼", 40 gm.	82.8	0	11.4	---	---	108	.02
Chickens, Hens and cocks, flesh only, light meat, stewed—1 sl., 3" x 3" x ¼", 40 gm.	72	0	12.88	---	---	52	.01
Chili con carne, canned, w/beans—½ cup, 115 gm.	167	9.8	7.5	3.45	3.45	69	.04
Chili con carne, canned, w/o beans—½ cup, 118 gm.	236	6.84	12.15	8.26	8.26	177	.02
Desiccated liver¹—1 heaping tbsp., 14 gm.	40	0	8.5	---	---	trace	.0375
Desiccated liver²—10½ grain tablet, ⅔ gm.	1.9	0	.4	---	---	trace	.0017
Deviled ham—see Sausages, Cold Cuts, and Luncheon Meats							
Duck, domesticated, flesh only, roasted—1 sl., 3½" x 2½" x ¼", 35 gm.	109	0	8	---	---	0	.03
Duck, roasted—½ duck, 8" x 4", 385 gm.	1,199	0	88	---	---	0	.33
Goose, domesticated, flesh and skin, roasted—1 sl., 3½" x 3" x ¾", 100 gm.	322	0	28.1	---	---	0	.09
Ham—see Pork							
Heart, beef, lean, cooked, braised—3" diam. x 3¼" piece, 100 gm.	188	.7	31.3	---	---	30	.25
Heart, beef, lean w/visible fat, cooked, braised—3" diam. x 3¼" piece, 105 gm.	390.6	.1	27.09	---	---	---	---
Knockwurst—see Sausages, Cold Cuts, and Luncheon Meats							
Kidneys, Beef, cooked, braised—½ cup diced, 155 gm.	390.6	1.24	51.15	---	---	1,782.5	.79
LAMB—RETAIL CUTS, CHOICE GRADE, LEAN ONLY							
Lamb, Breast cut, Lamb Breast—moist* cooked, 1 sl., 3" x 2" x ¼", 56 gm.	147.28	0	9.24	---	---	---	.08
Lamb, Breast cut, Lamb Stew meat—moist* cooked, 1" cube, 25 gm.	65.75	0	4.12	---	---	---	.03

¹ Also in desiccated liver—1 heaping tbsp.—Choline—140 mg.; Inositol—20 mg.; Biotin—13 mcg.; Peradoxine—100 mcg.   ² Also in desiccated liver—1 10½ grain tablet—Choline—6.6 mg.; Inositol—.952 mg.; Biotin—.619 mcg.; Peradoxine—4.76 mcg.
* Dry cooking: broiling, roasting—Moist cooking: stewing, braising.
** Pan fried—chicken fried in deep fat has vitamin value of 0.

Food and Amount	Riboflavin B₂ mg.	Niacin mg.	B₆ mg.	Folic Acid mg.	PABA mg.	Pantothenic Acid mg.	B₁₂ mcg.
Chicken, thigh, edible portion, broiled—3¼" x 2½", 58 gm.	.11	5.1	.1885	.00174	NA	.58	.23
Chicken, thigh, edible portion, fried**—3" x 2½", 42 gm.	.2	2.85	---	---	NA	---	---
Chicken, canned, meat only, boned—1 tbsp., 15 gm.	.032	1.7	.045	---	NA	.1275	.11
Chicken, potted—see Sausage, Cold Cuts, and Luncheon Meats							
Chicken potpie, home-prepared, baked—½ pie, 2" sq. serving, 116 gm.	.068	2.3	---	---		---	---
Chickens, Capon, flesh and skin, roasted—1 sl., 3" x 3" x ¼", 32 gm.	---	---	---	---	NA	---	---
Chickens, Hens and cocks, flesh and skin, cooked, stewed—1 sl., 3" x 3" x ¼", 45 gm.	.06	3.96	---	---	NA	---	---
Chickens, Hens and cocks, flesh only, cooked, stewed—1 sl., 3" x 3" x ¼", 40 gm.	.06	2.4	---	---	NA	---	---
Chickens, Hens and cocks, flesh only, dark meat, stewed—1 sl., 3" x 3" x ¼", 40 gm.	.08	3.32	---	---	NA	---	---
Chickens, Hens and cocks, flesh only, light meat, stewed—1 sl., 3" x 3" x ¼", 40 gm.	.03	4.4	---	---	NA	---	---
Chili con carne, canned, w/beans—½ cup, 115 gm.	.09	2.5	.11845	NA	NA	.161	---
Chili con carne, canned, w/o beans—½ cup, 118 gm.	.14	2.95	NA	NA	NA	NA	NA
Desiccated liver[1]—1 heaping tbsp., 14 gm.	.7	3.5	NA	.085	.042	1.5	15
Desiccated liver[2]—10½ grain tablet, ⅔ gm.	.032	.166	NA	.004	.002	.071	.71
Deviled ham—see Sausages, Cold Cuts, and Luncheon Meats							
Duck, domesticated, flesh only, roasted—1 sl., 3½" x 2½" x ¼", 35 gm.	.04	2.69	NA	NA	NA	NA	NA
Duck, roasted—½ duck, 8" x 4", 385 gm.	.44	29.59	NA	NA	NA	NA	NA
Goose, domesticated, flesh and skin, roasted—1 sl., 3½" x 3" x ¾", 100 gm.	.16	8.9	NA	NA	NA	NA	NA
Ham—see Pork							
Heart, beef, lean, cooked, braised—3" diam. x 3¼" piece, 100 gm.	1.22	7.6	.25 (raw)	NA	NA	2.5 (raw)	11 (raw)
Heart, beef, lean w/visible fat, cooked, braised—3" diam. x 3¼" piece, 105 gm.	---	---	---	NA	NA	---	---
Knockwurst—see Sausages, Cold Cuts, and Luncheon Meats							
Kidneys, Beef, cooked, braised—½ cup diced, 155 gm.	7.47	16.58	NA	NA	NA	NA	NA
LAMB—RETAIL CUTS, CHOICE GRADE, LEAN ONLY							
Lamb, Breast cut, Lamb Breast—moist* cooked, 1 sl., 3" x 2" x ¼", 56 gm.	.11	2.68	.154 (raw)	.00168	NA	.308 (raw)	1.2 (raw)
Lamb, Breast cut, Lamb Stew meat—moist* cooked, 1" cube, 25 gm.	.05	1.2	.0687 (raw)	.00075	NA	.1375 (raw)	.53 (raw)

[1] Also in desiccated liver—1 heaping tbsp.—Choline—140 mg.; Inositol—20 mg.; Biotin—13 mcg.; Peradoxine—100 mcg.   [2] Also in desiccated liver—1 10½ grain tablet—Choline—6.6 mg.; Inositol—.952 mg.; Biotin—.619 mcg.; Peradoxine—4.76 mcg.
* Dry cooking: broiling, roasting—Moist cooking: stewing, braising.
** Pan fried—chicken fried in deep fat has vitamin value of 0.

Vitamin C mg	Vitamin D IU	Vitamin E IU	Calcium mg.	Iodine mg.	Iron mg.	Magnesium mg.	Phosphorus mg.	Potassium mg.	Sodium mg.
---	NA	---	5.22	NA	.98	---	116.58	158.92	38.28
---	NA	---	5.46	NA	.96	---	99.12	---	---
---	---	---	2	NA	.25	---	23	20.7	---
6	NA	NA	19	NA	1.2	---	118	171.68	296.96
---	NA	---	---	NA	---	---	---	---	---
0	NA	---	4.95	NA	.67	8.55	60.3	---	---
0	NA	---	6	NA	.6	---	59.6	108.8	22
0	NA	---	5.2	NA	.72	---	55.2	95.6	25.6
0	NA	---	4.4	NA	.52	---	64	122.4	19.2
---	0	NA	44	NA	1.6	---	175	267.95	610.65
---	0	NA	44.84	NA	1.65	---	179.36	---	---
trace	NA	NA	NA	2.25	NA	NA	NA	NA	NA
trace	NA	NA	NA	.107	.166	NA	NA	NA	NA
0	NA	NA	7	NA	2.0	---	81	99.75	25.9
0	NA	NA	77	NA	22	---	891	1,097.25	284.9
0	NA	NA	10	NA	4.6	---	265	---	---
1	0	NA	6	NA	5.9	---	181	232	104
---	0	NA	---	NA	---	---	177.45	---	---
---	0	NA	27.9	NA	20.3	---	378.2	502.2	392.15
---	0	.08	5.6	NA	.67	11.76	82.32	---	---
---	0	.04	2.5	NA	.3	5.25	36.75	---	---

Food and Amount	Calories	Carbo-hydrate gm.	Protein gm.	Sat. Fatty Acids gm.	Unsat. Fatty Acids gm.	Vitamin A IU	Thiamin B1 mg.
Lamb, Breast Cut, Lamb Patties—dry* cooked, 2″ diam., 55 gm.	102.3	0	15.78	---	---	---	.08
Lamb, Shoulder Cut, Rolled Lamb Shoulder—dry* cooked, 1 sl., 3″ x 3″ x ½″, 50 gm.	102.5	0	13.4	3	2	0	.07
Lamb, Shoulder Cut, Boneless Shoulder Chops—dry* cooked, 1¾″ x 1½″ x ¾″, 52 gm.	106.6	0	13.93	3.12	2.08	0	.07
Lamb, Shoulder Cut, Arm Lamb Chop—dry* cooked, 1 chop, 3″ x 1½″ x ¾″, 57 gm.	144	0	14.6	3.42	2.28	0	.109
Lamb, Shoulder Cut, Blade Lamb Chop—dry* cooked, 3¼″ x 1¾″ x 1″, 93 gm.	260	0	25.4	5.58	3.72	0	.183
Lamb, Shoulder Cut, Cubes for Shish-kabob—dry* cooked, 1″ cube, 25 gm.	51.25	0	6.7	1.5	1	0	.03
Lamb, Rack, Lamb Crown Roast—dry* cooked, 1¾″ x 1¾″ x ¾″, 41 gm.	119	0	10.5	2.66	1.64	0	.086
Lamb, Rack, Rib Lamb Chop—dry* cooked, 1¾″ x 1¾″ x ¾″, 41 gm.	119	0	10.5	2.66	1.64	0	.086
Lamb, Rack, French Rib Lamb Chop—dry* cooked, 1¾″ x 1¾″ x ¾″, 41 gm.	119	0	10.5	2.66	1.64	0	.086
Lamb, Loin, Loin Lamb Chop—dry* cooked, 1¾″ x 1¾″ x ¾″, 46 gm.	103	0	12.5	1.97	1.47	0	.095
Lamb, Loin, English Lamb Chop—dry* cooked, 1½″ x 1½″ x ¾″, 40 gm.	75.2	0	11.28	1.72	1.28	0	.06
Lamb, Leg, Frenched Leg—dry* cooked, 1 sl., 4″ x 3″ x ½″, 61 gm.	107	0	17.6	2.44	1.83	0	.14
Lamb, Leg, Leg of Lamb—dry* cooked, 1 sl., 4″ x 3″ x ¼″, 98 gm.	192	0	27.6	3.92	2.94	0	.221
END OF LAMB RETAIL CUTS							
Liver, Beef, cooked, fried—1 sl., 3″ x 2¼″ x ⅜″, 37 gm.	86	5.6	8.8	---	---	18,658	.09
Liver, Calf, cooked, fried—1 sl., 3″ x 2¼″ x ⅜″, 36 gm.	74	1.7	8.1	---	---	9,565	.063
Liver, Chicken, cooked, simmered—½ cup, 90 gm.	148.5	2.79	23.85	---	---	11,070	.15
Liver, Hog, cooked, fried—1 sl., 3″ x 2¼″ x ⅜″, 37 gm.	85	3.8	8.8	1.11	2.22	6,035	.126
Liver, Lamb, cooked, broiled—1 sl., 3″ x 2¼″ x ⅜″, 37 gm.	86	4.3	9.3	---	---	21,465	.131
Liver paste—see Pâté de foie gras							
Liver sausage—see Sausages, Cold Cuts, and Luncheon Meats							
Meatloaf—see Sausage, Cold Cuts, and Luncheon Meats							
Pâté de foie gras, canned—1 rd. tbsp., 20 gm.	92.4	.96	2.28	---	---	---	.01
PORK, FRESH—RETAIL CUTS, MEDIUM FAT CLASS, LEAN ONLY, SEPARABLE FAT REMOVED							
Pork, Butt, Lard—see Fats and Oils							
Pork, Butt, Blade Pork Steaks—moist* cooked, 1 sl., 3″ x 1½″ x ½″, 54 gm.	150	0	15.7	3.24	4.48	0	.367

* Dry cooking: broiling, roasting—Moist cooking: stewing, braising.

Riboflavin B₂ mg.	Niacin mg.	B₆ mg.	Folic Acid mg.	PABA mg.	Pantothenic Acid mg.	B₁₂ mcg.	Vitamin C mg.	Vitamin D IU	Vitamin E IU	Calcium mg.	Iodine mg.
.16	3.41	.15125 (raw)	.00165	NA	.3025 (raw)	1.18 (raw)	0	0	.08	7.15	NA
.14	2.85	.1375 (raw)	.0015	NA	.275 (raw)	1.07 (raw)	0	0	.08	6	NA
.14	2.96	.143 (raw)	.00156	NA	.286 (raw)	1.11 (raw)	0	0	.08	6.24	.0075 (raw) Ohio
.172	4.1	.15675 (raw)	.00171	NA	.3135 (raw)	1.22 (raw)	0	0	.09	4	.0083 (raw) Ohio
.287	6.9	.25575 (raw)	.00279	NA	.5115 (raw)	1.99 (raw)	0	0	.14	11	.0135 (raw) Ohio
.07	1.42	.06875 (raw)	.00075	NA	.1375 (raw)	.53 (raw)	0	0	.04	3	NA
.135	3.2	.11275 (raw)	.00123	NA	.2255 (raw)	.88 (raw)	0	0	.06	3	.0059 (raw) Ohio
.135	3.2	.11275 (raw)	.00123	NA	.2255 (raw)	.88 (raw)	0	0	.06	3	.0059 (raw) Ohio
.135	3.2	.11275 (raw)	.00123	NA	.2255 (raw)	.88 (raw)	0	0	.06	3	.0059 (raw) Ohio
.149	3.6	.1265 (raw)	.00138	NA	.253 (raw)	.98 (raw)	0	0	.07	4	.0067 (raw) Ohio
.11	2.44	.11 (raw)	.0012	NA	.22 (raw)	.86 (raw)	0	0	.06	4.8	.0058 (raw) Ohio
.189	4.5	.16775 (raw)	.00183	NA	.3355 (raw)	1.31 (raw)	0	0	.09	5	NA
.298	7	.2695 (raw)	.00294	NA	.539 (raw)	2.1 (raw)	0	0	.15	8	NA
1.283	5.1	.3108 (raw)	.10878 (raw)	.37 (raw)	2.849 (raw)	29.6 (raw)	10	19	.23 (broiled)	4	NA
1.193	5.9	.2412 (raw)	NA	.07 (raw)	2.88 (raw)	21.6 (raw)	8	5	NA	3	NA
2.42	10.53	NA	NA	NA	NA	NA	14.4	---	NA	9.9	NA
1.148	6.2	.2405 (raw)	.08177	NA	2.368 (raw)	11.84 (raw)	5	19	NA	5	NA
1.265	6.2	---	NA	NA	---	---	7	9	NA	4	NA
.06	.5	NA	NA	NA	NA	NA	---	NA	NA	---	NA
.173	2.9	NA	NA	.16 (raw)	NA	NA	0	0	NA	4	NA

Food and Amount	Iron mg.	Mag-nesium mg.	Phos-phorus mg.	Potas-sium mg.	Sodium mg.
Lamb, Breast Cut, Lamb Patties—dry* cooked, 2″ diam., 55 gm.	1.21	11.55	130.9	159.5	38.5
Lamb, Shoulder Cut, Rolled Lamb Shoulder—dry* cooked, 1 sl., 3″ x 3″ x ½″, 50 gm.	.95	10.5	109.5	145	35
Lamb, Shoulder Cut, Boneless Shoulder Chops—dry* cooked, 1¾″ x 1½″ x ¾″, 52 gm.	.98	10.92	113.88	150.8	36.4
Lamb, Shoulder Cut, Arm Lamb Chop— dry* cooked, 1 chop, 3″ x 1½″ x ¾″, 57 gm.	1.3	14	135	252	43
Lamb, Shoulder Cut, Blade Lamb Chop —dry* cooked, 3¼″ x 1¾″ x 1″, 93 gm.	2.8	22	226	422	72
Lamb, Shoulder Cut, Cubes for Shish-kabob—dry* cooked, 1″ cube, 25 gm.	.47	5.25	54.75	72.5	17.5
Lamb, Rack, Lamb Crown Roast— dry* cooked, 1¾″ x 1¾″ x ¾″, 41 gm.	1.2	8	90	199	34
Lamb, Rack, Rib Lamb Chop— dry* cooked, 1¾″ x 1¾″ x ¾″, 41 gm.	1.2	8	90	199	34
Lamb, Rack, French Rib Lamb Chop— dry* cooked, 1¾″ x 1¾″ x ¾″, 41 gm.	1.2	8	90	199	34
Lamb, Loin, Loin Lamb Chop— dry* cooked, 1¾″ x 1¾″ x ¾″, 46 gm.	1.4	11	98	218	37
Lamb, Loin, English Lamb Chop— dry* cooked, 1½″ x 1½″ x ¾″, 40 gm.	.8	8.4	87.6	116	28
Lamb, Leg, Frenched Leg—dry* cooked, 1 sl., 4″ x 3″ x ½″, 61 gm.	1.9	14	134	312	52
Lamb, Leg, Leg of Lamb—dry* cooked, 1 sl., 4″ x 3″ x ¼″, 98 gm.	3	24	210	492	82
END OF LAMB RETAIL CUTS					
Liver, Beef, cooked, fried—1 sl., 3″ x 2¼″ x ⅜″, 37 gm.	2.9	8	156	143	34
Liver, Calf, cooked, fried—1 sl., 3″ x 2¼″ x ⅜″, 36 gm.	4.5	9	146	147	44
Liver, Chicken, cooked, simmered— ½ cup, 90 gm.	7.65	NA	143.1	135.9	54.9
Liver, Hog, cooked, fried—1 sl., 3″ x 2¼″ x ⅜″, 37 gm.	7.8	8.88	158	---	---
Liver, Lamb, cooked, broiled—1 sl., 3″ x 2¼″ x ⅜″, 37 gm.	5.5	8.51	158	---	---
Liver paste—see Pâté de foie gras					
Liver sausage—see Sausages, Cold Cuts, and Luncheon Meats					
Meatloaf—see Sausage, Cold Cuts, and Luncheon Meats					
Pâté de foie gras, canned—1 rd. tbsp., 20 gm.	---	---	---	---	---
PORK, FRESH—RETAIL CUTS, MEDIUM FAT CLASS, LEAN ONLY, SEPARABLE FAT REMOVED					
Pork, Butt, Lard—see Fats and Oils					
Pork, Butt, Blade Pork Steaks—moist* cooked, 1 sl., 3″ x 1½″ x ½″, 54 gm.	2.4	13	123	275	39

*Dry cooking: broiling, roasting—Moist cooking: stewing, braising.

Food and Amount	Calories	Carbo-hydrate gm.	Protein gm.	Sat. Fatty Acids gm.	Unsat. Fatty Acids gm.	Vitamin A IU	Thiamin B_1 mg.
Pork, Butt, Boston-Style Butt—dry* cooked, 1 sl., 3″ x 2″ x ½″, 58 gm.	164	0	14.7	3.48	4.81	0	.394
Pork, Butt, Rolled Boston Style Butt—dry* cooked, 1 sl., 3″ x 2″ x ½″, 58 gm.	164	0	14.7	3.48	4.81	0	.394
Pork, Loin, Lard—see Fats and Oils							
Pork, Loin, Loin Roast, Shoulder End—dry* cooked, 3¼″ x 3″ x ⅓″, 100 gm.	362	0	24.5	6	8.8	0	.92
Pork, Loin, Crown Pork Roast—dry* cooked, 2″ x 2″ x ½″, 40 gm.	101.6	0	11.76	2.4	3.52	0	.45
Pork, Loin, Loin Roast, Center Cut—dry* cooked, 3¼″ x 3″ x ⅓″, 100 gm.	362	0	24.5	6	8.8	0	.92
Pork, Loin, Loin Roast, Ham End—dry* cooked, 3¼″ x 3″ x ⅓″, 105 gm.	380.1	0	25.72	6.3	9.24	0	.96
Pork, Loin, Rib Chop—dry* cooked, 2″ x 2″ x ½″, 40 gm.	101.6	0	11.76	2.4	3.52	0	.45
Pork, Loin, Canadian Style Bacon—see Bacon, Canadian							
Pork, Loin, Loin Pork Chop—dry* cooked, 1 chop, 2″ x 1½″ x ¾″, 44 gm.	111.76	0	12.93	2.64	3.87	0	.49
Pork, Loin, Sirloin Pork Roast—dry* cooked, 1 sl., 2½″ x 1″ x ½″, 24 gm.	54	0	7.1	1 44	2.11	0	.301
Pork, Loin, Pork Tenderloin, frenched or whole—dry* cooked, 2½″ x 2″ x ½″, 45 gm.	114.3	0	13.23	2.7	3.96	0	.5
Pork, Picnic, Fresh Shoulder Hock—moist* cooked, 2½″ x 2″ x ½″, 47 gm.	116	0	12.2	2.06	2.53	0	.319
Pork, Picnic, Rolled Picnic Shoulder—dry* cooked, 1 sl., 2½″ x 2″ x ½″, 47 gm.	116	0	12.2	2.06	2.53	0	.319
Pork, Picnic, Fresh Picnic Shoulder—dry* cooked, 1 sl., 2½″ x 2″ x ½″, 47 gm.	116	0	12.2	2.06	2.53	0	.319
Pork, Spareribs—dry* cooked, 1 piece, 4″ x 1″, 24 gm.	105.6	0	4.99	4 17	5.16	0	.1
Pork, Side, Bacon—see Bacon							
Pork, Side, Salt Pork—fried, 1 sl., 3″ x 1½″ x ½″, 50 gm.	341	0	6	16	22	0	.14
Pork, Ham, Fresh Ham Roast—dry* cooked, 1 sl., 2″ x 1½″ x 1″, 53 gm.	126	0	19.6	2.38	2.91	0	.347
Pork, Ham, Rolled Fresh Ham Roast—dry* cooked, 1 sl., 2″ x 1½″ x 1″, 53 gm.	126	0	19.6	2.38	2.91	0	.347
Pork, Ham, Ham Butt Slice—dry* cooked, 5″ x 5″ x ¼″, 100 gm.	374	0	23	4.5	5.5	0	.51
Pork, Ham, Ham Center Slice—dry* cooked, 5″ x 5″ x ¼″, 100 gm.	374	0	23	4.5	5.5	0	.51
Pork, Ham, Cured Ham Butt Portion—dry* cooked, 1 sl., 3″ x 2″ x ½″, 60 gm.	123	.2	15.1	2.7	3.3	0	.468
Pork, Ham, Cured Ham Shank Portion—dry* cooked, 1 sl., 2″ x 2″ x ½″, 39 gm.	91	.1	10	1.75	2.14	0	.304
Pork, Ham, Cured Ham, Canned—4½″ x 4″ x ⅜″, 100 gm.	193	.9	18.3	4	6	0	.53

* Dry cooking: broiling, roasting—Moist cooking: stewing, braising.

Food and Amount	Riboflavin B_2 mg.	Niacin mg.	B_6 mg.	Folic Acid mg.	PABA mg.	Pantothenic Acid mg.	B_{12} mcg.
Pork, Butt, Boston-Style Butt—dry* cooked, 1 sl., 3″ x 2″ x ½″, 58 gm.	.186	3.1	NA	NA	.17 (raw)	NA	NA
Pork, Butt, Rolled Boston Style Butt—dry* cooked, 1 sl., 3″ x 2″ x ½″, 58 gm.	.186	3.1	NA	NA	.17 (raw)	NA	NA
Pork, Loin, Lard—see Fats and Oils							
Pork, Loin, Loin Roast, Shoulder End—dry* cooked, 3¼″ x 3″ x ⅓″, 100 gm.	.26	5.6	---	.002	.3 (raw)	---	---
Pork, Loin, Crown Pork Roast—dry* cooked, 2″ x 2″ x ½″, 40 gm.	.13	2.72	---	.0008	.12 (raw)	---	---
Pork, Loin, Loin Roast, Center Cut—dry* cooked, 3¼″ x 3″ x ⅓″, 100 gm.	.26	5.6	---	.002	.3 (raw)	---	---
Pork, Loin, Loin Roast, Ham End—dry* cooked, 3¼″ x 3″ x ⅓″, 105 gm.	.27	5.88	---	.0021	.31 (raw)	---	---
Pork, Loin, Rib Chop—dry* cooked, 2″ x 2″ x ½″, 40 gm.	.13	2.72	---	.0008	.12 (raw)	---	---
Pork, Loin, Canadian Style Bacon—see Bacon, Canadian							
Pork, Loin, Loin Pork Chop—dry* cooked, 1 chop, 2″ x 1½″ x ¾″, 44 gm.	.14	2.99	---	.00088	.13 (raw)	---	---
Pork, Loin, Sirloin Pork Roast—dry* cooked, 1 sl., 2½″ x 1″ x ½″, 24 gm.	.08	1.1	---	.00048	.07 (raw)	---	---
Pork, Loin, Pork Tenderloin, frenched or whole—dry* cooked, 2½″ x 2″ x ½″, 45 gm.	.14	3.06	---	.0009	.13 (raw)	---	---
Pork, Picnic, Fresh Shoulder Hock—moist* cooked, 2½″ x 2″ x ½″, 47 gm.	.15	2.5	NA	NA	.14 (raw)	NA	NA
Pork, Picnic, Rolled Picnic Shoulder—dry* cooked, 1 sl., 2½″ x 2″ x ½″, 47 gm.	.150	2.5	NA	NA	.14 (raw)	NA	NA
Pork, Picnic, Fresh Picnic Shoulder—dry* cooked, 1 sl., 2½″ x 2″ x ½″, 47 gm.	.150	2.5	NA	NA	.14 (raw)	NA	NA
Pork, Spareribs—dry* cooked, 1 piece, 4″ x 1″, 24 gm.	.05	.81	NA	NA	.07 (raw)	NA	NA
Pork, Side, Bacon—see Bacon							
Pork, Side, Salt Pork—fried, 1 sl., 3″ x 1½″ x ½″, 50 gm.	.05	1	NA	NA	NA	NA	NA
Pork, Ham, Fresh Ham Roast—dry* cooked, 1 sl., 2″ x 1½″ x 1″, 53 gm.	.163	2.7	.212 (raw)	---	.15 (raw)	.35775 (raw)	.31 (raw)
Pork, Ham, Rolled Fresh Ham Roast—dry* cooked, 1 sl., 2″ x 1½″ x 1″, 53 gm.	.163	2.7	.212 (raw)	---	.15 (raw)	.35775 (raw)	.31 (raw)
Pork, Ham, Ham Butt Slice—dry* cooked, 5″ x 5″ x ¼″, 100 gm.	.23	4.6	.4 (raw)	---	.3 (raw)	.675 (raw)	.6 (raw)
Pork, Ham, Ham Center Slice—dry* cooked, 5″ x 5″ x ¼″, 100 gm.	.23	4.6	.4 (raw)	---	.3 (raw)	.675 (raw)	.6 (raw)
Pork, Ham, Cured Ham Butt Portion—dry* cooked, 1 sl., 3″ x 2″ x ½″, 60 gm.	.144	2.5	.24 (raw)	.0066	NA	.405 (raw)	.36 (raw)
Pork, Ham, Cured Ham Shank Portion—dry* cooked, 1 sl., 2″ x 2″ x ½″, 39 gm.	.94	1.6	.156 (raw)	.00429	NA	.26325 (raw)	.23 (raw)
Pork, Ham, Cured Ham, Canned—4½″ x 4″ x ⅜″, 100 gm.	.19	3.8	.36	NA	NA	---	---

* Dry cooking: broiling, roasting—Moist cooking: stewing, braising.

Vitamin C mg.	Vitamin D IU	Vitamin E IU	Calcium mg.	Iodine mg.	Iron mg.	Magnesium mg.	Phosphorus mg.	Potassium mg.	Sodium mg.
0	0	NA	4	NA	2.2	13	131	296	42
0	0	NA	4	NA	2.2	13	131	296	42
0	0	---	11	NA	3.2	29	256	390	65
0	0	---	5.2	NA	1.52	11.6	124	156	26
0	0	---	11	NA	3.2	29	256	390	65
0	0	---	11.55	NA	3.36	29.1	268.8	409.5	68.25
0	0	---	5.2	NA	1.52	11.6	124	156	26
0	0	.07 (fried)	5.72	NA	1.67	12.76	136.4	171.6	28.6
0	0	---	1.3	NA	1.06	5.8	62	120	13
0	0	---	5.85	NA	1.71	13.05	139.5	175.5	29.25
0	0	NA	3	NA	1.8	10	102	240	34
0	0	NA	3	NA	1.8	10	102	240	34
0	0	NA	3	NA	1.8	10	102	240	34
0	0	NA	2.16	NA	.62	---	29.04	93.6	15.6
0	0	NA	4	NA	.8	---	60	21	606
0	0	.08 (fried)	4	NA	1.2	15	146	260	37
0	0	.08 (fried)	4	NA	1.2	15	146	260	37
0	0	.16 (fried)	10	NA	3	15.37	236	390	65
0	0	.16 (fried)	10	NA	3	15.37	236	390	65
0	0	---	5	NA	1.5	13	123	239	518
0	0	---	3	NA	1.0	8	73	155	336
---	0	---	11	NA	2.7	17	156	340	1,100

Food and Amount	Calories	Carbo-hydrate gm.	Protein gm.	Sat. Fatty Acids gm.	Unsat. Fatty Acids gm.	Vitamin A IU	Thiamin B_1 mg.
Pork, Ham, Dry, long cure, medium fat, country style—1 sl., 3″ x 2″ x ½″, 60 gm.	233.4	.18	10.14	13	18	0	---
Quail, raw, total edible—1 sl., 2½″ x 2″ x ¼″, 24 gm.	40.32	0	6	NA	NA	---	---
Rabbits, domesticated, flesh only, cooked, stewed—1 sl., 3″ x 1″ x ½″, 38 gm.	82.08	0	11.13	NA	NA	---	.01
SAUSAGE, COLD CUTS, AND LUNCHEON MEATS							
Blood sausage or blood pudding—1 sl., 3″ x 3″ x ⅛″, 60 gm.	226	0	8.9	---	---	0	---
Bologna, all meat—1 sl., 4½″ x ⅛″, 30 gm.	66	1.1	4.4	---	---	0	.054
Bologna, with nonfat dry milk—1 sl., 4½″ x ⅛″, 30 gm.	---	---	4.02	---	---	---	---
Bologna, with cereal—1 sl., 4½″ x ⅛″, 30 gm.	78.6	1.17	4.26	---	---	---	---
Braunschweiger (Liverwurst)—1 sl., 3″ diam. x ¼″, 30 gm.	79	.5	5	3	4.2	1,725	.051
Brown and serve sausage, browned—3½″ x ⅝″, 24 gm.	101.28	.67	3.96	---	---	---	---
Capicola or Capacola—4″ x 3″ x ⅛″, 22 gm.	109.78	0	4.44	3.52	5.06	---	---
Cervelat, dry—1 sl. 3¾″ diam. x 3/16″, 30 gm.	125	0	7.1	---	---	0	.08
Cervelat, soft—1 sl., 3¾″ diam. x 3/16″, 32 gm.	98.24	.51	5.95	---	---	0	.03
Country-style sausage—2″ diam., 30 gm.	103.5	0	4.53	3.3	4.8	---	.06
Deviled ham, canned—1 tbsp. (rounded), 20 gm.	70.2	0	2.78	2.4	3.4	0	.02
Frankfurters, cooked, all samples, average—1 frankfurter, 7″ x ¾″, 60 gm.	182.4	.96	7.44	---	---	---	.09
Frankfurters, canned, all samples, average—1¾″ x ½″, 7 gm.	15.47	.01	.93	---	---	---	.002
Frankfurters, raw, all samples, average—1 frankfurter, 7″ x ¾″, 60 gm.	185.4	1.08	7.5	---	---	---	.09
Head cheese—1 slice, 4″ x 3″ x ⅛″, 60 gm.	148	0	9	4.8	6.6	0	.048
Knockwurst, fresh—4″ x 1″ diam., 84 gm.	233.52	1.84	11.84	---	---	---	.14
Liverwurst—see Braunschweiger							
Luncheon meat, boiled ham—4″ sq. x 1/16″, 15 gm.	35.1	0	2.85	.9	1.35	0	.06
Luncheon meat, Pork, cured ham or shoulder, chopped, spiced or unspiced, canned—3″ x 2″ x ¼″, 40 gm.	117.6	.52	6	3.6	5.2	0	.12
Meatloaf—(beef and pork), 1 sl., 4″ x 3″ x ⅜″, 70 gm.	264	11.5	10.4	---	---	50	.118
Meat, potted (incl. potted beef, chicken and turkey, canned—1 tbsp., 12 gm.	29.76	0	2.1	---	---	---	.008
Mortadella—5″ diam. x 1/16″, 20 gm.	63	.12	4.08	---	---	---	---

Ribo-flavin B₂ mg.	Niacin mg.	B₆ mg.	Folic Acid mg.	PABA mg.	Panto-thenic Acid mg.	B₁₂ mcg.	Vitamin C mg.	Vitamin D IU	Vitamin E IU	Calcium mg.	Iodine mg.
---	---	---	---	NA	---	---	---	0	---	---	NA
---	1 ---	NA	NA	NA	NA	NA	---	0	NA	---	NA
.02	4.29	NA	NA	NA	NA	NA	---	NA	NA	7.98	NA
---	---	NA	NA	NA	NA	NA	0	0	NA	5	NA
.057	.8	.030	---	NA	---	---	0	0	.01	3	NA
---	---	---	---	NA	---	---	---	NA	---	---	NA
---	---	---	---	NA	---	---	---	NA	---	---	NA
.336	1.4	NA	NA	NA	NA	NA	0	5	.1	3	NA
---	---	NA	NA	NA	NA	NA	---	NA	NA	---	NA
---	---	NA	NA	NA	NA	NA	---	NA	NA	---	NA
.09	1.2	NA	NA	NA	NA	NA	0	0	NA	4	NA
.08	1.34	NA	NA	NA	NA	NA	0	0	NA	3.52	NA
.05	.93	NA	NA	NA	NA	NA	---	NA	NA	2.7	NA
.02	.32	NA	NA	NA	NA	NA	---	NA	NA	1.6	NA
.12	1.50	---	---	NA	---	---	---	NA	NA	3	NA
.008	.16	NA	NA	NA	NA	NA	---	NA	NA	.63	NA
.12	1.62	.084	---	NA	.258	.78	---	NA	NA	4.2	NA
.072	.7	NA	NA	NA	NA	NA	0	0	NA	6	NA
.17	2.18	NA	NA	NA	NA	NA	---	NA	NA	6.72	NA
.02	.39	NA	NA	NA	NA	NA	---	NA	NA	1.65	NA
.08	1.2	NA	NA	NA	NA	NA	---	NA	NA	3.6	NA
.111	2.0	NA	NA	NA	NA	NA	0	2	NA	26	NA
.02	.14	NA	NA	NA	NA	NA	---	NA	NA	---	NA
---	---	NA	NA	NA	NA	NA	---	NA	NA	2.4	NA

Food and Amount	Iron mg.	Magnesium mg.	Phosphorus mg.	Potassium mg.	Sodium mg.
Pork, Ham, Dry, long cure, medium fat, country style—1 sl., 3″ x 2″ x ½″, 60 gm.	...	...	...	...	...
Quail, raw, total edible—1 sl., 2½″ x 2″ x ¼″, 24 gm.	...	...	...	...	...
Rabbits, domesticated, flesh only, cooked, stewed—1 sl., 3″ x 1″ x ½″, 38 gm.	.57	NA	98.42	139.84	15.58
SAUSAGE, COLD CUTS, AND LUNCHEON MEATS					
Blood sausage or blood pudding—1 sl., 3″ x 3″ x ⅛″, 60 gm.	1.3	NA	96	...	...
Bologna, all meat—1 sl., 4½″ x ⅛″, 30 gm.	.7	NA	34	69	390
Bologna, with nonfat dry milk—1 sl., 4½″ x ⅛″, 30 gm.	...	NA	...	...	...
Bologna, with cereal—1 sl., 4½″ x ⅛″, 30 gm.	...	NA	...	...	...
Braunschweiger (Liverwurst)—1 sl., 3″ diam. x ¼″, 30 gm.	1.6	NA	71	...	...
Brown and serve sausage, browned—3½″ x ⅜″, 24 gm.	...	NA	...	...	...
Capicola or Capacola—4″ x 3″ x ⅛″, 22 gm.	...	...	...	...	...
Cervelat, dry—1 sl. 3¾″ diam. x 3/16″, 30 gm.	1.1	NA	84	...	...
Cervelat, soft—1 sl., 3¾″ diam. x 3/16″, 32 gm.	.89	NA	68.48	...	...
Country-style sausage—2″ diam., 30 gm.	.69	NA	50.4	...	...
Deviled ham, canned—1 tbsp. (rounded), 20 gm.	.42	NA	18.4	...	...
Frankfurters, cooked, all samples, average—1 frankfurter, 7″ x ¾″, 60 gm.	.90	...	61.2	...	...
Frankfurters, canned, all samples, average—1¾″ x ½″, 7 gm.	.15	NA	10.15	...	...
Frankfurters, raw, all samples, average—1 frankfurter, 7″ x ¾″, 60 gm.	1.14	...	79.8	132	660
Head cheese—1 slice, 4″ x 3″ x ⅛″, 60 gm.	1.4	NA	96	...	...
Knockwurst, fresh—4″ x 1″ diam., 84 gm.	1.76	NA	129.36	...	...
Liverwurst—see Braunschweiger					
Luncheon meat, boiled ham—4″ sq. x 1/16″, 15 gm.	.42	NA	24.9	...	...
Luncheon meat, Pork, cured ham or shoulder, chopped, spiced or unspiced, canned—3″ x 2″ x ¼″, 40 gm.	.88	NA	43.2	88.8	493.6
Meatloaf—(beef and pork), 1 sl., 4″ x 3″ x ⅜″, 70 gm.	1.7	NA	99	...	...
Meat, potted (incl. potted beef, chicken and turkey, canned—1 tbsp., 12 gm.	...	...	...	...	...
Mortadella—5″ diam. x 1/16″, 20 gm.	.62	...	47.6	...	...

Food and Amount	Calories	Carbo-hydrate gm.	Protein gm.	Sat. Fatty Acids gm.	Unsat. Fatty Acids gm.	Vitamin A IU	Thiamin B₁ mg.
Polish-style sausage—1 sl., 1½" diam x 1", 30 gm.	83	0	4.9	---	---	0	.054
Pork and beef (chopped together)—1 link, 2¼" x 1½" diam., 60 gm.	252	0	6.8	---	---	0	---
Pork sausage, links or bulk, cooked—1 link, 3" x ½" diam., 20 gm.	94	0	3.5	3.2	4.6	0	.098
Pork sausage, canned, drained solids—1 patty, 2" diam., 50 gm.	190.5	.95	9.15	7	9.5	---	---
Pork sausage, link, smoked—see Country-style sausage							
Salami, dry—1 slice, 3¾" x ¼", 30 gm.	130	.36	7.2	---	---	0	.075
Salami, cooked—1 slice, 3¾" x ¼", 32 gm.	99.52	.44	5.6	---	---	0	.08
Scrapple—1 sl., 3½" x 2¼" x ¼", 57 gm.	209	26	4.7	---	---	100	.083
Thuringer—6" x 1¼" diam., 100 gm.	307	1.6	18.6	---	---	---	.11
Vienna sausage, canned—2" x ¾" diam., 17 gm.	40.8	.05	2.38	---	---	---	.01
END OF SAUSAGE, COLD CUTS, AND LUNCHEON MEATS							
Squab (pigeon), raw, flesh and skin—3" x 2" x ¾", 60 gm.	176.4	0	11.1	---	---	---	---
Suet (beef kidney fat), raw—1 tbsp., 10 gm.	85.4	0	.15	---	---	---	---
Sweetbreads (thymus), calf, cooked, braised—½ cup, 100 gm.	168	0	32.6	---	---	---	.06
Thuringer—see Sausage, Cold Cuts, and Luncheon Meats							
Tongue, Beef, medium-fat, cooked, braised—1 sl., 3" x 2" x ⅛", 21 gm.	51.24	.08	4.51	---	---	---	.01
Tongue, Beef, Smoked—1 sl., 3" x 2" x ⅛", 20 gm.	---	---	5.44	---	---	---	.008
Tongue, canned or cured (beef, lamb, etc.), whole, canned or pickled—1 sl., 3" x 2" x ⅜", 60 gm.	160	.2	11.6	---	---	0	.03
Tongue, canned or cured, potted or deviled—1 rd. tbsp., 20 gm.	58	.14	3.72	---	---	---	.008
Tripe, beef, commercial—1 pc., 5" x 2½" diam., 85 gm.	84	0	16.2	---	---	0	.009
Tripe, beef, pickled—1 piece, 4" x 2" diam., 62 gm.	38.44	0	7.31	---	---	---	---
Turkey, flesh and skin, cooked, roasted—1 sl., 3" x 3" x ¼", 42 gm.	93.6	0	13.4	1.26	2.52	---	.02
Turkey, light meat, cooked, roasted—1 sl., 3" x 3" x ¼", 40 gm.	70.4	0	13.16	---	---	---	.02
Turkey, dark meat, cooked, roasted—1 sl., 3" x 3" x ¼", 40 gm.	81.2	0	12	---	---	---	.01
Turkey, canned, meat only—1 tbsp., 12 gm.	24.24	0	2.5	---	---	15.6	.006
Turkey, potted—see Sausage, Cold Cuts, and Luncheon Meats							
Turkey potpie, home-prepared, baked—4¼" pie, 227 gm.	417	35.9	15.2	9.08	18.16	2,043	.23

Food and Amount	Riboflavin B_2 mg.	Niacin mg.	B_6 mg.	Folic Acid mg.	PABA mg.	Pantothenic Acid mg.	B_{12} mcg.
Polish-style sausage—1 sl., 1½" diam x 1", 30 gm.	.057	.8	NA	NA	NA	NA	NA
Pork and beef (chopped together)—1 link, 2¼" x 1½" diam., 60 gm.	...	...	NA	NA	NA	NA	NA
Pork sausage, links or bulk, cooked—1 link, 3" x ½" diam., 20 gm.	.048	.6	.033	.0024	NA	.1364	.1
Pork sausage, canned, drained solids—1 patty, 2" diam., 50 gm.	...	...	...	...	NA	...	...
Pork sausage, link, smoked—see Country-style sausage							
Salami, dry—1 slice, 3¾" x ¼", 30 gm.	.063	.9	NA	NA	NA	NA	NA
Salami, cooked—1 slice, 3¾" x ¼", 32 gm.	.07	1.31	NA	NA	NA	NA	NA
Scrapple—1 sl., 3½" x 2¼" x ¼", 57 gm.	.032	.5	NA	NA	NA	NA	NA
Thuringer—6" x 1¼" diam., 100 gm.	.26	4.2	NA	NA	NA	NA	NA
Vienna sausage, canned—2" x ¾" diam., 17 gm.	.02	.44	NA	NA	NA	NA	NA
END OF SAUSAGE, COLD CUTS, AND LUNCHEON MEATS							
Squab (pigeon), raw, flesh and skin—3" x 2" x ¾", 60 gm.	...	...	NA	NA	NA	NA	NA
Suet (beef kidney fat), raw—1 tbsp., 10 gm.	...	...	NA	NA	NA	NA	NA
Sweetbreads (thymus), calf, cooked, braised—½ cup, 100 gm.	.16	2.9	NA	NA	NA	NA	NA
Thuringer—see Sausage, Cold Cuts, and Luncheon Meats							
Tongue, Beef, medium-fat, cooked, braised—1 sl., 3" x 2" x ⅛", 21 gm.	.06	.73	NA	NA	NA	NA	NA
Tongue, Beef, Smoked—1 sl., 3" x 2" x ⅛", 20 gm.	.04	.6	NA	NA	NA	NA	NA
Tongue, canned or cured (beef, lamb, etc.), whole, canned or pickled—1 sl., 3" x 2" x ⅜", 60 gm.	.13	1.5	NA	NA	NA	NA	NA
Tongue, canned or cured, potted or deviled—1 rd. tbsp., 20 gm.	.02	.26	NA	NA	NA	NA	NA
Tripe, beef, commercial—1 pc., 5" x 2½" diam., 85 gm.	.077	1.4	NA	NA	NA	NA	NA
Tripe, beef, pickled—1 piece, 4" x 2" diam., 62 gm.	...	...	NA	NA	NA	NA	NA
Turkey, flesh and skin, cooked, roasted—1 sl., 3" x 3" x ¼", 42 gm.	.06	3.4	...	...	NA	...	...
Turkey, light meat, cooked, roasted—1 sl., 3" x 3" x ¼", 40 gm.	.05	4.44	...	.0032	NA	.2364	...
Turkey, dark meat, cooked, roasted—1 sl., 3" x 3" x ¼", 40 gm.	.09	1.68	...	...	NA	.4512	...
Turkey, canned, meat only—1 tbsp., 12 gm.	.01	.56	...	...	NA	...	...
Turkey, potted—see Sausage, Cold Cuts, and Luncheon Meats							
Turkey potpie, home-prepared, baked—4¼" pie, 227 gm.	.23	3.9	...	...	NA	...	...

Vitamin C mg.	Vitamin D IU	Vitamin E IU	Calcium mg.	Iodine mg.	Iron mg.	Magnesium mg.	Phosphorus mg.	Potassium mg.	Sodium mg.
0	0	NA	3	NA	.7	NA	48	NA	NA
0	0	NA	4	NA	1.0	NA	73	NA	NA
0	0	.03 (fried)	2	NA	.4	3.2	35	---	---
---	0	---	5.5	NA	1.4	8	105	---	---
0	0	.03	4	NA	1.1	NA	78	---	---
0	0	---	3.2	NA	.83	NA	64	---	---
0	0	NA	4	NA	.6	NA	65	---	---
---	NA	NA	11	NA	2.8	NA	214	---	---
---	NA	NA	1.36	NA	.35	---	26.01	---	---
---	NA	NA	---	NA	---	NA	---	---	---
---	NA	NA	---	NA	---	NA	---	---	---
---	NA	NA	---	NA	---	---	---	---	---
---	NA	NA	1.47	NA	.46	3.36 (raw)	24.57	34.4	12.8
---	NA	NA	---	NA	---	---	---	---	---
0	0	NA	5	NA	1.5	9.6 (raw)	110	230	60
---	NA	NA	---	NA	---	3.2 (raw)	---	---	---
0	0	NA	59	NA	.8	NA	112	16	39
0	0	NA	---	NA	---	NA	---	11.78	28.52
---	NA	NA	---	NA	---	11.76	---	---	---
---	NA	NA	---	NA	.48	11.2	---	164.4	32.8
---	NA	NA	---	NA	.92	11.2	---	159.2	39.6
---	NA	NA	1.2	NA	.16	---	---	---	---
NA	NA	NA	22	NA	1.6	---	107	---	864

Food and Amount	Calories	Carbo-hydrate gm.	Protein gm.	Sat. Fatty Acids gm.	Unsat. Fatty Acids gm.	Vitamin A IU	Thiamin B₁ mg.
VEAL—RETAIL CUTS, CHOICE GRADE, LEAN ONLY, SEPARABLE FAT REMOVED							
Veal, Shank, Veal Patties—moist* cooked, 2″ diam., 52 gm.	112.32	0	14.92	2.7	2.7	0	.02
Veal, Breast, Veal Stew Meat—moist* cooked, w/onions and carrots, ½ cup, 119 gm.	121	3.6	8.8	12.61	12.61	1,627	.034
Veal, Breast—moist* cooked, 1 sl., 3″ x 2″ x ¼″, 35 gm.	82.25	0	9.76	3.71	3.71	0	.03
Veal, Shoulder, Blade Veal Roast—dry* cooked, 3″ x 3″ x ¼″, 42 gm.	163.8	0	9.74	2.68	2.68	0	.02
Veal, Shoulder, Rolled Veal Shoulder Roast—dry* cooked, 3″ x 3″ x ¼″, 42 gm.	163.8	0	9.74	2.68	2.68	0	.02
Veal, Rib, Veal Crown Roast—dry* cooked, 1¾″ sq. x ¾″, 40 gm.	107.6	0	10.88	3.4	3.36	0	.05
Veal, Rib, Frenched Veal Rib Chop— moist* cooked, 1¾″ sq. x ¾″, 40 gm.	107.6	0	10.88	3.4	3.36	0	.05
Veal, Rib, Veal Rib Roast—dry* cooked, 3″ x 2″ x ¼″, 38 gm.	102.2	0	10.33	3.23	3.19	0	.04
Veal, Loin, Loin Veal Chop—moist* cooked, 1½″ x 1¾″ x ½″, 30 gm.	70.2	0	7.92	2.01	2.01	0	.02
Veal, Loin, Sirloin Veal Steak—moist* cooked, 1 sl., 4″ x 2¼″ x ½″, 98 gm.	172	0	27.4	6.56	6.56	0	.168
Veal, Loin, Kidney Veal Chop—moist* cooked, 1¾″ x 1¾″ x ½″, 35 gm.	81.9	0	9.24	2.34	2.34	0	.02
Veal, Round, Veal Rump Roast— dry* cooked, 1 sl., 4″ x 2¼″ x ¼″, 48 gm.	84	0	14.7	2.68	2.64	0	.077
Veal, Round, Rolled Veal Rump Roast— dry* cooked, 1 sl., 4″ x 2¼″ x ¼″, 48 gm.	84	0	14.7	2.68	2.64	0	.077
Veal, Round, Veal Cutlet (Round Steak) —moist* cooked, 5″ x 3″ x ¼″, 70 gm.	151.2	0	18.97	3.92	3.85	0	.04
Veal, Round, Veal Round Roast— dry* cooked, 1 sl., 4″ x 3″ x ¼″, 56 gm.	120.96	0	15.17	3.13	3.08	0	.03
Veal, Round, Veal Scallops— moist* cooked, 1 sl., 3″ x 2″ x ¼″, 44 gm.	95.04	0	11.92	2.46	2.42	0	.03
Vienna Sausage—see Sausage, Cold Cuts, and Luncheon Meats							

*Dry cooking: broiling, roasting—Moist cooking: stewing, braising.

MISCELLANEOUS FOODS

Food and Amount	Calories	Carbo-hydrate gm.	Protein gm.	Sat. Fatty Acids gm.	Unsat. Fatty Acids gm.	Vitamin A IU	Thiamin B₁ mg.
Baking powder, home use, sodium aluminum sulfate and calcium sulfate —1 tsp., 1 gm.	1.04	.251	.001	NA	NA	0	0

Ribo-flavin B₂ mg.	Niacin mg.	B₆ mg.	Folic Acid mg.	PABA mg.	Panto-thenic Acid mg.	B₁₂ mcg.	Vitamin C mg.	Vitamin D IU	Vitamin E IU	Calcium mg.	Iodine mg.
.13	2.6	.208 (raw)	.0026	NA	.5512 (raw)	.91 (raw)	0	0	.02 (fried)	6.24	.003535 (raw) Ohio
.083	1.5	.476 (raw)	.00595	NA	1.2614 (raw)	2.08 (raw)	0	0	.05 (fried)	16	.00809 (raw) Ohio
.1	2.24	.14 (raw)	.00175	NA	.371 (raw)	.61 (raw)	0	0	.01 (fried)	4.2	.00238 (raw) Ohio
.09	1.76	.168 (raw)	---	NA	.4452 (raw)	.73 (raw)	0	0	.02 (fried)	4.62	.0028 (raw) Ohio
.09	1.76	.168 (raw)	---	NA	.4452 (raw)	.73 (raw)	0	0	.02 (fried)	4.62	.0028 (raw) Ohio
.12	3.12	.16 (raw)	---	NA	.424 (raw)	.7 (raw)	0	0	.02 (fried)	4.8	.0027 (raw) Ohio
.12	3.12	.16 (raw)	.002	NA	.424 (raw)	.7 (raw)	0	0	.02 (fried)	4.8	.0027 (raw) Ohio
.11	2.96	.152 (raw)	---	NA	.4028 (raw)	.66 (raw)	0	0	.01 (fried)	4.56	.00258 (raw) Ohio
.07	1.62	.12 (raw)	.0015	NA	.318 (raw)	.52 (raw)	0	0	.01 (fried)	3.3	.00204 (raw) Ohio
.244	8.2	.392 (raw)	.0049	NA	1.0388 (raw)	1.71 (raw)	0	0	.049 (fried)	8	.0066 (raw) Ohio
.08	1.89	.14 (raw)	.00175	NA	.371 (raw)	.61 (raw)	0	0	.01 (fried)	3.85	.00238 (raw) Ohio
.096	3.9	.192 (raw)	---	NA	.5088 (raw)	.84 (raw)	0	0	.02 (fried)	4	.00326 (raw) Ohio
.096	3.9	.192 (raw)	---	NA	.5088 (raw)	.84 (raw)	0	0	.02 (fried)	4	.00326 (raw) Ohio
.17	3.78	.28 (raw)	---	NA	.742 (raw)	1.22 (raw)	0	0	.03 (fried)	7.7	.00476 (raw) Ohio
.14	3.02	.224 (raw)	---	NA	.5936 (raw)	.98 (raw)	0	0	.03 (fried)	6.16	.0038 (raw) Ohio
.11	2.37	.176 (raw)	---	NA	.4664 (raw)	.77 (raw)	0	0	.02 (fried)	4.84	.0029 (raw) Ohio

MISCELLANEOUS FOODS

Ribo-flavin B₂ mg.	Niacin mg.	B₆ mg.	Folic Acid mg.	PABA mg.	Panto-thenic Acid mg.	B₁₂ mcg.	Vitamin C mg.	Vitamin D IU	Vitamin E IU	Calcium mg.	Iodine mg.
0	0	NA	NA	NA	NA	0	0	NA	NA	63.2	NA

Food and Amount	Iron mg.	Magnesium mg.	Phosphorus mg.	Potassium mg.	Sodium mg.
VEAL—RETAIL CUTS, CHOICE GRADE, LEAN ONLY, SEPARABLE FAT REMOVED					
Veal, Shank, Veal Patties—moist* cooked, 2" diam., 52 gm.	1.87	•••	80.08	260	41.6
Veal, Breast, Veal Stew Meat—moist* cooked, w/onions and carrots, ½ cup, 119 gm.	1.5	•••	96	•••	•••
Veal, Breast—moist* cooked, 1 sl., 3" x 2" x ¼", 35 gm.	1.22	•••	52.85	175	28
Veal, Shoulder, Blade Veal Roast—dry* cooked, 3" x 3" x ¼", 42 gm.	1.26	7.98	49.14	210	33.6
Veal, Shoulder, Rolled Veal Shoulder Roast—dry* cooked, 3" x 3" x ¼", 42 gm.	1.26	7.98	49.14	210	33.6
Veal, Rib, Veal Crown Roast—dry* cooked, 1¾" sq. x ¾", 40 gm.	1.36	7.6	99.2	200	32
Veal, Rib, Frenched Veal Rib Chop—moist* cooked, 1¾" sq. x ¾", 40 gm.	1.36	•••	99.2	200	32
Veal, Rib, Veal Rib Roast—dry* cooked, 3" x 2" x ¼", 38 gm.	1.29	7.22	94.24	190	30.4
Veal, Loin, Loin Veal Chop—moist* cooked, 1½" x 1¾" x ½", 30 gm.	.96	•••	67.5	150	24
Veal, Loin, Sirloin Veal Steak—moist* cooked, 1 sl., 4" x 2¼" x ½", 98 gm.	3.5	22	246	1,114	124
Veal, Loin, Kidney Veal Chop—moist* cooked, 1¾" x 1¾" x ½", 35 gm.	1.12	•••	78.75	175	28
Veal, Round, Veal Rump Roast—dry* cooked, 1 sl., 4" x 2¼" x ¼", 48 gm.	1.9	10	119	244	36
Veal, Round, Rolled Veal Rump Roast—dry* cooked, 1 sl., 4" x 2¼" x ¼", 48 gm.	1.9	10	119	244	36
Veal, Round, Veal Cutlet (Round Steak)—moist* cooked, 5" x 3" x ¼", 70 gm.	2.24	14	161.7	350	56
Veal, Round, Veal Round Roast—dry* cooked, 1 sl., 4" x 3" x ¼", 56 gm.	1.79	11.2	129.36	280	44.8
Veal, Round, Veal Scallops—moist* cooked, 1 sl., 3" x 2" x ¼", 44 gm.	1.4	8.8	101.64	220	35.2
Vienna Sausage—see Sausage, Cold Cuts, and Luncheon Meats					

* Dry cooking: broiling, roasting—Moist cooking: stewing, braising.

MISCELLANEOUS FOODS

Food and Amount	Iron mg.	Magnesium mg.	Phosphorus mg.	Potassium mg.	Sodium mg.
Baking powder, home use, sodium aluminum sulfate and calcium sulfate—1 tsp., 1 gm.	•••	NA	15.6	1.5	100

Food and Amount	Calories	Carbohydrate gm.	Protein gm.	Sat. Fatty Acids gm.	Unsat. Fatty Acids gm.	Vitamin A IU	Thiamin B₁ mg.
Barbeque sauce—see Sauces, barbeque							
Bouillon cubes or powder (meat extract) —1 cube, ½", 4 gm.	2	0	.2	NA	NA	---	---
Cornstarch—1 tbsp., 8 gm.	29	7	0	NA	NA	0	0
Cucumber pickles—see Pickles							
Gelatin, unflavored, dry—1 tbsp., 10 gm.	34	0	8.6	NA	NA	0	0
Granola—1 cup, 110 gm.	520	---	14	---	---	NA	.78
Horseradish, prepared—1 tsp., 6 gm.	1.9	.48	.06	NA	NA	---	---
Horseradish, raw—1 tsp., 5 gm.	4	.98	.16	NA	NA	---	.003
Mustard, prepared, brown—1 tsp., 5 gm.	4	.3	.3	NA	NA	---	---
Mustard, prepared, yellow—1 tsp., 5 gm.	3.75	.32	.23	NA	NA	---	---
Olives, pickled, canned or bottled, green —4 med., 3 large, or 2 giant, 1½", 16 gm.	15	trace	trace	trace	2	40	---
Olives, pickled, canned or bottled, ripe, Ascolano—1 olive, ⅞", 3 gm.	3.87	.07	.03	---	---	1.8	trace
Olives, pickled, canned or bottled, ripe, Manzanilla—1 large, 1", 4 gm.	5.16	.1	.04	---	---	2.4	trace
Olives, pickled, canned or bottled, ripe, Mission—3 sml. or 2 large, 1", 10 gm.	15	.32	trace	trace	2	10	trace
Olives, pickled, canned or bottled, ripe, Sevillano—1 olive, 1", 4 gm.	3.72	.1	.04	---	---	2.4	trace
Olives, pickled, canned or bottled, ripe, salt-cured, oil-coated, Greek style— 1", 5 gm.	16.9	.11	.43	.2	1.5	---	---
Pickles, cucumber, dill—1 pickle, 4" x 1¾" diam., 135 gm.	15	2.8	.9	---	---	420	trace
Pickles, cucumber, fresh (as bread and butter pickles)—1 slice, 1½" diam., ¼" thick, 7.5 gm.	5	1.5	trace	---	---	10	trace
Pickles, cucumber, sour—1 pickle, 1¾" diam. x 4", 136 gm.	13.6	2.72	.68	---	---	136	trace
Pickles, cucumber, sweet—1 pickle, 2½" long, ¾" diam., 15 gm.	20	6	trace	---	---	10	trace
Pickles, chow-chow*, sour—1 tbsp., 25 gm.	7.25	1.02	.35	---	---	---	---
Pickles, chow-chow*, sweet—1 tbsp., 25 gm.	29	6.75	.37	---	---	---	---
Pickles, Relish, finely cut or chopped, sour—1 tbsp., 15 gm.	2.85	.4	.10	---	---	---	---
Pickles, Relish, finely cut or chopped, sweet—1 tbsp., 15 gm.	20	5	trace	---	---	---	---
Pizza, w/cheese, home recipe, baked, cheese only—⅛ of 14" pie, 75 gm.	177	21.2	9	2.25	3.75	472	.04
Pizza, w/cheese, home recipe, baked, w/sausage—⅛ of 14" pie, 81 gm.	189	23.9	6.31	2.43	4.05	453	.07
Pizza, w/cheese, chilled, baked— ⅛ of 14" pie, 73 gm.	178	26.4	6.71	1.46	2.92	284	.04
Pizza, w/cheese, frozen, baked—⅛ of 14" pie, 73 gm.	178	25.8	6.9	1.46	2.19	321	.04
Salt, tablet†—1 tsp., 0.5 gm.	0	0	0	NA	NA	0	0

* Chow-chow—cucumber with added cauliflower, onion, and mustard.
† Iodized salt.

Food and Amount	Ribo-flavin B_2 mg.	Niacin mg.	B_6 mg.	Folic Acid mg.	PABA mg.	Panto-thenic Acid mg.	B_{12} mcg.
Barbeque sauce—see Sauces, barbeque							
Bouillon cubes or powder (meat extract) —1 cube, ½", 4 gm.	.072	1	NA	NA	NA	NA	NA
Cornstarch—1 tbsp., 8 gm.	0	0	NA	NA	NA	NA	0
Cucumber pickles—see Pickles							
Gelatin, unflavored, dry—1 tbsp., 10 gm.	0	0	.0007	NA	.001	---	---
Granola—1 cup, 110 gm.	NA	NA	NA	NA	NA	NA	NA
Horseradish, prepared—1 tsp., 6 gm.	---	---	NA	NA	NA	NA	0
Horseradish, raw—1 tsp., 5 gm.	---	---	NA	NA	NA	NA	0
Mustard, prepared, brown—1 tsp., 5 gm.	---	---	NA	NA	NA	NA	0
Mustard, prepared, yellow—1 tsp., 5 gm.	---	---	NA	NA	NA	NA	0
Olives, pickled, canned or bottled, green —4 med., 3 large, or 2 giant, 1½", 16 gm.	---	---	---	NA	NA	.00288	0
Olives, pickled, canned or bottled, ripe, Ascolano—1 olive, ⅞", 3 gm.	trace	---	---	---	NA	---	0
Olives, pickled, canned or bottled, ripe, Manzanilla—1 large, 1", 4 gm.	trace	---	.00064	.00002	NA	.0008	0
Olives, pickled, canned or bottled, ripe, Mission—3 sml. or 2 large, 1", 10 gm.	trace	---	.0014	.0001	NA	.0015	0
Olives, pickled, canned or bottled, ripe, Sevillano—1 olive, 1", 4 gm.	trace	---	---	---	NA	---	0
Olives, pickled, canned or bottled, ripe, salt-cured, oil-coated, Greek style— 1", 5 gm.	---	---	---	---	NA	---	NA
Pickles, cucumber, dill—1 pickle, 4"x 1¾" diam., 135 gm.	.081	.1	.00945	NA	NA	---	0
Pickles, cucumber, fresh (as bread and butter pickles)—1 slice, 1½" diam., ¼" thick, 7.5 gm.	trace	trace	NA	NA	NA	NA	0
Pickles, cucumber, sour—1 pickle, 1¾" diam. x 4", 136 gm.	.027	trace	NA	NA	NA	NA	0
Pickles, cucumber, sweet—1 pickle, 2½" long, ¾" diam., 15 gm.	trace	trace	NA	NA	NA	NA	0
Pickles, chow-chow*, sour—1 tbsp., 25 gm.	---	---	NA	NA	NA	NA	0
Pickles, chow-chow*, sweet—1 tbsp., 25 gm.	---	---	NA	NA	NA	NA	0
Pickles, Relish, finely cut or chopped, sour—1 tbsp., 15 gm.	---	---	NA	NA	NA	NA	0
Pickles, Relish, finely cut or chopped, sweet—1 tbsp., 15 gm.	---	---	NA	NA	NA	NA	0
Pizza, w/cheese, home recipe, baked, cheese only—⅛ of 14" pie, 75 gm.	.15	.75	NA	NA	NA	NA	NA
Pizza, w/cheese, home recipe, baked, w/sausage—⅛ of 14" pie, 81 gm.	.09	1.21	NA	NA	NA	NA	NA
Pizza, w/cheese, chilled, baked— ⅛ of 14" pie, 73 gm.	.11	.73	NA	NA	NA	NA	NA
Pizza, w/cheese, frozen, baked—⅛ of 14" pie, 73 gm.	.12	.73	NA	NA	NA	NA	NA
Salt, tablet†—1 tsp., 0.5 gm.	0	0	NA	NA	NA	NA	0

* Chow-chow—cucumber with added cauliflower, onion, and mustard.
† Iodized salt.

Vitamin C mg.	Vitamin D IU	Vitamin E IU	Calcium mg.	Iodine mg.	Iron mg.	Magnesium mg.	Phosphorus mg.	Potassium mg.	Sodium mg.
0	0	NA	---	NA	---	---	---	108	424
0	0	NA	0	NA	0	.16	0	trace	trace
0	0	NA	0	NA	0	.4	0	.2	11.2
NA	NA	NA	NA	NA	5.2	NA	NA	NA	NA
---	NA	NA	3.05	NA	.04	---	1.6	14.5	4.8
4.05	NA	NA	7	NA	.07	1.7	3.2	28	.40
---	---	---	5	NA	.1	2.4	6	6.5	65
---	NA	.08	4	NA	.1	2.4	3.6	6.5	62
---	NA	NA	8	NA	.2	3.52	2.7	8.8	384
---	NA	NA	2.52	NA	.04	---	.48	1.02	24.39
---	NA	NA	3.36	NA	.06	---	.64	1.36	32.52
---	NA	NA	9	NA	.1	---	1.7	2.7	75
---	NA	NA	2.96	NA	.06	---	.8	1.76	33.12
---	NA	NA	---	NA	---	---	1.45	---	164.4
8	0	NA	34	NA	1.6	16.2	27	270	1,890
.5	NA	NA	2.5	NA	.15	---	2.025	---	50.5
1	NA	NA	23	NA	4.35	---	20	---	1,840
1	NA	NA	2	NA	.2	.15	2.4	---	---
---	NA	NA	8	NA	.65	---	13.25	---	334.5
---	NA	NA	5.75	NA	.37	---	5.5	---	131.75
---	NA	NA	4.35	NA	.16	---	1.0	---	---
---	NA	NA	3	NA	.1	---	2.1	---	---
6	NA	NA	165	NA	.75	---	146	97	526
7	NA	NA	13.7	NA	.97	---	74	136	590
4	NA	NA	104	NA	.65	---	148	81.03	462
4	NA	NA	113	NA	.65	---	113	83.2	472
0	0	NA	1.265	.05	0	.595	0	.02	1.93

Food and Amount	Calories	Carbo-hydrate gm.	Protein gm.	Sat. Fatty Acids gm.	Unsat. Fatty Acids gm.	Vitamin A IU	Thiamin B₁ mg.
Sauce, Barbeque—1 cup, 250 gm.	230	20	4	2	14	900	.03
Sauce, Barbeque—1 tbsp., 15.625 gm.	14.375	1.25	.25	.125	.875	56.25	.001875
Sauce, Bordelaise—1 tbsp., 10 gm.	18	1.4	NA	---	---	NA	NA
Sauce, Champignon—1 tbsp., 12 gm.	12	1.4	NA	---	---	NA	NA
Sauce, Cheese—1 tbsp., 18.75 gm.	32.5	1.2	1.475	---	---	103	.0055
Sauce, Cheese—¼ cup, 75 gm.	130	4.8	5.9	---	---	412	.022
Sauce, Chili—see Vegetables and Vegetable Products, Peppers							
Sauce, Hollandaise—1 tbsp., 12.5 gm.	45	.1	.55	NA	NA	256.75	.00675
Sauce, Hollandaise—¼ cup, 50 gm.	180	.4	2.2	NA	NA	1,027	.027
Sauce, Marinara—½ cup, 110 gm.	84	11.4	NA	---	---	NA	NA
Sauce, Mint—1 tbsp., 8 gm.	16	4	NA	---	---	NA	NA
Sauce, Soy—see Nuts, Seeds, Sprouted Seeds, Dry Beans, and Related Products							
Sauce, Steak—1 tbsp., 7 gm.	21	4.8	NA	NA	NA	NA	NA
Sauce, Sweet and Sour—1 tbsp., 10 gm.	31.3	1.17	NA	---	---	NA	NA
Sauce, Tabasco—1 tsp., 2 gm.	1	0	NA	NA	NA	NA	NA
Sauce, Tartar—1 tbsp., 20 gm.	95	1.5	.2	---	---	55	.005
Sauce, White, thin—1 tbsp., 15.25 gm.	18.5	1.15	.6	---	---	53.25	.00425
Sauce, White, medium—1 tbsp., 16.5 gm.	26.75	1.525	.65	1.155	.66	82	.0055
Sauce, White, thick—1 tbsp., 17.5 gm.	34.65	1.925	.7	---	---	99.75	.0075
Sauce, White, thin—¼ cup, 61 gm.	74	4.6	2.4	---	---	213	.017
Sauce, White, medium—¼ cup, 66 gm.	107	6.1	2.6	4.62	2.64	328	.022
Sauce, White, thick—¼ cup, 70 gm.	138.6	7.7	2.8	---	---	399	.03
Sauce, Worcestershire—1 tsp., 5 gm.	4	.9	.1	NA	NA	---	---
Soups, commercial, canned, Asparagus, cream of[1]—1 cup, 240 gm.	64	10.08	2.4	NA	NA	312	.04
Soups, commercial, canned, Asparagus, cream of[2]—1 cup, 245 gm.	147	16.6	6.8	NA	NA	490	.07
Soups, commercial, canned, Bean w/pork[1]—1 cup, 250 gm.	170	22	8	1	4	650	.13
Soups, commercial, canned, Beef broth, bouillon and consomme[1]—1 cup, 240 gm.	30	3	5	---	---	trace	trace
Soups, commercial, canned, Beef noodle[1]—1 cup, 250 gm.	70	7	4	1	2	50	.05
Soups, commercial, canned, Celery, cream of[1]—1 cup, 240 gm.	86	8.8	1.68	NA	NA	192	.02
Soups, commercial, canned, Celery, cream of[2]—1 cup, 245 gm.	169	15.19	6.37	NA	NA	392	.04
Soups, commercial, canned, Chicken consomme[1]—1 cup, 240 gm.	21	1.92	3.36	NA	NA	---	---
Soups, commercial, canned, Chicken, cream of[1]—1 cup, 240 gm.	95	8	3	1	5	410	.02
Soups, commercial, canned, Chicken, cream of[2]—1 cup, 245 gm.	180	15	7	3	6	610	.05
Soups, commercial, canned, Chicken gumbo[1]—1 cup, 245 gm.	56	7.6	3	NA	NA	220	.02

[1] Prepared with equal volume of water.
[2] Prepared with equal volume of milk.

Ribo-flavin B₂ mg.	Niacin mg.	B₆ mg.	Folic Acid mg.	PABA mg.	Panto-thenic Acid mg.	B₁₂ mcg.	Vitamin C mg.	Vitamin D IU	Vitamin E IU	Calcium mg.	Iodine mg.
.03	.8	NA	NA	NA	NA	NA	13	NA	NA	53	NA
.001875	.05	NA	NA	NA	NA	NA	8.125	NA	NA	3.3125	NA
NA	NA	NA	NA	NA	NA	NA	NA	NA	NA	NA	NA
NA	NA	NA	NA	NA	NA	NA	NA	NA	NA	NA	NA
.03975	.025	NA	NA	NA	NA	NA	trace	NA	NA	44	NA
.159	.1	NA	NA	NA	NA	NA	trace	NA	NA	176	NA
.01075	trace	NA	NA	NA	NA	NA	trace	NA	NA	5.75	NA
.043	trace	NA	NA	NA	NA	NA	trace	NA	NA	23	NA
NA	NA	NA	NA	NA	NA	NA	NA	NA	NA	NA	NA
NA	NA	NA	NA	NA	NA	NA	NA	NA	NA	NA	NA
NA	NA	NA	NA	NA	NA	NA	NA	NA	NA	NA	NA
NA	NA	NA	NA	NA	NA	NA	NA	NA	NA	NA	NA
NA	NA	NA	NA	NA	NA	NA	NA	NA	NA	NA	NA
.006	trace	NA	NA	NA	NA	NA	1	NA	NA	4	NA
.02475	.025	NA	NA	NA	NA	NA	trace	NA	NA	18.25	NA
.026	.05	NA	NA	NA	NA	NA	trace	NA	NA	18.5	NA
.0275	.0525	NA	NA	NA	NA	NA	trace	NA	NA	18.725	NA
.099	.1	NA	NA	NA	NA	NA	trace	NA	NA	73	NA
.104	.2	NA	NA	NA	NA	NA	trace	NA	NA	74	NA
.11	.21	NA	NA	NA	NA	NA	trace	NA	NA	74.9	NA
---	---	NA	NA	NA	NA	NA	0	NA	NA	5	NA
.09	.72	NA	NA	NA	NA	NA	---	NA	NA	26	NA
.29	.73	NA	NA	NA	NA	NA	trace	NA	NA	176	NA
.08	1.0	NA	NA	NA	NA	NA	3	NA	NA	63	NA
.02	1.2	NA	NA	NA	NA	NA	---	NA	NA	trace	NA
.07	1.0	NA	NA	NA	NA	NA	trace	NA	NA	7	NA
.04	trace	NA	NA	NA	NA	NA	trace	NA	NA	48	NA
.26	.73	NA	NA	NA	NA	NA	2.45	NA	NA	198	NA
---	---	NA	NA	NA	NA	NA	---	NA	NA	12	NA
.05	.5	NA	NA	NA	NA	NA	trace	NA	NA	24	NA
.27	.7	NA	NA	NA	NA	NA	2	NA	NA	172	NA
.04	1.22	NA	NA	NA	NA	NA	5	NA	NA	19	NA

Food and Amount	Iron mg.	Magnesium mg.	Phosphorus mg.	Potassium mg.	Sodium mg.
Sauce, Barbeque—1 cup, 250 gm.	2	NA	50	435	2,037
Sauce, Barbeque—1 tbsp., 15.625 gm.	.125	NA	3.125	27.1875	127.3125
Sauce, Bordelaise—1 tbsp., 10 gm.	NA	NA	NA	NA	NA
Sauce, Champignon—1 tbsp., 12 gm.	NA	NA	NA	NA	NA
Sauce, Cheese—1 tbsp., 18.75 gm.	.05	NA	32.25	NA	NA
Sauce, Cheese—¼ cup, 75 gm.	.2	NA	129	NA	NA
Sauce, Chili—see Vegetables and Vegetable Products, Peppers					
Sauce, Hollandaise—1 tbsp., 12.5 gm.	.225	NA	19.5	NA	NA
Sauce, Hollandaise—¼ cup, 50 gm.	.9	NA	78	NA	NA
Sauce, Marinara—½ cup, 110 gm.	NA	NA	NA	NA	NA
Sauce, Mint—1 tbsp., 8 gm.	NA	NA	NA	NA	NA
Sauce, Soy—see Nuts, Seeds, Sprouted Seeds, Dry Beans, and Related Products					
Sauce, Steak—1 tbsp., 7 gm.	NA	NA	NA	NA	NA
Sauce, Sweet and Sour—1 tbsp., 10 gm.	NA	NA	NA	NA	NA
Sauce, Tabasco—1 tsp., 2 gm.	NA	NA	NA	NA	NA
Sauce, Tartar—1 tbsp., 20 gm.	.2	NA	10	15.6	141.4
Sauce, White, thin—1 tbsp., 15.25 gm.	.025	---	14.75	22.285	53.5275
Sauce, White, medium—1 tbsp., 16.5 gm.	.05	---	15.25	22.935	62.535
Sauce, White, thick—1 tbsp., 17.5 gm.	.0525	---	15.75	23.275	69.825
Sauce, White, thin—¼ cup, 61 gm.	.1	---	59	89.06	214.11
Sauce, White, medium—¼ cup, 66 gm.	.2	---	61	91.74	250.14
Sauce, White, thick—¼ cup, 70 gm.	.21	---	63	93.1	279.3
Sauce, Worcestershire—1 tsp., 5 gm.	.3	NA	3	NA	NA
Soups, commercial, canned, Asparagus, cream of[1]—1 cup, 240 gm.	.72	NA	38	120	984
Soups, commercial, canned, Asparagus, cream of[2]—1 cup, 245 gm.	.73	NA	156	301	1,068
Soups, commercial, canned, Bean w/pork[1]—1 cup, 250 gm.	2.3	---	127	395	1,007
Soups, commercial, canned, Beef broth, bouillon and consommé[1]—1 cup, 240 gm.	.5	--.-	31	129	782
Soups, commercial, canned, Beef noodle[1]—1 cup, 250 gm.	1.0	---	50	80	955
Soups, commercial, canned, Celery, cream of[1]—1 cup, 240 gm.	.48	NA	36	108	955
Soups, commercial, canned, Celery, cream of[2]—1 cup, 245 gm.	.73	NA	154	289	1,038
Soups, commercial, canned, Chicken consommé[1]—1 cup, 240 gm.	1.2	NA	72	---	722
Soups, commercial, canned, Chicken, cream of[1]—1 cup, 240 gm.	.5	NA	34	79	970
Soups, commercial, canned, Chicken, cream of[2]—1 cup, 245 gm.	.5	NA	152	260	1,053
Soups, commercial, canned, Chicken gumbo[1]—1 cup, 245 gm.	.49	NA	24	110	970

[1] Prepared with equal volume of water.
[2] Prepared with equal volume of milk.

Food and Amount	Calories	Carbo-hydrate gm.	Protein gm.	Sat. Fatty Acids gm.	Unsat. Fatty Acids gm.	Vitamin A IU	Thiamin B₁ mg.
Soups, commercial, canned, Chicken noodle[1]—1 cup, 245 gm.	63	8	3	NA	NA	49	.02
Soups, commercial, canned, Chicken w/rice[1]—1 cup, 245 gm.	49	5.8	3	NA	NA	147	trace
Soups, commercial, canned, Chicken vegetable[1]—1 cup, 248 gm.	76	9.6	4	NA	NA	2,182	.02
Soups, commercial, canned, Clam chowder††[1]—1 cup, 245 gm.	80	12	2	---	---	880	.02
Soups, commercial, canned, Minestrone[1]—1 cup, 245 gm.	105	14	5	---	---	2,350	.07
Soup, commercial, canned, Mushroom, cream of[1]—1 cup, 240 gm.	135	10	2	1	8	70	.02
Soup, commercial, canned, Mushroom, cream of[2]—1 cup, 245 gm.	215	16	7	4	9	250	.05
Soup, commercial, canned, Onion[1]—1 cup, 240 gm.	65	5	5	NA	NA	trace	trace
Soup, commercial, canned, Pea, green[1]—1 cup, 245 gm.	130	22	5	NA	NA	343	.04
Soup, commercial, canned, Pea, green[2]—1 cup, 248 gm.	210	29	10	NA	NA	520	.09
Soup, commercial, canned, Pea, split[1]—1 cup, 245 gm.	145	21	9	1	2	440	.25
Soup, commercial, canned, Tomato[1]—1 cup, 245 gm.	90	16	2	trace	2	1,000	.05
Soup, commercial, canned, Tomato[2]—1 cup, 250 gm.	175	23	7	3	3	1,200	.10
Soup, commercial, canned, Turkey noodle[1]—1 cup, 245 gm.	80	8	4	NA	NA	196	.04
Soup, commercial, canned, Vegetable beef[1]—1 cup, 245 gm.	80	10	5	---	---	2,700	.05
Soup, commercial, canned, Vegetable w/beef broth[1]—1 cup, 240 gm.	76	13	2.6	NA	NA	3,120	.04
Soup, commercial, canned, Vegetarian vegetable[1]—1 cup, 245 gm.	80	13	2	---	---	2,940	.05
Soup, dehydrated, Beef noodle, 2 oz. mix, 3 cups water—1 cup, 240 gm.	67	11	2.4	---	---	24	.09
Soup, dehydrated, Chicken noodle, 2 oz. mix, 4 cups water—1 cup, 240 gm.	52	7	1.9	---	---	48	.07
Soup, dehydrated, Chicken rice, 1½ oz. mix, 3 cups water—1 cup, 240 gm.	48	8	1.2	---	---	trace	trace
Soup, dehydrated, Onion, mix, dry form —1 pkg., 1½ oz., 43 gm.	150	23	6	1	3	30	.05
Soup, dehydrated, Onion, 1½ oz. mix, 4 cups water—1 cup, 240 gm.	36	5.5	1.44	---	---	trace	trace
Soup, dehydrated, Pea, green, 2 oz. mix, 3 cups water—1 cup, 240 gm.	120	20	7	---	---	48	.14
Soup, dehydrated, Tomato vegetable w/noodles, 2½ oz. mix, 4 cups water —1 cup, 240 gm.	65	12	1.44	---	---	480	.04
Soup, frozen, clam chowder††[1]—1 cup, 240 gm.	130	11	4	---	---	50	.05
Soup, frozen, clam chowder**[2]—1 cup, 245 gm.	210	16	9	---	---	250	.07

[1] Prepared with equal volume of water. [2] Prepared with equal volume of milk.
†† Manhattan clam chowder with tomatoes, without milk.
** New England clam chowder—with milk, without tomatoes.

Food and Amount	Riboflavin B₂ mg.	Niacin mg.	B₆ mg.	Folic Acid mg.	PABA mg.	Pantothenic Acid mg.	B₁₂ mcg.
Soups, commercial, canned, Chicken noodle[1]—1 cup, 245 gm.	.02	.73	NA	NA	NA	NA	NA
Soups, commercial, canned, Chicken w/rice[1]—1 cup, 245 gm.	.02	.73	NA	NA	NA	NA	NA
Soups, commercial, canned, Chicken vegetable[1]—1 cup, 248 gm.	.04	.99	NA	NA	NA	NA	NA
Soups, commercial, canned, Clam chowder††[1]—1 cup, 245 gm.	.02	1.0	NA	NA	NA	NA	NA
Soups, commercial, canned, Minestrone[1]—1 cup, 245 gm.	.05	1.0	NA	NA	NA	NA	NA
Soup, commercial, canned, Mushroom, cream of[1]—1 cup, 240 gm.	.12	.7	NA	NA	NA	NA	NA
Soup, commercial, canned, Mushroom, cream of[2]—1 cup, 245 gm.	.34	.7	NA	NA	NA	NA	NA
Soup, commercial, canned, Onion[1]—1 cup, 240 gm.	.02	trace	NA	NA	NA	NA	NA
Soup, commercial, canned, Pea, green[1]—1 cup, 245 gm.	.04	.98	NA	NA	NA	NA	NA
Soup, commercial, canned, Pea, green[2]—1 cup, 248 gm.	.27	1.24	NA	NA	NA	NA	NA
Soup, commercial, canned, Pea, split[1]—1 cup, 245 gm.	.15	1.5	NA	NA	NA	NA	NA
Soup, commercial, canned, Tomato[1]—1 cup, 245 gm.	.05	1.2	NA	NA	NA	NA	NA
Soup, commercial, canned, Tomato[2]—1 cup, 250 gm.	.25	1.3	NA	NA	NA	NA	NA
Soup, commercial, canned, Turkey noodle[1]—1 cup, 245 gm.	.04	1.2	NA	NA	NA	NA	NA
Soup, commercial, canned, Vegetable beef[1]—1 cup, 245 gm.	.05	1.0	NA	NA	NA	NA	NA
Soup, commercial, canned, Vegetable w/beef broth[1]—1 cup, 240 gm.	.02	1.2	•••	NA	NA	.336	NA
Soup, commercial, canned, Vegetarian vegetable[1]—1 cup, 245 gm.	.05	1.0	NA	NA	NA	NA	NA
Soup, dehydrated, Beef noodle, 2 oz. mix, 3 cups water—1 cup, 240 gm.	.04	.72	NA	NA	NA	NA	NA
Soup, dehydrated, Chicken noodle, 2 oz. mix, 4 cups water—1 cup, 240 gm.	.04	.48	NA	NA	NA	NA	NA
Soup, dehydrated, Chicken rice, 1½ oz. mix, 3 cups water—1 cup, 240 gm.	trace	.24	NA	NA	NA	NA	NA
Soup, dehydrated, Onion, mix, dry form —1 pkg., 1½ oz., 43 gm.	.03	.3	NA	NA	NA	NA	NA
Soup, dehydrated, Onion, 1½ oz. mix, 4 cups water—1 cup, 240 gm.	trace	trace	NA	NA	NA	NA	NA
Soup, dehydrated, Pea, green, 2 oz. mix, 3 cups water—1 cup, 240 gm.	.14	1.44	NA	NA	NA	NA	NA
Soup, dehydrated, Tomato vegetable w/noodles, 2½ oz. mix, 4 cups water —1 cup, 240 gm.	.02	.48	NA	NA	NA	NA	NA
Soup, frozen, clam chowder††[1]—1 cup, 240 gm.	.10	.5	NA	NA	NA	NA	NA
Soup, frozen, clam chowder**[2]—1 cup, 245 gm.	.29	.5	NA	NA	NA	NA	NA

[1] Prepared with equal volume of water.　[2] Prepared with equal volume of milk.
†† Manhattan clam chowder with tomatoes, without milk.
** New England clam chowder—with milk, without tomatoes.

Vitamin C mg.	Vitamin D IU	Vitamin E IU	Calcium mg.	Iodine mg.	Iron mg.	Magnesium mg.	Phosphorus mg.	Potassium mg.	Sodium mg.
trace	NA	NA	9.8	NA	.49	---	36	56	999
---	NA	NA	7.3	NA	.24	NA	24	100	935
---	NA	NA	17	NA	.49	NA	39	99	1,046
---	NA	NA	34	NA	1.0	NA	46	183	938
---	NA	NA	37	NA	1.0	---	59	313	995
trace	NA	NA	41	NA	.5	NA	50	98	955
1	NA	NA	191	NA	.5	---	169	279	1,039
---	NA	NA	29	NA	.48	NA	26	103	1,051
7	NA	NA	44	NA	.98	---	112	196	899
10	NA	NA	196	NA	.99	NA	233	379	974
1	NA	NA	.29	NA	1.5	NA	149	269	940
12	NA	NA	15	NA	.7	22.05	34	230	970
15	NA	NA	168	NA	.8	NA	155	417	1,055
trace	NA	NA	14	NA	.73	NA	44	78	1,019
---	NA	NA	12	NA	.7	NA	49	161	1,046
---	NA	NA	19	NA	.72	---	38	235	828
---	NA	NA	20	NA	1.0	NA	39	171	838
trace	NA	NA	9.6	NA	.48	NA	26	40	420
trace	NA	NA	7.2	NA	.24	NA	19	19	578
---	NA	NA	7.2	NA	trace	NA	9.6	9.6	621
6	NA	NA	42	NA	.6	NA	48	237	2,870
2.4	NA	NA	9.6	NA	.24	NA	12	57	688
trace	NA	NA	19	NA	1.9	NA	103	288	780
4.8	NA	NA	7.2	NA	.24	NA	19	29	1,024
---	NA	NA	91	NA	1.0	NA	81	220	1,044
trace	NA	NA	240	NA	1.0	NA	201	406	1,129

Food and Amount	Calories	Carbohydrate gm.	Protein gm.	Sat. Fatty Acids gm.	Unsat. Fatty Acids gm.	Vitamin A IU	Thiamin B₁ mg.
Soup, frozen, Pea, green w/ham[1]— 1 cup, 245 gm.	140	19	9	NA	NA	221	.19
Soup, frozen, Potato, cream of[1]— 1 cup, 240 gm.	105	12	3	3	2	410	.05
Soup, frozen, Potato, cream of[2]—1 cup, 245 gm.	185	18	8	5	3	590	.10
Soup, frozen, Shrimp, cream of[1]—1 cup, 240 gm.	160	8	5	---	---	120	.05
Soup, frozen, Shrimp, cream of[2]—1 cup, 245 gm.	245	15	9	---	---	290	.07
Soup, frozen, Vegetable w/beef[1]—1 cup, 240 gm.	84	8	6	NA	NA	2,640	.04
Vinegar, cider—1 tbsp., 15 gm.	2	.8	0	---	---	---	---
Vinegar, distilled—1 tbsp., 15 gm.	2	.75	---	NA	NA	---	---
Vinegar, cider—1 tsp., 5 gm.	.66	.26	0	---	---	---	---
Vinegar, distilled—1 tsp., 5 gm.	.66	.25	---	NA	NA	---	---
Yeast, Baker's compressed—1 cake, 1½" sq., 12 gm.	10	1.3	1.4	---	---	trace	.085
Yeast, Brewer's, debittered—1 tbsp., 9.5 gm.	27	3.6	3.7	---	---	trace	1.484
Yogurt, Flavored (vanilla and coffee)[3]—1 cup, 245 gm.	200	32.7	8	2	1	---	---
Yogurt, Fruit (with preserves)[3]—1 cup, 245 gm.	260	48.8	7	1.8	1	---	---

[1] Prepared with equal volume of water.
[2] Prepared with equal volume of milk.
[3] Yogurt—see also entries on page 246.

NONALCOHOLIC BEVERAGES AND MIXERS

Food and Amount	Calories	Carbohydrate gm.	Protein gm.	Sat. Fatty Acids gm.	Unsat. Fatty Acids gm.	Vitamin A IU	Thiamin B₁ mg.
Carbonated water, sweetened, Quinine water—1 cup, 230 gm.	71	18	0	NA	NA	0	0
Carbonated water, unsweetened, Club Soda—1 cup, 230 gm.	0	0	0	NA	NA	0	0
Cola-type carbonated beverages—1 cup, 230 gm.	90	23	0	NA	NA	0	0
Coffee, instant, water-soluble solids, dry powder—1 tsp., 2 gm.	2.3	.66	trace	NA	NA	0	0
Coffee, instant, water-soluble solids, dry powder—1 tbsp., 6 gm.	7	2	trace	NA	NA	0	0
Cream sodas—1 cup, 230 gm.	99	25	0	NA	NA	0	0
Fruit flavored sodas (citrus, cherry, grape, strawberry, Tom Collins mixer, other) (10–13% sugar)—1 cup, 230 gm.	105	0	0	NA	NA	0	0
Ginger ale, pale dry, and golden— 1 cup, 230 gm.	80	20.7	---	NA	NA	0	0
Root beer—1 cup, 230 gm.	94	24.1	0	NA	NA	0	0
Tea, instant, water-soluble solids, carbohydrate added, dry powder— 1 tbsp., 6 gm.	17	4.8	---	NA	NA	---	---
Tea, regular, clear, no sugar—1 cup, 200 gm.	2	.4	.1	NA	NA	0	0

Riboflavin B2 mg.	Niacin mg.	B6 mg.	Folic Acid mg.	PABA mg.	Pantothenic Acid mg.	B12 mcg.	Vitamin C mg.	Vitamin D IU	Vitamin E IU	Calcium mg.	Iodine mg.
.07	1.22	NA	NA	NA	NA	NA	---	NA	NA	29	NA
.05	.5	NA	NA	NA	NA	NA	---	NA	NA	58	NA
.27	.5	NA	NA	NA	NA	NA	trace	NA	NA	208	NA
.05	.5	NA	NA	NA	NA	NA	---	NA	NA	38	NA
.27	.5	NA	NA	NA	NA	NA	trace	NA	NA	189	NA
.09	1.9	NA	NA	NA	NA	NA	---	NA	NA	26	NA
---	---	NA	NA	NA	NA	0	---	0	NA	1	NA
---	---	NA	NA	NA	NA	0	---	0	NA	---	NA
---	---	NA	NA	NA	NA	0	---	0	NA	.3	NA
---	---	NA	NA	NA	NA	0	---	0	NA	---	NA
.198	1.3	.072	NA	.57	.420	0	trace	NA	NA	2	NA
.406	3.6	.02375	.19209	4.94	1.140	0	trace	NA	NA	20	NA
---	---	---	NA	NA	---	---	---	NA	NA	NA	NA
.4	---	.1177	NA	NA	---	.26	---	NA	NA	298	NA

NONALCOHOLIC BEVERAGES AND MIXERS

Riboflavin B2 mg.	Niacin mg.	B6 mg.	Folic Acid mg.	PABA mg.	Pantothenic Acid mg.	B12 mcg.	Vitamin C mg.	Vitamin D IU	Vitamin E IU	Calcium mg.	Iodine mg.
0	0	NA	NA	NA	NA	0	0	NA	NA	---	NA
0	0	NA	NA	NA	NA	0	0	NA	NA	---	NA
0	0	NA	NA	NA	NA	0	0	NA	NA	---	NA
.003	.6	.0006	NA	NA	.008	0	0	NA	NA	3.3	NA
.01	1.8	.00192	NA	NA	.024	0	0	NA	NA	10	NA
0	0	NA	NA	NA	NA	0	0	NA	NA	---	NA
0	0	NA	NA	NA	NA	0	0	NA	NA	---	NA
0	0	NA	NA	NA	NA	0	0	NA	NA	---	NA
0	0	NA	NA	NA	NA	0	0	NA	NA	---	NA
.05	.53	NA	NA	NA	NA	0	---	NA	NA	.66	NA
.04	.1	NA	NA	NA	NA	0	1	NA	NA	5	NA

Food and Amount	Iron mg.	Magnesium mg.	Phosphorus mg.	Potassium mg.	Sodium mg.
Soup, frozen, Pea, green w/ham[1]— 1 cup, 245 gm.	1.96	NA	125	245	919
Soup, frozen, Potato, cream of[1]— 1 cup, 240 gm.	1.0	NA	62	221	1,176
Soup, frozen, Potato, cream of[2]—1 cup, 245 gm.	1.0	NA	181	406	1,264
Soup, frozen, Shrimp, cream of[1]—1 cup, 240 gm.	.5	NA	48	57	1,032
Soup, frozen, Shrimp, cream of[2]—1 cup, 245 gm.	.5	NA	166	237	1,117
Soup, frozen, Vegetable w/beef[1]—1 cup, 240 gm.	.96	NA	76	172	950
Vinegar, cider—1 tbsp., 15 gm.	.1	NA	2	15	.2
Vinegar, distilled—1 tbsp., 15 gm.	---	.15	---	2.25	.15
Vinegar, cider—1 tsp., 5 gm.	.03	NA	.66	5	.06
Vinegar, distilled—1 tsp., 5 gm.	---	.05	---	.75	.05
Yeast, Baker's compressed—1 cake, 1½″ sq., 12 gm.	.6	7	47	73	2
Yeast, Brewer's, debittered—1 tbsp., 9.5 gm.	1.6	22	166	180	12
Yogurt, Flavored (vanilla and coffee)[3]— 1 cup, 245 gm.	---	---	---	---	---
Yogurt, Fruit (with preserves)[3]—1 cup, 245 gm.	.3	---	231.8	367.6	127.4

[1] Prepared with equal volume of water.
[2] Prepared with equal volume of milk.
[3] Yogurt—see also entries on page 246.

NONALCOHOLIC BEVERAGES AND MIXERS

Food and Amount	Iron mg.	Magnesium mg.	Phosphorus mg.	Potassium mg.	Sodium mg.
Carbonated water, sweetened, Quinine water—1 cup, 230 gm.	---	NA	---	---	---
Carbonated water, unsweetened, Club Soda—1 cup, 230 gm.	---	NA	---	---	---
Cola-type carbonated beverages—1 cup, 230 gm.	---	NA	---	---	---
Coffee, instant, water-soluble solids, dry powder—1 tsp., 2 gm.	.11	9.12	7.66	65	1.33
Coffee, instant, water-soluble solids, dry powder—1 tbsp., 6 gm.	.33	27.36	23	195	4
Cream sodas—1 cup, 230 gm.	---	NA	---	---	---
Fruit flavored sodas (citrus, cherry, grape, strawberry, Tom Collins mixer, other) (10–13% sugar)—1 cup, 230 gm.	---	NA	---	---	---
Ginger ale, pale dry, and golden— 1 cup, 230 gm.	---	NA	---	1	18
Root beer—1 cup, 230 gm.	---	NA	---	---	---
Tea, instant, water-soluble solids, carbohydrate added, dry powder— 1 tbsp., 6 gm.	.09	23.7	---	271	---
Tea, regular, clear, no sugar—1 cup, 200 gm.	.2	44	4	NA	NA

Food and Amount	Calories	Carbohydrate gm.	Protein gm.	Sat. Fatty Acids gm.	Unsat. Fatty Acids gm.	Vitamin A IU	Thiamin B₁ mg.
Almonds, shelled, dried, whole— 1 cup, 142 gm. .	850	28	26	6	67	0	.34
Almonds, shelled, roasted and salted —1 cup, 135 gm.	846	77	25	6.75	68.85	0	.06
Almonds, sugar-coated—1 cup, 140 gm.	638	98	10.9	1.4	22.4	0	.07
Almond extract—1 teaspoon, 5 gm.	NA	NA	NA	NA	NA	NA	NA
Almond meal, partially defatted— 2 tbsp., 25 gm. .	102	7.2	9.8	.25	4	0	.08
Bean Sprouts—see Mung Beans—Vegetables section, Soybeans—this section							
Broad beans, mature seeds, dry— ½ cup, 75 gm.	253	43.6	1.27	NA	NA	52.5	.37
Butternuts, shelled—1 nut, 3 gm.	19	.25	.71	NA	NA	---	---
Cashew nuts, roasted—1 cup, 140 gm.	785	41	24	11	49	140	.6
Coconut cream (liquid from grated coconut meat)—1 tbsp., 14 gm.	46	1.16	.61	3.92	.28	0	.002
Coconut meat, fresh—1 piece, 2″ x 2″ x ½″, 45 gm.	155	4	2	14	1	0	.02
Coconut meat, fresh, grated—1 cup (firmly packed), 130 gm.	450	12	5	39	3	0	.07
Coconut meat, dried, unsweetened— 1 tbsp., 8 gm.	53	1.8	.57	4.48	.4	0	.004
Coconut meat, dried, sweetened, shredded—1 cup, 62 gm.	339	33	2.23	21.08	1.86	0	.02
Coconut milk (liquid from mixture of grated coconut meat and water)— 1 cup, 244 gm.	614	12.6	7.8	53.68	4.88	0	.07
Coconut water (liquid from coconuts) —1 cup, 245 gm.	54	11.5	.73	NA	NA	0	trace
Filberts, shelled—10 nuts, 15 gm.	95	2.5	1.89	.45	6.6	---	.06
Hazelnuts—see Filberts							
Hickory nuts, shelled—1 nut, 1 gm.	6.7	.12	.13	.06	.59	---	---
Lichees, raw—6 nuts, 18 gm.	11	2.95	.16	NA	NA	---	---
Lichees, dried—6 nuts, 15 gm.	41	10.6	.57	NA	NA	---	---
Macadamia nuts, shelled—14 nuts, 30 gm.	207	4.77	2.34	NA	NA	0	.10
Peanuts, raw, with skins—¼ cup, 60 gm.	336	11.16	15.6	6	20.4	---	.68
Peanuts, raw, without skins—¼ cup, 60 gm.	340	10.56	15.6	6	20.4	0	.56
Peanuts, boiled—½ cup, 60 gm.	225	8.7	9.3	4.2	13.8	---	.28
Peanuts, roasted with skins—1 tbsp., 15 gm.	87	3.09	3.9	1.65	5.25	---	.04
Peanuts, roasted and salted, halves— 1 cup, 144 gm.	840	27	37	16	52	---	.46
Peanut butter, sml. amts. added fat, salt—1 tbsp., 16 gm.	93	2.75	4.4	1.44	6.24	---	.02
Peanut butter, sml. amts. added fat, sweetener, salt—1 tbsp., 16 gm.	93	3.12	4.08	1.44	6.24	---	.01
Peanut butter, mod. amts. added fat, sweetener, salt—1 tbsp., 16 gm.	94	3.0	4.03	1.44	6.24	---	.01
Peanut flour, defatted—1 cup, 80 gm.	297	25.2	38.32	1.6	5.6	---	.60

Food and Amount	Ribo-flavin B₂ mg.	Niacin mg.	B₆ mg.	Folic Acid mg.	PABA mg.	Panto-thenic Acid mg.	B₁₂ mcg.
Almonds, shelled, dried, whole— 1 cup, 142 gm.	1.31	5.0	.142	.0639	NA	.6674	0
Almonds, shelled, roasted and salted —1 cup, 135 gm.	1.24	4.7	.12825	NA	NA	.3375	0
Almonds, sugar-coated—1 cup, 140 gm.	.37	1.4	---	NA	NA	---	0
Almond extract—1 teaspoon, 5 gm.	NA	NA	NA	NA	NA	NA	NA
Almond meal, partially defatted— 2 tbsp., 25 gm.	.42	1.57	NA	NA	NA	NA	0
Bean Sprouts—see Mung Beans—Vegetables section, Soybeans—this section							
Broad beans, mature seeds, dry— ½ cup, 75 gm.	.22	1.87	NA	NA	NA	NA	0
Butternuts, shelled—1 nut, 3 gm.	---	---	NA	NA	NA	NA	0
Cashew nuts, roasted—1 cup, 140 gm.	.35	2.5	---	---	NA	1.82	0
Coconut cream (liquid from grated coconut meat)—1 tbsp., 14 gm.	.001	.07	NA	NA	NA	NA	0
Coconut meat, fresh—1 piece, 2″ x 2″ x ½″, 45 gm.	.01	.2	.0198	.0126	NA	.09	0
Coconut meat, fresh, grated—1 cup (firmly packed), 130 gm.	.03	.7	.0572	.0364	NA	.26	0
Coconut meat, dried, unsweetened— 1 tbsp., 8 gm.	.003	.04	NA	NA	NA	NA	0
Coconut meat, dried, sweetened, shredded—1 cup, 62 gm.	.01	.24	NA	NA	NA	NA	0
Coconut milk (liquid from mixture of grated coconut meat and water)— 1 cup, 244 gm.	trace	1.95	NA	NA	NA	NA	0
Coconut water (liquid from coconuts) —1 cup, 245 gm.	trace	.24	NA	NA	NA	NA	0
Filberts, shelled—10 nuts, 15 gm.	---	.13	---	.00999	NA	.17	0
Hazelnuts—see Filberts							
Hickory nuts, shelled—1 nut, 1 gm.	---	---	NA	NA	NA	NA	0
Lichees, raw—6 nuts, 18 gm.	.009	---	NA	NA	NA	NA	0
Lichees, dried—6 nuts, 15 gm.	---	---	NA	NA	NA	NA	0
Macadamia nuts, shelled—14 nuts, 30 gm.	.03	.39	NA	NA	NA	NA	0
Peanuts, raw, with skins—¼ cup, 60 gm.	.04	10.32	NA	NA	1	NA	0
Peanuts, raw, without skins—¼ cup, 60 gm.	.04	9.48	NA	NA	1	NA	0
Peanuts, boiled—⅓ cup, 60 gm.	.04	6	NA	NA	NA	NA	0
Peanuts, roasted with skins—1 tbsp., 15 gm.	.01	2.56	.060	.0085	NA	.315	0
Peanuts, roasted and salted, halves— 1 cup, 144 gm.	.19	24.7	---	---	NA	---	0
Peanut butter, sml. amts. added fat, salt—1 tbsp., 16 gm.	.02	2.51	.0528	.00904	NA	.4	0
Peanut butter, sml. amts. added fat, sweetener, salt—1 tbsp., 16 gm.	.01	2.44	.0528	.00904	NA	.4	0
Peanut butter, mod. amts. added fat, sweetener, salt—1 tbsp., 16 gm.	.01	2.35	---	---	NA	---	0
Peanut flour, defatted—1 cup, 80 gm.	.17	22.24	NA	NA	NA	NA	0

Vitamin C mg.	Vitamin D IU	Vitamin E IU	Calcium mg.	Iodine mg.	Iron mg.	Magnesium mg.	Phosphorus mg.	Potassium mg.	Sodium mg.
trace	NA	NA	332	.00284	6.7	383.4	715	1,097	5.68
0	NA	NA	317	---	6.3	---	680	1,043	267
0	NA	NA	140	NA	2.6	NA	232	357	28
NA	NA	NA	NA	NA	NA	NA	NA	NA	NA
NA	NA	NA	106	NA	2.1	NA	228	350	1.75
---	NA	NA	76	NA	5.3	NA	293	---	---
---	NA	NA	---	NA	.02	NA	---	---	---
---	---	NA	53	NA	5.3	173.8	522	649	21
.14	0	NA	2.1	NA	.25	NA	17	45	.56
1	0	NA	6	NA	.8	20.7	42	115	10.3
4	0	NA	17	NA	2.2	59.8	123.5	332.8	29.9
0	0	NA	2.08	NA	.26	7.2	15	47	---
0	0	NA	9.92	NA	1.24	47.74	69	218	---
4.8	0	NA	39	NA	3.9	NA	244	---	---
4.9	0	NA	49	NA	.73	68.6	31	360	61
trace	0	NA	31	.00022	.51	27.6	50	105	.30
---	0	NA	trace	NA	.02	1.6	3.6	---	---
7.5	NA	NA	1.4	NA	.07	NA	7.5	30	.54
---	0	NA	4.9	NA	.25	NA	27	165	.45
0	0	NA	14.4	NA	.60	NA	48	79	---
0	0	NA	41.2	NA	1.24	124	240	404	3
0	0	NA	35.4	NA	1.2	123.6	244	404	3
0	0	NA	25.8	NA	.78	NA	108	277	2.4
0	0	4.65	10.8	NA	.33	26.25	61	105	.75
0	0	44.64	107	NA	3.0	252	577	970	602
0	0	NA	10	NA	.32	27.68	65	107	97
0	0	NA	9.76	NA	.32	27.68	63	104	97
0	0	NA	9.44	NA	.30	NA	61	100	97
0	0	NA	83.2	NA	2.8	288	576	949	7.2

Food and Amount	Calories	Carbo-hydrate gm.	Protein gm.	Sat. Fatty Acids gm.	Unsat. Fatty Acids gm.	Vitamin A IU	Thiamin B₁ mg.
Peas, mature seeds, split, dry, raw—½ cup, 125 gm.	435	78.3	30.25	NA	NA	150	.92
Peas, mature seeds, split, dry, cooked —1 cup, 250 gm.	290	52	20	---	---	100	.37
Pecans, halves—1 cup, 108 gm.	740	16	10	5	63	140	.93
Pigeon peas, raw, immature seeds—½ cup, 100 gm.	117	21.3	7.2	---	---	140	.4
Pigeon peas, raw, mature seeds, dry—½ cup, 100 gm.	342	63.9	20.4	---	---	80	.32
Pilinuts, shelled—2 tbsp., 15 gm.	100	1.26	1.71	NA	NA	6	.13
Pistachio nuts, shelled—2 nuts, 1 gm.	5.9	.19	.19	.05	.45	2.3	.0067
Pumpkin and squash seed kernels, dry—1 tbsp., 5 gm.	27.65	.75	1.45	.4	1.85	3.5	.01
Safflower seed kernels, dry—1 tbsp., 4 gm.	24.6	.49	.76	.2	2.08	---	---
Safflower seed meal, partially defatted—1 cup, 200 gm.	710	73	79.2	---	---	---	2.24
Sesame seeds, dry, whole—1 tbsp., 4 gm.	22.52	.86	.74	.28	1.6	1.2	.03
Sesame seeds, dry, decorticated—1 tbsp., 4 gm.	23.28	.7	.72	.28	1.68	---	.009
Soybeans, immature seeds, raw—½ cup, 75 gm.	134	9.9	8.17	.75	3	517	.33
Soybeans, immature seeds, cooked, boiled, drained—1 cup, 135 gm.	159	13.6	13.2	1.35	5.4	291	.41
Soybeans, immature seeds, canned, solids and liquid—1 cup, 135 gm.	101	8.5	8.77	1.35	5.4	459	.08
Soybeans, mature seeds, dry, raw—½ cup, 100 gm.	403	33.5	34.1	3	13	80	1.10
Soybeans, mature seeds, dry, cooked—½ cup, 100 gm.	130	10.8	11.0	1	4	30	.21
Soybeans, sprouted seeds (beansprouts), raw—½ cup, 50 gm.	23	2.65	3.10	---	---	40	.115
Soybeans, sprouted seeds, cooked, boiled, drained—½ cup, 70 gm.	26	2.59	3.71	---	---	56	.11
Soybean curd (tofu)—1 cake, 2¾″ x 2½″ x 1″, 120 gm.	86	2.88	9.36	1.2	3.6	0	.07
Soybean flour, full-fat—1 cup stirred, 72 gm.	303	21.9	26.4	2.16	10.8	79	.61
Soybean flour, high-fat—1 cup stirred, 88 gm.	334	29.3	36.2	1.76	7.04	---	.78
Soybean flour, low-fat—1 cup stirred, 100 gm.	356	36.6	43.4	1	4	80	.83
Soybean flour, defatted—1 cup stirred, 138 gm.	450	52.6	64.9	---	---	55	1.5
Soybean milk, fluid—1 cup, 240 gm.	79	5.28	8.16	---	---	96	.19
Soybean milk, powder—1 tbsp., 6 gm.	25.74	1.68	2.5	---	---	---	---
Soybean milk products, sweetened, liquid concentrate—1 cup, 245 gm.	308	30.13	11.76	2.45	12.25	trace	.14
Soy sauce—1 tbsp., 15 gm.	10	1.42	.84	---	---	0	.003
Squash seeds—see Pumpkin seeds							

Riboflavin B_2 mg.	Niacin mg.	B_6 mg.	Folic Acid mg.	PABA mg.	Pantothenic Acid mg.	B_{12} mcg.	Vitamin C mg.	Vitamin D IU	Vitamin E IU	Calcium mg.	Iodine mg.
.36	3.75	.1625	.06375	NA	2.5	0	---	NA	NA	41.2	.008125 Calif.
.22	2.2	.05	NA	NA	.55	0	---	NA	NA	28	NA
.14	1.0	.19764	.02916	NA	1.84356	0	2	0	NA	79	NA
.17	2.2	NA	NA	NA	NA	0	.39	NA	NA	42	NA
.16	3	NA	NA	NA	NA	0	NA	NA	NA	107	NA
.01	.07	NA	NA	NA	NA	0	trace	NA	NA	21	NA
---	.0014	NA	NA	NA	NA	0	0	NA	NA	1.31	NA
.009	.12	NA	NA	NA	NA	0	---	NA	NA	2.55	NA
---	---	NA	NA	NA	NA	0	---	NA	NA	---	NA
.8	4.4	NA	NA	NA	NA	0	0	NA	NA	150	NA
.0096	.21	NA	NA	NA	NA	0	0	NA	NA	46.4	NA
.0089	.21	NA	NA	NA	NA	0	0	NA	NA	4.4	NA
.12	1.05	NA	NA	NA	NA	0	21.75	NA	NA	50	NA
.17	1.62	NA	NA	NA	NA	0	22.95	NA	NA	81	NA
---	---	NA	NA	NA	NA	0	2.7	NA	NA	90	NA
.31	2.2	---	---	NA	---	0	---	NA	NA	226	NA
.09	.6	.64	.224	NA	1.68	0	0	NA	NA	73	NA
.10	.4	NA	NA	NA	NA	0	6.5	NA	NA	24	NA
.10	.49	NA	NA	NA	NA	0	2.8	NA	NA	30	NA
.036	.12	NA	NA	NA	NA	0	0	NA	NA	153	NA
.22	1.5	.4723	.30672	NA	1.2	0	0	NA	NA	143	NA
.32	2	.57728	.37488	NA	1.47	0	0	NA	NA	211	NA
.36	2.6	.656	.426	NA	1.68	0	0	NA	NA	263	NA
.47	3.6	.90528	.58788	NA	2.31	0	0	NA	NA	366	NA
.07	.48	NA	NA	NA	NA	0	0	NA	NA	50	NA
---	---	NA	NA	NA	NA	0	---	NA	NA	16.5	NA
.07	.49	NA	NA	NA	NA	0	0	NA	NA	73.5	NA
.03	.06	NA	NA	NA	NA	0	0	NA	NA	12.3	NA

Food and Amount	Iron mg.	Mag- nesium mg.	Phos- phorus mg.	Potas- sium mg.	Sodium mg.
Peas, mature seeds, split, dry, raw— ½ cup, 125 gm.	6.3	225	335	1,118	50
Peas, mature seeds, split, dry, cooked —1 cup, 250 gm.	4.2	---	222	740	32
Pecans, halves—1 cup, 108 gm.	2.6	153.36	312	651	trace
Pigeon peas, raw, immature seeds— ½ cup, 100 gm.	1.6	NA	127	552	5
Pigeon peas, raw, mature seeds, dry— ½ cup, 100 gm.	8	121	316	981	26
Pilinuts, shelled—2 tbsp., 15 gm.	.51	NA	83	73	.45
Pistachio nuts, shelled—2 nuts, 1 gm.	.0073	1.58	5	9.72	---
Pumpkin and squash seed kernels, dry—1 tbsp., 5 gm.	.56	NA	57.2	---	---
Safflower seed kernels, dry— 1 tbsp., 4 gm.	---	NA	---	---	---
Safflower seed meal, partially defatted—1 cup, 200 gm.	---	NA	1,240	---	---
Sesame seeds, dry, whole— 1 tbsp., 4 gm.	.42	7.24	24.64	29	2.4
Sesame seeds, dry, decorticated— 1 tbsp., 4 gm.	.09	---	23.68	---	---
Soybeans, immature seeds, raw— ½ cup, 75 gm.	2.10	---	168	---	---
Soybeans, immature seeds, cooked, boiled, drained—1 cup, 135 gm.	3.37	---	257	---	---
Soybeans, immature seeds, canned, solids and liquid—1 cup, 135 gm.	3.78	---	154	---	318
Soybeans, mature seeds, dry, raw— ½ cup, 100 gm.	8.4	265	554	1,677	5
Soybeans, mature seeds, dry, cooked— ½ cup, 100 gm.	2.7	---	179	540	2
Soybeans, sprouted seeds (beansprouts), raw—½ cup, 50 gm.	.5	---	33.5	---	---
Soybeans, sprouted seeds, cooked, boiled, drained—½ cup, 70 gm.	.49	---	35	---	---
Soybean curd (tofu)—1 cake, 2¾″ x 2½″ x 1″, 120 gm.	2.28	133.2	151	50	8
Soybean flour, full-fat—1 cup stirred, 72 gm.	6	178	402	1,195	1
Soybean flour, high-fat—1 cup stirred, 88 gm.	7.9	239	572	1,562	1
Soybean flour, low-fat—1 cup stirred, 100 gm.	9.1	289	634	1,859	1
Soybean flour, defatted—1 cup stirred, 138 gm.	15.3	427.8	904	2,512	1
Soybean milk, fluid—1 cup, 240 gm.	1.92	---	115	---	---
Soybean milk, powder—1 tbsp., 6 gm.	---	NA	---	---	---
Soybean milk products, sweetened, liquid concentrate—1 cup, 245 gm.	1.96	---	144	580	105
Soy sauce—1 tbsp., 15 gm.	.72	---	15.6	55	1,098
Squash seeds—see Pumpkin seeds					

¼ Food and Amount	Calories	Carbo-hydrate gm.	Protein gm.	Sat. Fatty Acids gm.	Unsat. Fatty Acids gm.	Vitamin A IU	Thiamin B_1 mg.
Sunflower seed kernels, dry—1 tbsp., 5 gm.	28	.99	1.2	.3	1.95	2.5	.09
Sunflower seed flour, partially defatted—1 cup, 110 gm.	372.9	41.47	49.72	trace	3.3	...	3.96
Walnuts, Black, shelled, chopped—1 cup, 126 gm.	790	19	26	4	62	380	.28
Walnuts, Persian or English, shelled—1 cup, halves, 100 gm.	651	15.8	14.8	4	50	30	.33

CANDIES, SUGARS, DESSERTS, ETC.

Food and Amount	Calories	Carbo-hydrate gm.	Protein gm.	Sat. Fatty Acids gm	Unsat. Fatty Acids gm.	Vitamin A IU	Thiamin B_1 mg.
Apple brown betty—½ cup, 140 gm.	211	41.6	2.2	1.4	1.4	140	.08
Blancmange—see Puddings, vanilla							
Bread pudding w/raisins—1 cup, 220 gm.	411	62.48	12.3	6.6	4.4	660	.13
Cake, from mix, Angelfood, made w/water, flavorings—1 piece, 1/12 of 10" cake, 53 gm.	135	32	3	...	...	0	trace
Cake, Chocolate malt, from mix, with eggs, water, uncooked white icing—1 piece, 1/16 of 8" cake, 70 gm.	242	46.6	2.38	3.5	4.9	133	.02
Cake, Coffee cake, from mix, with enriched flour, egg, milk—1 piece, 3" x 1½", 28 gm.	90	14	1.7	.84	2.24	45	.05
Cake, cupcake, from mix, w/eggs, milk—2½" cupcake, 25 gm.	90	14	1	1	2	40	.01
Cake, Devil's Food, from mix, with eggs, water, choc. icing—1 piece, 1/16 of 9" cake, 69 gm.	235	40	3	3	5	100	.02
Cake, Gingerbread, from mix, w/water—1 piece, 1/9 of 8" sq., 63 gm.	175	32	2	1	3	trace	.02
Cake, Honeyspice, from mix, w/eggs, water, caramel icing—1 sl., 3" x 3" x ½", 52 gm.	183.04	31.66	2.13	...	...	83.2	.01
Cake, Marble, from mix, w/eggs, water, boiled white icing—1 piece, 1/16 of 9" cake, 70 gm.	231	43	3	3.5	4.9	63	.01
Cake, White, from mix, w/egg whites, water, chocolate icing—1 piece, 1/16 of 9" cake, 71 gm.	250	45	3	3	4	40	.01
Cake, Yellow, from mix, w/eggs, water, chocolate icing—1 piece, 1/16 of 9" cake, 71 gm.	239	41	2.9	3.55	4.97	99	.01
Cake Icing, home recipe, Caramel—1 cup, 200 gm.	720	153	2.6	...	...	560	.02
Cake Icing, Chocolate, home recipe—1 cup, 275 gm.	1,035	185	9	21	15	580	.06
Cake Icing, Coconut, home recipe—1 cup, 166 gm.	605	124	3	11	1	0	.02
Cake Icing, Chocolate Fudge, from mix—1 cup, 260 gm.	982.8	174.2	5.72	15.6	20.8	702	.02

¼ Food and Amount	Riboflavin B_2 mg.	Niacin mg.	B_6 mg.	Folic Acid mg.	PABA mg.	Pantothenic Acid mg.	B_{12} mcg.
Sunflower seed kernels, dry—1 tbsp., 5 gm.	.01	.27	NA	NA	NA	NA	0
Sunflower seed flour, partially defatted—1 cup, 110 gm.	.5	30.03	NA	NA	NA	NA	0
Walnuts, Black, shelled, chopped—1 cup, 126 gm.	.14	.9	---	.09702	NA	---	0
Walnuts, Persian or English, shelled—1 cup, halves, 100 gm.	.13	.9	.73	.077	NA	.9	0

CANDIES, SUGARS, DESSERTS, ETC.

Food and Amount	Riboflavin B_2 mg	Niacin mg.	B_6 mg.	Folic Acid mg.	PABA mg.	Pantothenic Acid mg.	B_{12} mcg.
Apple brown betty—½ cup, 140 gm.	.06	.6	NA	NA	NA	NA	NA
Blancmange—see Puddings, vanilla							
Bread pudding w/raisins—1 cup, 220 gm.	.41	.22	NA	NA	NA	NA	NA
Cake, from mix, Angelfood, made w/water, flavorings—1 piece, 1/12 of 10″ cake, 53 gm.	.06	.1	NA	NA	NA	NA	NA
Cake, Chocolate malt, from mix, with eggs, water, uncooked white icing—1 piece, 1/16 of 8″ cake, 70 gm.	.04	.14	NA	NA	NA	NA	NA
Cake, Coffee cake, from mix, with enriched flour, egg, milk—1 piece, 3″ x 1½″, 28 gm.	.04	.39	NA	NA	NA	NA	NA
Cake, cupcake, from mix, w/eggs, milk—2½″ cupcake, 25 gm.	.03	.1	NA	NA	NA	NA	NA
Cake, Devil's Food, from mix, with eggs, water, choc. icing—1 piece, 1/16 of 9″ cake, 69 gm.	.06	.2	NA	NA	NA	NA	NA
Cake, Gingerbread, from mix, w/water—1 piece, 1/9 of 8″ sq., 63 gm.	.06	.5	NA	NA	NA	NA	NA
Cake, Honeyspice, from mix, w/eggs, water, caramel icing—1 sl., 3″ x 3″ x ½″, 52 gm.	.04	.1	NA	NA	NA	NA	NA
Cake, Marble, from mix, w/eggs, water, boiled white icing—1 piece, 1/16 of 9″ cake, 70 gm.	.05	.14	NA	NA	NA	NA	NA
Cake, White, from mix, w/egg whites, water, chocolate icing—1 piece, 1/16 of 9″ cake, 71 gm.	.06	.1	NA	NA	NA	NA	NA
Cake, Yellow, from mix, w/eggs, water, chocolate icing—1 piece, 1/16 of 9″ cake, 71 gm.	.05	.14	NA	NA	NA	NA	NA
Cake Icing, home recipe, Caramel—1 cup, 200 gm.	.12	trace	NA	NA	NA	NA	NA
Cake Icing, Chocolate, home recipe—1 cup, 275 gm.	.28	.6	NA	NA	NA	NA	NA
Cake Icing, Coconut, home recipe—1 cup, 166 gm.	.07	.3	NA	NA	NA	NA	NA
Cake Icing, Chocolate Fudge, from mix—1 cup, 260 gm.	.1	.52	NA	NA	NA	NA	NA

Vitamin C mg.	Vitamin D IU	Vitamin E IU	Calcium mg.	Iodine mg.	Iron mg.	Magnesium mg.	Phosphorus mg.	Potassium mg.	Sodium mg.
---	NA	NA	6	NA	.35	1.9	41.85	46	1.5
---	NA	NA	382.8	NA	14.52	---	987.8	1,188	61.6
---	0	NA	trace	.00378 (dried)	7.6	239.4	718	579	3.78
2	0	NA	99	.003 (dried)	3.1	131	380	450	2

CANDIES, SUGARS, DESSERTS, ETC.

Vitamin C mg.	Vitamin D IU	Vitamin E IU	Calcium mg.	Iodine mg.	Iron mg.	Magnesium mg.	Phosphorus mg.	Potassium mg.	Sodium mg.
1	NA	NA	25	NA	.8	7	31	140	214
2.2	NA	NA	239	NA	2.42	---	251	473	442
0	NA	NA	50	NA	.2	NA	63	32	77
trace	NA	NA	44	NA	.49	NA	116	56	222
trace	NA	NA	17	NA	.44	NA	48	30	120
trace	NA	NA	40	NA	.1	NA	49	29	83
trace	NA	NA	41	NA	.6	NA	72	90	181
trace	NA	NA	57	NA	1.0	NA	63	172	191
trace	NA	NA	36.92	NA	.41	NA	100.36	42.64	127.4
trace	NA	NA	54	NA	.56	NA	119	85	181
trace	NA	NA	70	NA	.4	NA	127	82	161
trace	NA	NA	64	NA	.42	NA	129	77	161
trace	NA	NA	204	NA	4	NA	126	104	166
1	NA	NA	165	NA	3.3	NA	105	536	167
0	NA	NA	10	NA	.8	NA	50	277	196
0	NA	NA	41.6	NA	.25	NA	171.6	163.8	405.6

Food and Amount	Calories	Carbo-hydrate gm.	Protein gm.	Sat. Fatty Acids gm.	Unsat. Fatty Acids gm.	Vitamin A IU	Thiamin B_1 mg.
Cake Icing, Creamy Fudge, from mix, w/water—1 cup, 245 gm.	830	183	7	5	11	trace	.05
Cake Icing, Creamy Fudge, from mix, w/water, table fat—1 cup, 250 gm.	957	164	6.5	17.5	20	975	.05
Cake Icing, White, uncooked, home recipe—1 cup, 158 gm.	594.08	128.92	.79	...	...	426.6	trace
Cake Icing, White, boiled, home recipe—1 cup, 94 gm.	300	76	1	...	...	0	trace
Candy, Butterscotch—¾″ sq. x ⅜″, 5 gm.	20	4.74	trace	.1	.05	7	0
Candy, Candy corn—see Fondant							
Candy, Caramels, plain or chocolate—⅞″ sq. x ½″, 10 gm.	40	7.66	.4	.5	.6	1.0	.003
Candy, Caramels, plain or chocolate w/nuts—⅞″ sq. x ½″, 12 gm.	51	8.46	.54	.72	1.08	2.4	.01
Candy, Caramels, chocolate-flavored roll—2″ x ½″ roll, 20 gm.	79	16.5	.44	1	1.2	trace	.004
Candy, Chocolate, Bittersweet—¾″ x 1½″ x ¼″, 6 gm.	28	2.8	.47	1.2	.84	2.4	.01
Candy, Chocolate, Semisweet—1 cup small pieces, 170 gm.	860	97	7	34	23	30	.02
Candy, Chocolate, sweet—1 square, 1 ounce, 28 gm.	133	17.8	.6	5.6	3.92	9	.009
Candy, Milk Chocolate, plain—¾″ x 1½″ x ¼″, 6 gm.	31	3.41	.46	1.2	.84	16	.003
Candy, Milk Chocolate, w/almonds—¾″ x 1½″ x ¼″, 6 gm.	32	3.07	.55	.42	2.1	13.8	.004
Candy, Milk Chocolate, w/peanuts—¾″ x 1½″ x ¼″, 6 gm.	32.5	2.67	.84	...	...	10.8	.01
Candy, Chocolate-coated Almonds—1 piece, 2 gm.	11	.79	.24	.14	.7	trace	.002
Candy, Chocolate-coated Chocolate Fudge—2″ sq. x ⅝″, 46 gm.	198	33.6	1.74	2.76	4.14	trace	.01
Candy, Chocolate-coated Chocolate Fudge w/nuts—2″ sq. x ⅝″, 46 gm.	208	31	2.25	2.76	4.14	trace	.02
Candy, Chocolate-coated Coconut center—1 piece, ¾″ diam., 17 gm.	74	12	.47	1.7	1.02	0	.003
Candy, Chocolate-coated Fondant—1″ sq. x ⅝″, 8 gm.	32	6	.13	.4	.48	trace	.002
Candy, Chocolate-coated Caramel, Fudge, and peanuts—2″ x 1″, 40 gm.	173.2	25.64	3.08	...	...	trace	.06
Candy, Chocolate-coated, honeycombed hard candy w/peanut butter—1 piece, 1″ cube, 18 gm.	83.34	12.7	1.18	...	...	trace	.006
Candy, Chocolate-coated Nougat and Caramel—1 piece, 1″ sq. x ½″, 20 gm.	83.2	14.56	.8	...	...	8	.01
Candy, Chocolate-coated Peanuts—1 nut, 2 gm.	11	.78	.32	.22	.58	trace	.007
Candy, Chocolate-coated Raisins—1 raisin, 1 gm.	4.2	.70	.05	.10	.06	1.50	.0008
Candy, Chocolate-coated Vanilla creams—1¼″ diam. x ¾″, 14 gm.	61	9.8	.53	.84	1.26	trace	.007
Candy, Fondant—1″ sq. x ⅝″, 8 gm.	29	7.1	.008	.16	.08	0	trace
Candy, Chocolate Fudge—2″ sq. x ⅝″, 45 gm.	180	33.75	1.21	2.25	2.7	trace	.009

Riboflavin B2 mg.	Niacin mg.	B6 mg.	Folic Acid mg.	PABA mg.	Pantothenic Acid mg.	B12 mcg.	Vitamin C mg.	Vitamin D IU	Vitamin E IU	Calcium mg.	Iodine mg.
.2	.7	NA	NA	NA	NA	NA	trace	NA	NA	96	NA
.17	.75	NA	NA	NA	NA	NA	trace	NA	NA	92	NA
.03	trace	NA	NA	NA	NA	NA	trace	NA	NA	23.7	NA
.03	trace	NA	NA	NA	NA	NA	0	NA	NA	2	NA
trace	trace	NA	NA	NA	NA	NA	0	0	NA	.85	NA
.017	.02	NA	NA	NA	NA	NA	trace	---	NA	15	NA
.02	.02	NA	NA	NA	NA	NA	trace	---	NA	16	NA
.01	.02	NA	NA	NA	NA	NA	trace	NA	NA	13	NA
.01	.06	NA	NA	NA	NA	NA	0	---	NA	3.4	.00033
.14	.9	NA	NA	NA	NA	NA	0	48	NA	51	.00935
.043	.2	NA	NA	NA	NA	NA	0	0	NA	18	.00154
.02	.01	NA	NA	NA	NA	NA	trace	5	.06	13	.00033
.02	.04	NA	NA	NA	NA	NA	trace	5	---	13	NA
.01	.30	NA	NA	NA	NA	NA	trace	NA	---	10	NA
.01	.03	NA	NA	NA	NA	NA	trace	.71	NA	4	NA
.05	.09	NA	NA	NA	NA	NA	0	NA	NA	46	NA
.05	.09	NA	NA	NA	NA	NA	trace	NA	NA	46	NA
.011	.03	NA	NA	NA	NA	NA	0	---	NA	8	NA
.004	.008	NA	NA	NA	NA	NA	trace	---	NA	4.5	NA
.08	.76	NA	NA	NA	NA	NA	trace	---	NA	71.6	NA
.01	.52	NA	NA	NA	NA	NA	trace	NA	NA	14.4	NA
.03	.04	NA	NA	NA	NA	NA	trace	NA	NA	25.4	NA
.003	.14	NA	NA	NA	NA	NA	trace	NA	NA	2.32	NA
.002	.004	NA	NA	NA	NA	NA	trace	NA	NA	1.52	NA
.009	.01	NA	NA	NA	NA	NA	trace	NA	NA	18	NA
trace	trace	NA	NA	NA	NA	NA	0	NA	NA	1.12	NA
.04	.09	NA	NA	NA	NA	NA	trace	NA	NA	34.65	NA

Food and Amount	Iron mg.	Magnesium mg.	Phosphorus mg.	Potassium mg.	Sodium mg.
Cake Icing, Creamy Fudge, from mix, w/water—1 cup, 245 gm.	2.7	NA	218	237	568
Cake Icing, Creamy Fudge, from mix, w/water, table fat—1 cup, 250 gm.	2.5	NA	202	222	802
Cake Icing, White, uncooked, home recipe—1 cup, 158 gm.	trace	NA	18.96	28.44	77.42
Cake Icing, White, boiled, home recipe—1 cup, 94 gm.	trace	NA	1.8	17	134
Candy, Butterscotch—¾" sq. x ⅜", 5 gm.	.07	NA	.30	.10	3.30
Candy, Candy corn—see Fondant					
Candy, Caramels, plain or chocolate —⅞" sq. x ½", 10 gm.	.14	•••	12	19	22
Candy, Caramels, plain or chocolate w/nuts—⅞" sq. x ½", 12 gm.	.18	•••	16	28	24
Candy, Caramels, chocolate-flavored roll—2" x ½" roll, 20 gm.	.36	NA	23	24	39
Candy, Chocolate, Bittersweet—¾" x 1½" x ¼", 6 gm.	.30	NA	17	37	.18
Candy, Chocolate, Semisweet—1 cup small pieces, 170 gm.	4.4	NA	9	19	.12
Candy, Chocolate, sweet—1 square, 1 ounce, 28 gm.	.8	29.96	81	64	9.8
Candy, Milk Chocolate, plain—¾" x 1½" x ¼", 6 gm.	.06	3.48	14	23	5.6
Candy, Milk Chocolate, w/almonds—¾" x 1½" x ¼", 6 gm.	.09	•••	16	26	4.8
Candy, Milk Chocolate, w/peanuts—¾" x 1½" x ¼", 6 gm.	.08	•••	17	29	3.96
Candy, Chocolate-coated Almonds—1 piece, 2 gm.	.05	NA	7	11	1.18
Candy, Chocolate-coated Chocolate Fudge—2" sq. x ⅝", 46 gm.	.59	NA	50	88	105
Candy, Chocolate-coated Chocolate Fudge w/nuts—2" sq. x ⅝", 46 gm.	.69	NA	60	100	94
Candy, Chocolate-coated Coconut center—1 piece, ¾" diam., 17 gm.	.18	NA	13	28	33
Candy, Chocolate-coated Fondant—1" sq. x ⅝", 8 gm.	.08	NA	4.3	7.2	14
Candy, Chocolate-coated Caramel, Fudge, and peanuts—2" x 1", 40 gm.	.56	•••	74.4	120.4	81.6
Candy, Chocolate-coated, honeycombed hard candy w/peanut butter—1 piece, 1" cube, 18 gm.	.32	•••	24.3	40.5	29.34
Candy, Chocolate-coated Nougat and Caramel—1 piece, 1" sq. x ½", 20 gm.	.32	NA	24.6	42.2	34.6
Candy, Chocolate-coated Peanuts—1 nut, 2 gm.	.03	NA	6	10	1.2
Candy, Chocolate-coated Raisins—1 raisin, 1 gm.	.02	NA	1.74	6.03	.64
Candy, Chocolate-coated Vanilla creams—1¼" diam. x ¾", 14 gm.	.08	NA	15	25	25
Candy, Fondant—1" sq. x ⅝", 8 gm.	.08	NA	.48	.40	17
Candy, Chocolate Fudge—2" sq. x ⅝", 45 gm.	.45	•••	37.8	66	85

Food and Amount	Calories	Carbo-hydrate gm.	Protein gm.	Sat. Fatty Acids gm.	Unsat. Fatty Acids gm.	Vitamin A IU	Thiamin B1 mg.
Candy, Chocolate Fudge w/nuts—2″ sq. x ⅝″, 45 gm.	191	31	1.75	2.7	4.95	trace	.01
Candy, Vanilla Fudge—2″ sq. x ⅝″, 45 gm.	179	33.6	1.35	2.25	2.7	trace	.009
Candy, Vanilla Fudge w/nuts—2″ sq. x ⅝″, 45 gm.	190	31	1.89	2.25	2.7	trace	.02
Candy, Gumdrops (starch jelly)—1 drop, ⅞″ diam., 10 gm.	33	8.6	0	...	...	0	0
Candy, Hard—1 piece, 1″ x 1½″, 10 gm.	38	9.9	0	...	...	0	0
Candy, Jelly beans—1 bean, ½″ diam., 2 gm.	7.3	1.86	trace	...	...	0	0
Candy, Marshmallows—1 marshmallow, 1¼″ diam., 6 gm.	19	4.82	.12	...	...	0	0
Candy, Mints, uncoated—1 mint, ¾″, 2 gm.	7.2	1.79	.002	...	...	0	trace
Candy, Peanut bars—1 bar, 2″ x 1″ x ¼″, 45 gm.	231.75	21.24	7.87	...	...	0	.19
Candy, Peanut brittle—1 piece, 2½″ x 2½″ x ⅜″, 25 gm.	110	18.2	2.1	.5	1.75	7	.022
Candy, Sugar-coated Almonds—see Nuts, Seeds, Sprouted Seeds, Dry Beans, and Related Products							
Candy, Sugar-coated, Chocolate discs—1 disc, ½″ diam., 1 gm.	4.66	.72	.05	.1	.06	1	.0006
Chewing gum—1 stick, 3 gm.	9.51	2.85	...	...	...	0	0
Chocolate, Bitter or baking—1 square, 1 ounce, 28 gm.	142	8.3	1.6	8.4	5.88	17	.014
Chocolate—see Candy, chocolate							
Chocolate syrup, thin type—1 tbsp., 19 gm.	46.5	11.9	.43	.19	.19	trace	.003
Chocolate syrup, Fudge type—1 tbsp., 19 gm.	62.7	10.2	.96	1.33	.95	28.5	.007
Cocoa drink powder and nonfat dry milk—1 tbsp., 7 gm.	25.13	4.95	1.3	.14	.07	1.4	.009
Cocoa drink powder w/o milk—1 tbsp., 7 gm.	24.29	6.25	.28	.07	.07	...	.001
Cocoa mix for hot chocolate—1 tbsp., 7 gm.	27.44	5.17	.65	.42	.28	.70	.005
Cocoa, dry powder, high-fat or breakfast, plain—1 tbsp., 7 gm.	20.93	3.38	1.17	.91	.63	2.10	.007
Cream puffs w/custard filling—1 avg., 3″ diam., 105 gm.	296	15	3.9	...	...	1,120	.07
Custard, baked—1 custard, 4 from 1 qt. milk, 157 gm.	205	22.8	8.8	...	...	607	.08
Custard, baked—1 cup, 265 gm.	305	29	14	7.95	5.3	927	.10
Custard, frozen—see Ice Cream, Egg and Dairy Products, and Related Products							
Custard dessert mix—see Pudding mixes							
Eclairs w/custard filling and chocolate icing—1 eclair, 4″ long, 110 gm.	316	39.1	7.6	4.4	8.8	730	.12
Frosting—see Cake Icings							
Gelatin desserts, made w/water—1 cup, 240 gm.	140	34	4	...	...	...	...
Honey, strained or extracted—1 tbsp., 21 gm.	65	17	trace	...	...	0	trace

Food and Amount	Riboflavin B_2 mg.	Niacin mg.	B_6 mg.	Folic Acid mg.	PABA mg.	Pantothenic Acid mg.	B_{12} mcg.
Candy, Chocolate Fudge w/nuts—2" sq. x ⅝", 45 gm.	.04	.13	NA	NA	NA	NA	NA
Candy, Vanilla Fudge—2" sq. x ⅝", 45 gm.	.05	.04	NA	NA	NA	NA	NA
Candy, Vanilla Fudge w/nuts—2" sq. x ⅝", 45 gm.	.05	.04	NA	NA	NA	NA	NA
Candy, Gumdrops (starch jelly)—1 drop, ⅞" diam., 10 gm.	0	0	NA	NA	NA	NA	NA
Candy, Hard—1 piece, 1" x 1½", 10 gm.	0	0	NA	NA	NA	NA	NA
Candy, Jelly beans—1 bean, ½" diam., 2 gm.	trace	trace	NA	NA	NA	NA	NA
Candy, Marshmallows—1 marshmallow, 1¼" diam., 6 gm.	trace	trace	NA	NA	NA	NA	NA
Candy, Mints, uncoated—1 mint, ¾", 2 gm.	trace	trace	NA	NA	NA	NA	NA
Candy, Peanut bars—1 bar, 2" x 1" x ¼", 45 gm.	.03	4.23	NA	NA	NA	NA	NA
Candy, Peanut brittle—1 piece, 2½" x 2½" x ⅜", 25 gm.	.012	1.2	NA	NA	NA	NA	NA
Candy, Sugar-coated Almonds—see Nuts, Seeds, Sprouted Seeds, Dry Beans, and Related Products							
Candy, Sugar-coated, Chocolate discs—1 disc, ½" diam., 1 gm.	.002	.003	NA	NA	NA	NA	NA
Chewing gum—1 stick, 3 gm.	0	0	NA	NA	NA	NA	0
Chocolate, Bitter or baking—1 square, 1 ounce, 28 gm.	.068	.3	.0098	.0281	NA	.0532	0
Chocolate—see Candy, chocolate							
Chocolate syrup, thin type—1 tbsp., 19 gm.	.01	.07	NA	NA	NA	NA	0
Chocolate syrup, Fudge type—1 tbsp., 19 gm.	.04	.07	NA	NA	NA	NA	0
Cocoa drink powder and nonfat dry milk—1 tbsp., 7 gm.	.05	.04	NA	NA	NA	NA	NA
Cocoa drink powder w/o milk—1 tbsp., 7 gm.	.006	.03	NA	NA	NA	NA	NA
Cocoa mix for hot chocolate—1 tbsp., 7 gm.	.02	.03	NA	NA	NA	NA	NA
Cocoa, dry powder, high-fat or breakfast, plain—1 tbsp., 7 gm.	.03	.16	NA	NA	NA	NA	NA
Cream puffs w/custard filling—1 avg., 3" diam., 105 gm.	.12	.3	NA	NA	NA	NA	NA
Custard, baked—1 custard, 4 from 1 qt. milk, 157 gm.	.32	.1	NA	NA	NA	NA	NA
Custard, baked—1 cup, 265 gm.	.50	.26	NA	NA	NA	NA	NA
Custard, frozen—see Ice Cream, Egg and Dairy Products, and Related Products							
Custard dessert mix—see Pudding mixes							
Eclairs w/custard filling and chocolate icing—1 eclair, 4" long, 110 gm.	.24	1	NA	NA	NA	NA	NA
Frosting—see Cake Icings							
Gelatin desserts, made w/water—1 cup, 240 gm.	---	---	NA	NA	NA	NA	NA
Honey, strained or extracted—1 tbsp., 21 gm.	.01	.1	.0042	.00063	NA	.042	0

Vitamin C mg.	Vitamin D IU	Vitamin E IU	Calcium mg.	Iodine mg.	Iron mg.	Magnesium mg.	Phosphorus mg.	Potassium mg.	Sodium mg.
trace	NA	NA	35.55	NA	.54	---	51.3	79.6	77
trace	NA	NA	50.4	NA	.22	---	37.3	57.1	93.6
trace	NA	NA	50	NA	.36	NA	50.85	51.3	84
0	NA	NA	0	NA	0	NA	0	.50	3.5
0	0	NA	0	NA	0	trace	0	.40	3.2
0	NA	NA	.24	NA	.02	NA	.08	.02	.24
0	NA	NA	1.08	NA	.09	NA	.36	.36	2.34
0	NA	NA	.28	NA	.02	NA	.12	.10	4.24
0	NA	NA	19.8	NA	.81	---	122.85	201.6	4.5
0	NA	NA	10	NA	.5	---	31	37.75	7.75
trace	NA	NA	1.35	NA	.01	NA	1.4	2.5	.72
0	NA	NA	---	NA	---	NA	---	---	---
0	0	NA	28	.00168	1.2	81.76	126	232	1.1
0	NA	NA	1.23	NA	.30	11.97	17	53.5	9.88
trace	NA	NA	24.13	NA	.24	---	30.2	53.9	16.91
.21	NA	NA	41.23	NA	.12	NA	38.1	56	36.75
0	NA	NA	2.10	.000455 Ohio	.14	NA	11.97	35	18.76
.07	NA	NA	19.25	NA	.09	NA	20.30	42	26.74
0	NA	.21	9.31	NA	.74	29.4	45.36	106.54	.42
0	NA	NA	48	NA	.7	NA	70	127	87.15
0	NA	NA	163	NA	1.1	NA	189	229	124
trace	NA	NA	297	NA	1.06	---	310	387	209
0	NA	NA	90	NA	1.3	NA	150	---	---
---	NA	NA	---	NA	---	NA	---	---	122
trace	0	NA	1	NA	.1	.63	1.26	10.71	1.05

Food and Amount	Calories	Carbo-hydrate gm.	Protein gm.	Sat. Fatty Acids gm.	Unsat. Fatty Acids gm.	Vitamin A IU	Thiamin B_1 mg.
Ice cream—see Dairy Products							
Ice cream cones—1 cone, 5", 5 gm.	19	3.89	.50	.05	.05	trace	.002
Ice milk—see Dairy Products							
Ices, water—1 popsicle, twin bar, 128 gm.	95	23.7	trace	NA	NA	0	trace
Icings—see Cake Icings							
Jams and preserves—1 tbsp., 20 gm.	55	14	trace	---	---	trace	trace
Jellies—1 tbsp., 18 gm.	50	13	trace	---	---	trace	trace
Marmalade, citrus—1 tbsp., 20 gm.	51.4	14.02	.10	NA	NA	---	.004
Molasses, cane, Barbados—1 tbsp., 20 gm.	54	14	---	NA	NA	---	.012
Molasses, cane, blackstrap—1 tbsp., 20 gm.	43	11	---	NA	NA	---	.056
Molasses, cane, light—1 tbsp., 20 gm.	50	13	---	NA	NA	---	.014
Molasses, cane, medium—1 tbsp., 20 gm.	46	12	---	NA	NA	---	---
*Pie, Apple, home recipe, unenriched flour—4" sector, 135 gm.	350	51	3	4	10	40	.03
Pie, Banana custard, home recipe, unenriched flour—⅙ of 9" pie, 160 gm.	353	49.2	7.2	4.8	12.8	400	.06
Pie, Blackberry, home recipe, unenriched flour—⅙ of 9" pie, 160 gm.	389	55	4.2	4.8	12.8	144	.03
Pie, Blueberry, home recipe, unenriched flour—⅙ of 9" pie, 160 gm.	387	56	3.8	4.8	12.8	48	.03
Pie, Boston Cream—see Grain Products—Cakes							
*Pie, Butterscotch, home recipe, unenriched flour—4" sector, 130 gm.	350	50	6	5	8	340	.04
*Pie, Cherry, home recipe, unenriched flour—4" sector, 135 gm.	350	52	4	4	10	590	.03
Pie, Chocolate chiffon, home recipe, unenriched flour—⅙ of 9" pie, 160 gm.	525	70	10.9	4.8	12.8	496	.05
Pie, Chocolate meringue, home recipe, unenriched flour—⅙ of 9" pie, 150 gm.	378	50	7.2	4.5	12	286	.05
Pie, Coconut custard, home recipe, unenriched flour—⅙ of 9" pie, 155 gm.	365	38.5	9.4	4.65	12.4	357	.09
*Pie, Custard, home recipe, unenriched flour—4" sector, 130 gm.	285	30	8	5	8	300	.07
Pie, Lemon chiffon, home recipe, unenriched flour—⅙ of 9" pie, 107 gm.	335	46.9	7.5	3.21	8.56	182	.03
*Pie, Lemon meringue, home recipe, unenriched flour—4" sector, 120 gm.	305	45	4	4	8	200	.04
*Pie, Mince, home recipe, unenriched flour—4" sector, 135 gm.	365	56	3	4	11	trace	.09
Pie, Peach, home recipe, unenriched flour—⅙ of 9" pie, 165 gm.	421	63	4	4.95	13.2	1,200	.03
*Pie, Pecan, home recipe, unenriched flour—4" sector, 118 gm.	490	60	6	4	21	190	.19
Pie, Pineapple, home recipe, unenriched flour—⅙ of 9" pie, 160 gm.	404	61	3.5	4.8	12.8	32	.06
*Pie, Pineapple chiffon, home recipe, unenriched flour—4" sector, 93 gm.	265	36	6	3	7	320	.04
Pie, Pineapple custard, home recipe, unenriched flour—⅙ of 9" pie, 150 gm.	330	48.1	6.0	4.5	12	270	.06

*4" sector, ⅐ of 9" pie.

Riboflavin B₂ mg.	Niacin mg.	B₆ mg.	Folic Acid mg.	PABA mg.	Pantothenic Acid mg.	B₁₂ mcg.	Vitamin C mg.	Vitamin D IU	Vitamin E IU	Calcium mg.	Iodine mg.
.01	.02	NA	NA	NA	NA	NA	trace	NA	NA	7.80	NA
trace	trace	NA	NA	NA	NA	0	1.28	NA	NA	trace	NA
.01	trace	.005	NA	NA	---	0	trace	0	NA	4	NA
.01	trace*	NA	NA	NA	NA	0	1	0	NA	4	NA
.004	.02	NA	NA	NA	NA	0	1.2	0	NA	7	NA.
.04	---	NA	NA	.01	NA	0	---	0	NA	NA	NA
.05	.4	NA	---	.01	---	0	---	0	NA	116	NA
.012	trace	.04	.002	.01	.07	0	---	0	NA	33	NA
---	---	.054	.0019	.01	.092	0	---	0	NA	58	NA
.03	.5	---	NA	NA	.1485	0	1	NA	3.37	11	NA
.20	.5	NA	NA	NA	NA	NA	2	NA	NA	106	NA
.03	.5	NA	NA	NA	NA	NA	6	NA	NA	30	NA
.03	.5	NA	NA	NA	NA	NA	5	NA	4.99	18	NA
.13	.3	NA	NA	NA	NA	NA	trace	NA	NA	98	NA
.03	.7	NA	NA	NA	NA	NA	trace	NA	NA	19	NA
.16	.3	NA	NA	NA	NA	NA	0	NA	NA	38	NA
.18	.3	NA	NA	NA	NA	NA	trace	NA	NA	103	NA
.29	.47	NA	NA	NA	NA	NA	0	NA	NA	145	NA
.21	.4	---	NA	NA	1.2298	0	0	NA	NA	125	NA
.08	.2	NA	NA	NA	NA	NA	3	NA	NA	25	NA
.10	.2	NA	NA	NA	NA	NA	4	NA	NA	17	NA
.05	.5	NA	NA	NA	NA	NA	1	NA	NA	38	NA
.07	1.2	NA	NA	NA	NA	NA	5	NA	NA	16	NA
.08	.4	NA	NA	NA	NA	NA	trace	NA	NA	55	NA
.03	.6	NA	NA	NA	NA	NA	2	NA	NA	21	NA
.08	.4	NA	NA	NA	NA	NA	1	NA	NA	22	NA
.14	.6	NA	NA	NA	NA	NA	2	NA	NA	75	NA

Food and Amount	Iron mg.	Magnesium mg.	Phosphorus mg.	Potassium mg.	Sodium mg.
Ice cream—see Dairy Products					
Ice cream cones—1 cone, 5", 5 gm.	.02	NA	9.90	12.20	11.60
Ice milk—see Dairy Products					
Ices, water—1 popsicle, twin bar, 128 gm.	trace	NA	trace	3.84	trace
Icings—see Cake Icings					
Jams and preserves—1 tbsp., 20 gm.	.2	1	1.8	17.6	2.4
Jellies—1 tbsp., 18 gm.	.3	.72	1.26	13.5	3.06
Marmalade, citrus—1 tbsp., 20 gm.	.12	.8	1.8	6.6	2.8
Molasses, cane, Barbados—1 tbsp., 20 gm.	---	NA	10	---	---
Molasses, cane, blackstrap—1 tbsp., 20 gm.	2.3	51.6	17	585.4	19.2
Molasses, cane, light—1 tbsp., 20 gm.	.9	9.2	9	300	16
Molasses, cane, medium—1 tbsp., 20 gm.	1.2	16.2	14	212.6	7.4
*Pie, Apple, home recipe, unenriched flour—4" sector, 135 gm.	.4	---	29.7	108	406.3
Pie, Banana custard, home recipe, unenriched flour—⅙ of 9" pie, 160 gm.	.8	---	131	325	310
Pie, Blackberry, home recipe, unenriched flour—⅙ of 9" pie, 160 gm.	.8	---	42	160	429
Pie, Blueberry, home recipe, unenriched flour—⅙ of 9" pie, 160 gm.	1	---	37	104	429
Pie, Boston Cream—see Grain Products—Cakes					
*Pie, Butterscotch, home recipe, unenriched flour—4" sector, 130 gm.	1.2	---	105.3	123.5	278
*Pie, Cherry, home recipe, unenriched flour—4" sector, 135 gm.	.4	---	33.7	141.7	410
Pie, Chocolate chiffon, home recipe, unenriched flour—⅙ of 9" pie, 160 gm.	1.9	---	155	176	403
Pie, Chocolate meringue, home recipe, unenriched flour—⅙ of 9" pie, 150 gm.	1	---	147	209	385
Pie, Coconut custard, home recipe, unenriched flour—⅙ of 9" pie, 155 gm.	1.1	---	180	253	284
*Pie, Custard, home recipe, unenriched flour—4" sector, 130 gm.	.8	---	283	178	373
Pie, Lemon chiffon, home recipe, unenriched flour—⅙ of 9" pie, 107 gm.	1.0	---	89	87	279
*Pie, Lemon meringue, home recipe, unenriched flour—4" sector, 120 gm.	.6	---	58.8	60	338
*Pie, Mince, home recipe, unenriched flour—4" sector, 135 gm.	1.4	---	51	240	604
Pie, Peach, home recipe, unenriched flour—⅙ of 9" pie, 165 gm.	.8	---	48	245	246
*Pie, Pecan, home recipe, unenriched flour—4" sector, 118 gm.	3.3	---	121	145	260
Pie, Pineapple, home recipe, unenriched flour—⅙ of 9" pie, 160 gm.	.8	---	34	115	434
*Pie, Pineapple chiffon, home recipe, unenriched flour—4" sector, 93 gm.	.8	---	70	91	238
Pie, Pineapple custard, home recipe, unenriched flour—⅙ of 9" pie, 150 gm.	.6	---	98	145	279

*4" sector, ⅐ of 9" pie.

Food and Amount	Calories	Carbo-hydrate gm.	Protein gm.	Sat. Fatty Acids gm.	Unsat. Fatty Acids gm.	Vitamin A IU	Thiamin B_1 mg.
*Pie, Pumpkin, home recipe, unenriched flour—4″ sector, 130 gm.	275	32	5	5	8	3,210	.04
Pie, Raisin, home recipe, unenriched flour—⅙ of 9″ pie, 120 gm.	325	32.5	3.1	3.6	9.6	trace	.04
Pie, Rhubarb, home recipe, unenriched flour—⅙ of 9″ pie, 160 gm.	405	61.2	4.0	4.8	12.8	80	.03
Pie, Strawberry, home recipe, unenriched flour—⅙ of 9″ pie, 115 gm.	228	35.6	2.2	3.45	9.2	46	.02
Pie, Sweet potato, home recipe, unenriched flour—⅙ of 9″ pie, 160 gm.	342	37.8	7.2	4.8	12.8	3,840	.08
Pie, Apple, frozen, baked—⅙ of 9″ pie, 160 gm.	407	64	3.0	3.2	9.6	16	.03
Pie, Cherry, frozen, baked—⅙ of 9″ pie, 160 gm.	465	71	3.5	3.2	9.6	465	.03
Pie, Coconut Custard, frozen, baked—⅙ of 9″ pie, 160 gm.	398	47.2	9.6	3.2	9.6	256	.06
Pie, Coconut Custard, from mix, baked w/egg yolk and milk—⅙ of 9″ pie, 160 gm.	325	46.56	6.88	4.8	6.4	336	.04
Piecrust—see Grain Products							
Prune whip—1 cup, 136 gm.	212.16	50.184	5.5	---	---	625.60	.0272
Puddings, Chocolate, starch base, from home recipe—1 cup, 260 gm.	385	67	8	7	4	390	.05
Pudding, Vanilla (blancmange), starch base, from home recipe—1 cup, 255 gm.	285	41	9	5	3	410	.08
Pudding, Chocolate, from regular mix, starch base, cooked w/milk—1 cup, 255 gm.	316	58	8.6	5.1	2.55	331	.05
Pudding, Chocolate, from instant mix, starch base, made w/milk—1 cup, 255 gm.	319	62	7.65	5.1	2.55	331	.07
Pudding, custard dessert, cooked from mix, w/vegetable gum base—1 cup, 260 gm.	340	58	8.06	5.2	2.6	364	.05
Rennin tablet (salts, starch, rennin enzyme)—1 tablet, 0.5 gm.	.535	.121	.0005	NA	NA	0	0
Rennin dessert, home prepared, w/tablet—1 cup, 250 gm.	222.5	29	7.75	NA	NA	350	.07
Rennin dessert, Chocolate, from mix, made w/milk—1 cup, 250 gm.	255	35.25	8.5	NA	NA	350	.07
Rennin dessert, other flavors, fruit or vanilla, from mix, made w/milk—1 cup, 250 gm.	237.5	32	8	NA	NA	375	.07
Rice pudding with raisins—1 cup, 192 gm.	280	51	6.91	3.84	1.92	211	.05
Sherbet, all types—1 cup, 193 gm.	260	59	2	---	---	120	.02
Sugar, Beet or Cane, Brown, firmly packed—1 cup, 220 gm.	820	212	0	0	0	0	.02
Sugar, Beet or Cane, Brown, firmly packed—1 tbsp., 14 gm.	52	13	0	0	0	0	.001
Sugar, Beet or Cane, White, granulated—1 tbsp., 11 gm.	40	11	0	0	0	0	0
Sugar, Beet or Cane, White, powdered, stirred—1 tbsp., 8 gm.	30.	7.96	0	0	0	0	0

*4″ sector ⅐ of 9″ pie.

Food and Amount	Riboflavin B_2 mg.	Niacin mg.	B_6 mg.	Folic Acid mg.	PABA mg.	Pantothenic Acid mg.	B_{12} mcg.
*Pie, Pumpkin, home recipe, unenriched flour—4" sector, 130 gm.	.13	.7	---	NA	NA	.6747	---
Pie, Raisin, home recipe, unenriched flour—⅙ of 9" pie, 120 gm.	.04	.4	NA	NA	NA	NA	NA
Pie, Rhubarb, home recipe, unenriched flour—⅙ of 9" pie, 160 gm.	.06	.5	NA	NA	NA	NA	NA
Pie, Strawberry, home recipe, unenriched flour—⅙ of 9" pie, 115 gm.	.05	.4	NA	NA	NA	NA	NA
Pie, Sweet potato, home recipe, unenriched flour—⅙ of 9" pie, 160 gm.	.19	.5	NA	NA	NA	NA	NA
Pie, Apple, frozen, baked—⅙ of 9" pie, 160 gm.	.03	.3	NA	NA	NA	NA	NA
Pie, Cherry, frozen, baked—⅙ of 9" pie, 160 gm.	.03	.3	NA	NA	NA	NA	NA
Pie, Coconut Custard, frozen, baked—⅙ of 9" pie, 160 gm.	.26	.3	NA	NA	NA	NA	NA
Pie, Coconut Custard, from mix, baked w/egg yolk and milk—⅙ of 9" pie, 160 gm.	.22	.32	NA	NA	NA	NA	NA
Piecrust—see Grain Products							
Prune whip—1 cup, 136 gm.	.19	.680	NA	NA	NA	NA	0
Puddings, Chocolate, starch base, from home recipe—1 cup, 260 gm.	.36	.3	NA	NA	NA	NA	NA
Pudding, Vanilla (blancmange), starch base, from home recipe—1 cup, 255 gm.	.41	.3	NA	NA	NA	NA	NA
Pudding, Chocolate, from regular mix, starch base, cooked w/milk—1 cup, 255 gm.	.38	.25	NA	NA	NA	NA	NA
Pudding, Chocolate, from instant mix, starch base, made w/milk—1 cup, 255 gm.	.38	.25	NA	NA	NA	NA	NA
Pudding, custard dessert, cooked from mix, w/vegetable gum base—1 cup, 260 gm.	.36	.26	NA	NA	NA	NA	NA
Rennin tablet (salts, starch, rennin enzyme)—1 tablet, 0.5 gm.	0	0	NA	NA	NA	NA	NA
Rennin dessert, home prepared, w/tablet—1 cup, 250 gm.	.37	.25	NA	NA	NA	NA	NA
Rennin dessert, Chocolate, from mix, made w/milk—1 cup, 250 gm.	.37	.25	NA	NA	NA	NA	NA
Rennin dessert, other flavors, fruit or vanilla, from mix, made w/milk—1 cup, 250 gm.	.4	.25	NA	NA	NA	NA	NA
Rice pudding with raisins—1 cup, 192 gm.	.26	.38	NA	NA	NA	NA	NA
Sherbet, all types—1 cup, 193 gm.	.06	trace	NA	NA	NA	NA	0
Sugar, Beet or Cane, Brown, firmly packed—1 cup, 220 gm.	.07	.4	NA	NA	NA	NA	0
Sugar, Beet or Cane, Brown, firmly packed—1 tbsp., 14 gm.	.004	.02	NA	NA	NA	NA	0
Sugar, Beet or Cane, White, granulated—1 tbsp., 11 gm.	0	0	NA	NA	NA	NA	0
Sugar, Beet or Cane, White, powdered, stirred—1 tbsp., 8 gm.	0	0	NA	NA	NA	NA	0

*4" sector ⅐ of 9" pie.

Vitamin C mg.	Vitamin D IU	Vitamin E IU	Calcium mg.	Iodine mg.	Iron mg.	Magnesium mg.	Phosphorus mg.	Potassium mg.	Sodium mg.
trace	NA	NA	66	NA	.7	---	90	208	278
1	NA	NA	22	NA	1.1	---	48	231	342
5	NA	NA	102	NA	1.1	---	42	254	432
29	NA	NA	18	NA	.8	---	29	138	227
6	NA	NA	110	NA	.8	---	134	261	349
trace	NA	NA	13	NA	.5	NA	34	115	341
3	NA	NA	19	NA	.5	NA	37	131	366
trace	NA	NA	152	NA	1.0	NA	184	275	403
trace	NA	NA	149	NA	.64	NA	165	246	376
2.72	0	NA	29.92	NA	1.768	NA	44.88	394.40	223.04
1	NA	NA	250	NA	1.3	---	255	444	145
2	NA	NA	298	NA	trace	---	232	352	165
trace	NA	NA	260	NA	.76	---	242	347	329
trace	NA	NA	367	NA	1.27	---	232	329	316
trace	NA	NA	275	NA	trace	NA	213	335	257
0	---	NA	17.5	NA	---	---	1.0	---	111
2.5	---	NA	277.5	NA	trace	---	207.5	315	205
2.5	---	NA	305	NA	trace	---	240	312.5	130
2.5	---	NA	292.5	NA	trace	---	230	320	115
trace	NA	NA	188	NA	.76	---	180	340	136
4	NA	NA	31	NA	trace	---	NA	NA	NA
0	0	NA	187	.03564	7.5	---	41.8	756	66
0	0	NA	12	.002268	.47	---	2.66	48	4.2
0	0	NA	0	.001782	trace	trace	0	.33	.11
0	0	NA	0	.001296	.008	trace	0	.24	.08

Food and Amount	Calories	Carbo-hydrate gm.	Protein gm.	Sat. Fatty Acids gm.	Unsat. Fatty Acids gm.	Vitamin A IU	Thiamin B₁ mg.
Sugar, Beet or Cane, White, granulated —1 cup, 200 gm.	770	199	0	0	0	0	0
Sugar, Beet or Cane, White, powdered, stirred—1 cup, 120 gm.	460	11.9	0	0	0	0	0
Sugar, Dextrose, Anhydrous—1 tbsp., 9 gm.	32.94	8.95	0	0	0	0	0
Sugar, Maple—1 piece, 1¼″ x 1″ x ½″, 15 gm.	52	13.5	---	NA	NA	---	---
Syrup, Cane—1 tbsp., 20 gm.	52	13.6	0	NA	NA	0	.02
Syrup, Chocolate (see Chocolate)							
Syrup, Maple—1 tbsp., 20 gm.	50	12.8	0	NA	NA	0	---
Syrup, Sorghum—1 tbsp., 21 gm.	55	14	---	---	---	---	---
Syrup, Table blend, light and dark corn —1 tbsp., 21 gm.	60	15	0	---	---	0	0
Syrup, Table blend, cane and maple— 1 tbsp., 20 gm.	50	13	0	NA	NA	0	0
Tapioca, dry—1 cup, 152 gm.	535	131	1	---	---	0	0
Tapioca dessert, apple tapioca—1 cup, 250 gm.	295	74	1	---	---	30	trace
Tapioca cream pudding—1 cup, 165 gm.	220	28	8	4	3	480	.07

VEGETABLES AND VEGETABLE PRODUCTS

Food and Amount	Calories	Carbo-hydrate gm.	Protein gm.	Sat. Fatty Acids gm.	Unsat. Fatty Acids gm.	Vitamin A IU	Thiamin B₁ mg.
Artichokes, globe or French, cooked, boiled, drained—1 heart of 3″ diam. artichoke, 25 gm.	7	2.47	.70	---	---	37.5	.01
Artichokes, globe or French, raw— 3″ diam., 50 gm.	14	5.30	1.45	---	---	80	.04
Asparagus, green, canned, solids and liquid, regular pack—1 cup, 244 gm.	45	7	5	---	---	1,240	.15
Asparagus, white, canned, solids and liquid, regular pack—1 cup, 244 gm.	44	8.05	3.9	---	---	122	.122
Asparagus, green, cooked spears, boiled, drained—spears, ½″ diam. at base, 1 spear, 15 gm.	3	.54	3.3	---	---	13.5	.024
Asparagus, green, cooked, boiled, drained—pieces, 1½″ and 2″ lengths, 1 cup, 145 gm.	30	5	3	---	---	1,310	.23
Asparagus, green, raw spears— 6″ stalk, 13 gm.	3	.65	.32	---	---	117	.02
Bamboo shoots, raw—1 cup, 135 gm.	36.45	7.02	3.51	---	---	27	.2025
Beans, common, mature seeds, dry, white, raw—½ cup, 90 gm.	306	55.17	20.07	---	---	0	.585
Beans, common, mature seeds, dry, white, cooked—½ cup, 85 gm.	100.3	18.02	6.63	---	---	0	.119
Beans, common, mature seeds, dry, white, canned (no pork), solids and liquid—½ cup, 125 gm.	150	28.75	7.87	---	---	75	.08
Beans, common, mature seeds, dry, red, raw—½ cup, 100 gm.	343	61.9	22.5	---	---	20	.51

Riboflavin B2 mg.	Niacin mg.	B6 mg.	Folic Acid mg.	PABA mg.	Pantothenic Acid mg.	B12 mcg.	Vitamin C mg.	Vitamin D IU	Vitamin E IU	Calcium mg.	Iodine mg.
0	0	NA	NA	NA	NA	0	0	0	NA	0	.0324
0	0	NA	NA	NA	NA	0	0	0	NA	0	.01944
0	0	NA	NA	NA	NA	0	0	0	NA	---	NA
---	---	NA	NA	NA	NA	0	---	0	NA	27	NA
.01	.02	NA	NA	NA	NA	0	0	0	NA	12	NA
---	---	NA	NA	NA	NA	0	0	0	NA	.33	NA
.02	trace	NA	NA	NA	NA	0	---	0	NA	35	NA
0	0	NA	NA	NA	NA	0	0	0	NA	9	NA
0	0	NA	NA	NA	NA	0	0	0	NA	3.2	NA
0	0	NA	.00912	NA	NA	NA	0	0	NA	15	.001824
trace	trace	NA	---	NA	NA	NA	trace	NA	NA	8	---
.3	.2	NA	---	NA	NA	NA	2	NA	NA	173	---

VEGETABLES AND VEGETABLE PRODUCTS

Riboflavin B2 mg.	Niacin mg.	B6 mg.	Folic Acid mg.	PABA mg.	Pantothenic Acid mg.	B12 mcg.	Vitamin C mg.	Vitamin D IU	Vitamin E IU	Calcium mg.	Iodine mg.
.01	.17	NA	NA	NA	NA	0	2	NA	NA	12.75	NA
.025	.50	NA	NA	NA	NA	0	6	NA	NA	25.5	NA
.22	2.0	.1342	.0658	---	.4758	0	37	NA	NA	44	NA
.1464	1.708	NA	NA	NA	NA	0	36.6	NA	NA	36.6	NA
.027	.21	---	.016	---	---	0	3.9	NA	NA	3.15	trace Ohio
.26	2.0	---	.158	---	---	0	38	NA	NA	30	.00074 Ohio
.02	.19	.01768	.01417	---	.08	0	4.3	NA	NA	2.86	NA
.0945	.810	NA	NA	NA	NA	0	5.4	NA	NA	17.55	NA
.198	2.16	.504	.1125	NA	.6525	0	---	NA	.42	129.6	NA
.0595	.595	---	---	NA	---	0	0	NA	---	42.5	NA
.05	.75	---	---	NA	---	0	2.5	NA	---	85	.01443 Miss.
.20	2.3	.374	.153	NA	.425	0	---	NA	NA	110	NA

Food and Amount	Iron mg.	Magnesium mg.	Phosphorus mg.	Potassium mg.	Sodium mg.
Sugar, Beet or Cane, White, granulated —1 cup, 200 gm.	.2	trace	0	6	2
Sugar, Beet or Cane, White, powdered, stirred—1 cup, 120 gm.	.1	trace	0	3.6	1.2
Sugar, Dextrose, Anhydrous—1 tbsp., 9 gm.	---	NA	---	---	---
Sugar, Maple—1 piece, 1¼″ x 1″ x ½″, 15 gm.	.5	NA	2	36	2 .
Syrup, Cane—1 tbsp., 20 gm.	.72	NA	5.8	85	---
Syrup, Chocolate (see Chocolate)					
Syrup, Maple—1 tbsp., 20 gm.	.6	NA	3	26	3
Syrup, Sorghum—1 tbsp., 21 gm.	2.6	NA	5	---	---
Syrup, Table blend, light and dark corn —1 tbsp., 21 gm.	.8	NA	3.3	.84	14
Syrup, Table blend, cane and maple— 1 tbsp., 20 gm.	trace	NA	.20	5.2	.40
Tapioca, dry—1 cup, 152 gm.	.6	4.56	27	27	4.5
Tapioca dessert, apple tapioca—1 cup, 250 gm.	.5	---	10	65	127
Tapioca cream pudding—1 cup, 165 gm.	.7	---	180	222	257

VEGETABLES AND VEGETABLE PRODUCTS

Food and Amount	Iron mg.	Magnesium mg.	Phosphorus mg.	Potassium mg.	Sodium mg.
Artichokes, globe or French, cooked, boiled, drained—1 heart of 3″ diam. artichoke, 25 gm.	.27	NA	17	75	7.5
Artichokes, globe or French, raw— 3″ diam., 50 gm.	.65	NA	44	215	21.5
Asparagus, green, canned, solids and liquid, regular pack—1 cup, 244 gm.	4.1	---	104.92	405.04	575.8
Asparagus, white, canned, solids and liquid, regular pack—1 cup, 244 gm.	2.196	NA	80.52	341.6	575.8
Asparagus, green, cooked spears, boiled, drained—spears, ½″ diam. at base, 1 spear, 15 gm.	.09	3	7.5	27.45	.15
Asparagus, green, cooked, boiled, drained—pieces, 1½″ and 2″ lengths, 1 cup, 145 gm.	.9	29	72.5	265.35	1.45
Asparagus, green, raw spears— 6″ stalk, 13 gm.	.13	2.6	8	36	.26
Bamboo shoots, raw—1 cup, 135 gm.	.675	NA	79.65	719.55	---
Beans, common, mature seeds, dry, white, raw—½ cup, 90 gm.	7.02	153	382.5	1,076.4	17.1
Beans, common, mature seeds, dry, white, cooked—½ cup, 85 gm.	2.295	---	125.8	353.6	5.95
Beans, common, mature seeds, dry, white, canned (no pork), solids and liquid—½ cup, 125 gm.	2.5	46.25	151.25	335	422.5
Beans, common, mature seeds, dry, red, raw—½ cup, 100 gm.	6.9	138	406	984	10

Food and Amount	Calories	Carbohydrate gm.	Protein gm.	Sat. Fatty Acids gm.	Unsat. Fatty Acids gm.	Vitamin A IU	Thiamin B₁ mg.
Beans, common, mature seeds, dry, red, cooked—1 cup, 250 gm.	295	53.5	19.5	•••	•••	trace	.27
Beans, common, mature seeds, dry, red, solids and liquid, canned—½ cup, 90 gm.	81	14.76	5.13	•••	•••	trace	.04
Beans, common, mature seeds, dry, pinto, calico, and red Mexican, raw—1 cup, 150 gm.	523	95.55	34.35	•••	•••	•••	1.26
Beans, common, mature seeds, dry; other, incl. black, brown, and Bayo; raw—1 cup, 150 gm.	508.5	91.8	33.45	•••	•••	45	.82
Beans, lima, immature seeds, raw—1 cup, 150 gm.	184	33	12.6	•••	•••	435	.36
Beans, lima, immature seeds, cooked, boiled, drained—1 cup, 170 gm.	190	34	13	•••	•••	480	.31
Beans, lima, immature seeds, canned, regular pack, solids and liquid—½ cup, 130 gm.	92	17	5.3	•••	•••	169	.05
Beans, lima, immature seeds, frozen, thick-seeded types (Fordhooks), cooked, boiled, drained—1 cup, 160 gm.	158	30.56	9.6	•••	•••	368	.11
Beans, lima, immature seeds, frozen, thin-seeded types (Baby Limas), cooked, boiled, drained—1 cup, 160 gm.	188	35.68	11.84	•••	•••	trace	.14
Beans, lima, mature seeds, dry, raw—½ cup, 100 gm.	345	64.0	20.4	•••	•••	trace	.48
Beans, lima, mature seeds, dry, cooked (baked)—1 cup, 184 gm.	254	47.1	15.08	•••	•••	•••	.23
Beans, mung, mature seeds, dry, raw—½ cup, 105 gm.	357	63.31	25.41	•••	•••	84	.39
Beans, mung sprouted seeds (Beansprouts), uncooked—½ cup, 45 gm.	15	2.97	1.71	•••	•••	9	.05
Beans, mung, sprouted seeds (Beansprouts), cooked, boiled, drained—1 cup, 125 gm.	35	7	4	•••	•••	30	.11
Beans, snap, green, raw—1 cup of 1″ pieces, 100 gm.	32	7	1.9	•••	•••	600	.08
Beans, snap, green, cooked, boiled, drained—1 cup, 125 gm.	30	7	2	•••	•••	680	.09
Beans, snap, green, canned, reg. pack, solids and liquid—1 cup, 239 gm.	45	10	2	•••	•••	690	.07
Beans, snap, green, frozen, cut, cooked, boiled, drained—½ cup, 80 gm.	20	4.56	1.3	•••	•••	44	.05
Beans, snap, green, frozen, French style, cooked, boiled, drained—½ cup, 85 gm.	22	5.1	1.3	•••	•••	450	.05
Beans, snap, yellow or wax, raw—1 cup, 1″ pieces, 100 gm.	27	6	1.7	•••	•••	250	.08
Beans, snap, yellow or wax, cooked, boiled, drained—1 cup, 125 gm.	30	6	2	•••	•••	290	.09
Beans, snap, yellow or wax, canned, solids and liquid—1 cup, 239 gm.	45	10	2	•••	•••	140	.07
Beans, snap, yellow or wax, frozen, cut, cooked, boiled, drained—½ cup, 85 gm.	23	5.27	1.44	•••	•••	85	.05

Food and Amount	Ribo-flavin B₂ mg.	Niacin mg.	B₆ mg.	Folic Acid mg.	PABA mg.	Panto-thenic Acid mg.	B₁₂ mcg.
Beans, common, mature seeds, dry, red, cooked—1 cup, 250 gm.	.15	1.75	---	---	NA	---	0
Beans, common, mature seeds, dry, red, solids and liquid, canned— ½ cup, 90 gm.	.03	.54	---	---	NA	---	0
Beans, common, mature seeds, dry, pinto, calico, and red Mexican, raw— 1 cup, 150 gm.	.31	3.30	NA	NA	NA	NA	0
Beans, common, mature seeds, dry; other, incl. black, brown, and Bayo; raw—1 cup, 150 gm.	.3	3.3	NA	NA	NA	NA	0
Beans, lima, immature seeds, raw— 1 cup, 150 gm.	.18	2.1	.255	.051	NA	.67	0
Beans, lima, immature seeds, cooked, boiled, drained—1 cup, 170 gm.	.17	2.2	---	.0578	NA	---	0
Beans, lima, immature seeds, canned, regular pack, solids and liquid— ½ cup, 130 gm.	.05	.65	.1053	.0169	NA	.14	0
Beans, lima, immature seeds, frozen, thick-seeded types (Fordhooks), cooked, boiled, drained—1 cup, 160 gm.	.08	1.6	.240	.0544	NA	.384	0
Beans, lima, immature seeds, frozen, thin-seeded types (Baby Limas), cooked, boiled, drained—1 cup, 160 gm.	.08	1.92	---	---	NA	---	0
Beans, lima, mature seeds, dry, raw— ½ cup, 100 gm.	.17	1.9	.580	.103	NA	.975	0
Beans, lima, mature seeds, dry, cooked (baked)—1 cup, 184 gm.	.11	1.28	---	.235	NA	---	0
Beans, mung, mature seeds, dry, raw—½ cup, 105 gm.	.22	2.73	---	---	NA	---	0
Beans, mung sprouted seeds (Bean-sprouts), uncooked—½ cup, 45 gm.	.05	.36	NA	---	NA	NA	0
Beans, mung, sprouted seeds (Bean-sprouts), cooked, boiled, drained— 1 cup, 125 gm.	.13	.9	NA	.181	NA	NA	0
Beans, snap, green, raw—1 cup of 1″ pieces, 100 gm.	.11	.5	.063	.0275	NA	.2	0
Beans, snap, green, cooked, boiled, drained—1 cup, 125 gm.	.11	.6	.10	.035	NA	.237	0
Beans, snap, green, canned, reg. pack, solids and liquid—1 cup, 239 gm.	.10	.7	.096	.029	NA	.179	0
Beans, snap, green, frozen, cut, cooked, boiled, drained—½ cup, 80 gm.	.07	.32	.056	.022	NA	.108	0
Beans, snap, green, frozen, French style, cooked, boiled, drained— ½ cup, 85 gm.	.06	.25	---	---	NA	---	0
Beans, snap, yellow or wax, raw— 1 cup, 1″ pieces, 100 gm.	.11	.5	---	---	NA	---	0
Beans, snap, yellow or wax, cooked, boiled, drained—1 cup, 125 gm.	.11	.6	---	.040	NA	.312	0
Beans, snap, yellow or wax, canned, solids and liquid—1 cup, 239 gm.	.10	.7	.100	---	NA	---	0
Beans, snap, yellow or wax, frozen, cut, cooked, boiled, drained— ½ cup, 85 gm.	.06	.34	---	---	NA	---	0

Vitamin C mg.	Vitamin D IU	Vitamin E IU	Calcium mg.	Iodine mg.	Iron mg.	Mag- nesium mg.	Phos- phorus mg.	Potas- sium mg.	Sodium mg.
---	NA	NA	95	NA	6	---	350	850	7.5
---	NA	NA	26.1	NA	1.62	---	98.1	237.6	2.7
---	NA	NA	202	NA	9.60	---	685	1,476	15
---	NA	NA	202.5	NA	11.85	---	630	1,557	37.5
43	NA	NA	78	NA	4.2	100.5	213	975	3
29	NA	NA	80	NA	4.3	114	205.7	717.4	1.7
9.1	NA	NA	34	NA	3.12	---	87	288	307
27.2	NA	NA	32	NA	2.72	77	144	681.6	161.6
19.2	NA	NA	56	NA	4.16	---	201.6	630.4	206.4
---	NA	NA	72	.0005 Md.	7.8	180	385	1,529	4
---	NA	NA	53.36	NA	5.7	---	283.36	1,126	3.68
---	NA	NA	123.9	NA	8.08	---	357	1,079	6.3
8	NA	NA	8.55	NA	.58	---	28.8	100	2.25
8	NA	NA	21	NA	1.1	---	60	195	5
19	NA	---	56	.00026 Penn.	.8	32	44	243	7
15	NA	---	63	NA	.8	40	46	189	5
10	NA	.07	81	NA	2.9	33	50	227	564
4	NA	.08	32	NA	.56	17	26	122	.8
5.95	NA	---	32	NA	.76	---	25	115	1.7
20	NA	NA	56	NA	.8	---	43	243	7
16	NA	NA	63	NA	.8	---	46	189	3.75
12	NA	NA	81	NA	2.9	---	50	227	564
5	NA	NA	30	NA	.59	---	26	139	.85

Food and Amount	Calories	Carbo-hydrate gm.	Protein gm.	Sat. Fatty Acids gm.	Unsat. Fatty Acids gm.	Vitamin A IU	Thiamin B₁ mg.
Beets, common, red, cooked, boiled, drained—1 beet, 2" diam., 50 gm.	15	3.5	.5	---	---	10	.015
Beets, common, red, cooked, boiled, drained, peeled, diced or sliced—1 cup, 170 gm.	55	12	2	---	---	30	.05
Beets, common, red, canned, solids and liquid, reg. pack—1 cup, 246 gm.	85	19	2	---	---	20	.02
Beet greens, common, raw—1 cup, 100 gm.	24	4.6	2.2	NA	NA	6,100	.10
Beet greens, common, cooked, boiled, drained, leaves and stems—1 cup, 145 gm.	25	5	3	---	---	7,400	.10
Blackeye peas (see Cowpeas)							
Broadbeans, raw, immature seeds—1 cup, 150 gm.	157	26.7	12.6	---	---	330	.42
Broadbeans, raw, mature seeds, dry—see Nuts, Seeds, Sprouted Seeds, Dry Beans, and Related Products							
Broccoli, raw spears—1 stalk, 5½" long, 100 gm.	32	5.9	3.6	---	---	2,500	.10
Broccoli, cooked spears, boiled, drained—1 spear, 180 gm.	45	8	6	---	---	4,500	.16
Broccoli, cooked, boiled, drained—spears cut into ½" pieces, 1 cup, 155 gm.	40	7	5	---	---	3,880	.14
Broccoli, frozen, chopped, cooked, boiled, drained—1 cup, 182 gm.	47	8.37	5.27	---	---	4,732	.10
Brussels sprouts, cooked, boiled, drained—1¼-1½" diam., 7-8 per cup, 1 cup, 155 gm.	55	10	7	---	---	810	.12
Brussels sprouts, frozen, cooked, boiled, drained—1½" diam., 1 sprout, 19 gm.	6.2	1.23	.6	---	---	108	.01
Cabbage, common varieties, raw, coarsely shredded or sliced—1 cup, 70 gm.	15	4	1	---	---	90	.04
Cabbage, common varieties, raw, finely shredded or chopped—1 cup, 90 gm.	20	5	1	---	---	120	.05
Cabbage, common varieties, cooked, drained—1 cup, 145 gm.	30	6	2	---	---	190	.06
Cabbage, red, raw, coarsely shredded—1 cup, 70 gm.	20	5	1	---	---	30	.06
Cabbage, savoy, raw, coarsely shredded—1 cup, 70 gm.	15	3	2	---	---	140	.04
Cabbage, celery or Chinese, raw—1 cup of 1" pieces, 75 gm.	10	2	1	---	---	110	.04
Cabbage, spoon (pakchoy), cooked, boiled, drained—1 cup, 170 gm.	25	4	2	---	---	5,270	.07
Carrots, canned, regular pack, solids and liquid—1 cup, 250 gm.	70	16	1.5	---	---	25,000	.05
Carrots, cooked, boiled, diced—1 cup, 145 gm.	45	10	1	---	---	15,220	.08
Carrots, raw—1 whole, 5½" x 1", 50 gm.	20	5	1	---	---	5,500	.03
Carrots, raw, grated—1 cup, 110 gm.	45	11	1	---	---	12,100	.06
Cauliflower, cooked, flower buds—1 cup, 120 gm.	25	5	3	---	---	70	.11

Riboflavin B2 mg.	Niacin mg.	B6 mg.	Folic Acid mg.	PABA mg.	Pantothenic Acid mg.	B12 mcg.	Vitamin C mg.	Vitamin D IU	Vitamin E IU	Calcium mg.	Iodine mg.
.02	.15	.027	.007	NA	.075	0	3	NA	.1	7	.0105
.07	.5	.093	.024	NA	.255	0	10	NA	.34	24	.0357
.05	.2	.123	.007	NA	.246	0	7	NA	NA	34	.00093 Ohio
.22	.4	.1	.06	NA	.25	0	30	NA	NA	119	NA
.22	.4	---	.087	NA	---	0	22	NA	NA	144	NA
.25	2.4	NA	NA	NA	NA	0	45	NA	NA	40	NA
.23	.9	.171	.0535	NA	1.29	0	113	NA	---	103	NA
.36	1.4	---	.097	NA	---	0	162	NA	---	158	.00067 Ohio
.31	1.2	---	.083	NA	---	0	140	NA	---	136	.00057 Ohio
.21	.91	.309	.098	NA	.955	0	104	NA	---	98	NA
.22	1.2	.271	.076	NA	651	0	135	NA	2.63	50	NA
.01	.11	.03325	---	NA	.0798	0	15	NA	---	4	NA
.04	.2	.112	.022	---	.143	0	33	NA	.49	34	NA
.05	.3	.144	.028	---	.185	0	42	NA	.63	44	NA
.06	.4	NA	NA	NA	NA	0	48	NA	1.01	64	.00029 Ohio
.04	.3	NA	NA	NA	NA	0	43	NA	.14	29	NA
.06	.2	NA	NA	NA	NA	0	39	NA	.14	47	NA
.03	.5	NA	NA	NA	NA	0	19	NA	NA	32	.00016 Ohio
.14	1.2	NA	NA	NA	NA	0	26	NA	NA	252	NA
.05	1.0	.075	.007	NA	.325	0	5	NA	.27	62.5	NA
.07	.7	---	---	NA	---	0	9	NA	2.17	48	.00016 Ohio
.03	.3	.075	.004	.19	.140	0	4	NA	.05	18	.019
.06	.7	.165	.009	.41	.308	0	9	NA	.12	41	.0418
.10	.7	---	---	NA	---	0	66	NA	NA	25	NA

Food and Amount	Iron mg.	Mag- nesium mg.	Phos- phorus mg.	Potas- sium mg.	Sodium mg.
Beets, common, red, cooked, boiled, drained—1 beet, 2" diam., 50 gm.	.25	12.5	11.5	104	21.5
Beets, common, red, cooked, boiled, drained, peeled, diced or sliced— 1 cup, 170 gm.	.9	42.5	39	353	73
Beets, common, red, canned, solids and liquid, reg. pack—1 cup, 246 gm.	1.5	37	42	411	580
Beet greens, common, raw—1 cup, 100 gm.	3.3	106	40	570	130
Beet greens, common, cooked, boiled, drained, leaves and stems—1 cup, 145 gm.	2.8	NA	16.25	481	110
Blackeye peas (see Cowpeas)					
Broadbeans, raw, immature seeds— 1 cup, 150 gm.	3.3	NA	235	706	6
Broadbeans, raw, mature seeds, dry—see Nuts, Seeds, Sprouted Seeds, Dry Beans, and Related Products					
Broccoli, raw spears—1 stalk, 5½" long, 100 gm.	1.1	24	78	382	15
Broccoli, cooked spears, boiled, drained—1 spear, 180 gm.	1.4	NA	111	480	18
Broccoli, cooked, boiled, drained— spears cut into ½" pieces, 1 cup, 155 gm.	1.2	NA	87	329	23
Broccoli, frozen, chopped, cooked, boiled, drained—1 cup, 182 gm.	1.27	38	102	386	27
Brussels sprouts, cooked, boiled, drained—1¼–1½" diam., 7–8 per cup, 1 cup, 155 gm.	1.7	45	95	457	21.7
Brussels sprouts, frozen, cooked, boiled, drained—1½" diam., 1 sprout, 19 gm.	.15	3.99	11.59	56	2.6
Cabbage, common varieties, raw, coarsely shredded or sliced— 1 cup, 70 gm.	.3	9	20	163	14
Cabbage, common varieties, raw, finely shredded or chopped—1 cup, 90 gm.	.4	11.7	26	210	18
Cabbage, common varieties, cooked, drained—1 cup, 145 gm.	.4	---	29	236	20
Cabbage, red, raw, coarsely shredded— 1 cup, 70 gm.	.6	NA	24.5	188	18
Cabbage, savoy, raw, coarsely shredded—1 cup, 70 gm.	.6	NA	37.8	188	15
Cabbage, celery or Chinese, raw— 1 cup of 1" pieces, 75 gm.	.5	10	30	190	17
Cabbage, spoon (pakchoy), cooked, boiled, drained—1 cup, 170 gm.	1.0	NA	56.1	364	30.6
Carrots, canned, regular pack, solids and liquid—1 cup, 250 gm.	1.75	---	50	300	590
Carrots, cooked, boiled, diced— 1 cup, 145 gm.	.9	---	44.9	322	47.85
Carrots, raw—1 whole, 5½" x 1", 50 gm.	.4	11	18	171	23.5
Carrots, raw, grated—1 cup, 110 gm.	.8	25	39.6	375	51.7
Cauliflower, cooked, flower buds— 1 cup, 120 gm.	.8	---	50.4	247	10.8

Food and Amount	Calories	Carbo-hydrate gm.	Protein gm.	Sat. Fatty Acids gm.	Unsat. Fatty Acids gm.	Vitamin A IU	Thiamin B₁ mg.
Cauliflower, frozen, cooked, boiled, drained—1 cup, 115 gm.	20.7	3.79	2.18	---	---	34.5	.04
Cauliflower, raw—1 cup flower pieces, 100 gm.	27	5.2	2.7	---	---	60	.11
Celery, raw—1 stalk, 8" x 1½" at root end, 40 gm.	5	2	trace	---	---	100	.01
Celery, raw, diced—1 cup, 100 gm.	15	4	1	---	---	240	.03
Chervil, raw—1 cup, 60 gm.	34	6.9	2.04	---	---	---	---
Chickpeas (garbanzos), mature seeds, dry, raw—½ cup, 100 gm.	360	61	20.5	---	---	50	.31
Chicory, Witloof (French or Belgian endive), bleached head, raw— 10 sml. inner leaves, 25 gm.	3.75	.80	.25	---	---	trace	---
Chicory greens, raw—35 inner leaves, 95 gm.	19	3.61	1.71	---	---	3,800	.05
Chives, raw—1 tbsp. chopped, 10 gm.	2.8	.58	.18	---	---	580	.008
Coleslaw, commercial French dressing—1 cup, 108 gm.	102.6	8.2	1.29	1.08	6.48	118.8	.04
Coleslaw, homemade French dressing —1 cup, 110 gm.	141.9	5.61	1.21	2.2	9.9	121	.04
Coleslaw, mayonnaise—1 cup, 120 gm.	172.8	5.76	1.56	2.4	12	192	.06
Coleslaw, mayonnaise-type salad dressing—1 cup, 120 gm.	119	8.5	1.44	1.2	7.2	180	.06
Collards, cooked—1 cup, 190 gm.	55	9	5	---	---	10,260	.27
Corn, sweet, canned, regular pack, white and yellow, cream style, solids and liquid—½ cup, 125 gm.	103	25	2.62	---	---	412	.03
Corn, sweet, canned, whole kernel, yellow, vacuum pack, solids and liquid—1 cup, 242 gm.	200.86	49.61	6.05	---	---	847	.07
Corn, sweet, canned, whole kernel, white and yellow, wet pack, solids and liquid—1 cup, 256 gm.	170	40	5	---	---	690*	.07
Corn, sweet, cooked, boiled, drained, white and yellow kernels, cooked on cob—1 ear, 5" x 1¾", 140 gm.	70	16	3	---	---	310*	.09
Corn, sweet, frozen, kernels, cut off cob bef. cooking, cooked, boiled, drained —½ cup, 90 gm.	71	17	2.7	---	---	315	.08
Corn, sweet, frozen, cooked on cob (kernels), cooked, boiled, drained— ½ cup (3" cob), 85 gm.	79.9	18.36	2.97	---	---	297.5	.11
Cowpeas, immature seeds, cooked, boiled, drained—1 cup, 160 gm.	175	29	13	---	---	560	.49
Cowpeas, immature seeds, canned, solids and liquid—½ cup, 100 gm.	70	12.4	5	---	---	60	.09
Cowpeas (blackeye peas only), frozen, cooked, boiled, drained—1 cup, 165 gm.	136	24.67	9.3			179	.42
Cowpeas, young pods w/seeds, cooked, boiled, drained—1 cup, 140 gm.	48	9.8	3.64			1,960	.12
Cowpeas, mature seeds, dry, cooked— ½ cup, 125 gm.	95	17.25	6.37	---	---	125	.20
Cress, garden, raw—6 sprigs, 10 gm.	3.2	.55	.26	---	---	930	NA

*Yellow varieties; white varieties contain only trace amounts.

Food and Amount	Ribo-flavin B₂ mg.	Niacin mg.	B₆ mg.	Folic Acid mg.	PABA mg.	Panto-thenic Acid mg.	B₁₂ mcg.
Cauliflower, frozen, cooked, boiled, drained—1 cup, 115 gm.	.05	.46	.218	---	NA	.621	0
Cauliflower, raw—1 cup flower pieces, 100 gm.	.10	.7	.210	.022	NA	1.0	0
Celery, raw—1 stalk, 8″ x 1½″ at root end, 40 gm.	.01	.1	.024	.003	NA	.171	0
Celery, raw, diced—1 cup, 100 gm.	.03	.3	.060	.007	NA	.429	0
Chervil, raw—1 cup, 60 gm.	---	---	NA	NA	NA	NA	0
Chickpeas (garbanzos), mature seeds, dry, raw—½ cup, 100 gm.	.15	2	NA	NA	NA	NA	0
Chicory, Witloof (French or Belgian endive), bleached head, raw— 10 sml. inner leaves, 25 gm.	---	---	NA	NA	NA	NA	0
Chicory greens, raw—35 inner leaves, 95 gm.	.09	.47	.04275	.0266	NA	---	0
Chives, raw—1 tbsp. chopped, 10 gm.	.013	.05	NA	NA	NA	NA	0
Coleslaw, commercial French dressing—1 cup, 108 gm.	.04	.32	NA	NA	NA	NA	0
Coleslaw, homemade French dressing —1 cup, 110 gm.	.04	.33	NA	NA	NA	NA	0
Coleslaw, mayonnaise—1 cup, 120 gm.	.06	.36	NA	NA	NA	NA	0
Coleslaw, mayonnaise-type salad dressing—1 cup, 120 gm.	.06	.36	NA	NA	NA	NA	0
Collards, cooked—1 cup, 190 gm.	.37	2.4	---	.194	NA	---	0
Corn, sweet, canned, regular pack, white and yellow, cream style, solids and liquid—½ cup, 125 gm.	.06	1.25	.25	.01	NA	.275	0
Corn, sweet, canned, whole kernel, yellow, vacuum pack, solids and liquid—1 cup, 242 gm.	.14	2.66	.47	.02	NA	.52	0
Corn, sweet, canned, whole kernel, white and yellow, wet pack, solids and liquid—1 cup, 256 gm.	.12	2.3	.512	.02048	NA	.5632	0
Corn, sweet, cooked, boiled, drained, white and yellow kernels, cooked on cob—1 ear, 5″ x 1¾″, 140 gm.	.08	1.0	---	.039	NA	---	0
Corn, sweet, frozen, kernels, cut off cob bef. cooking, cooked, boiled, drained —½ cup, 90 gm.	.05	1.35	---	---	NA	---	0
Corn, sweet, frozen, cooked on cob (kernels), cooked, boiled, drained— ½ cup (3″ cob), 85 gm.	.06	1.44	---	---	NA	---	0
Cowpeas, immature seeds, cooked, boiled, drained—1 cup, 160 gm.	.18	2.3	---	.065	NA	---	0
Cowpeas, immature seeds, canned, solids and liquid—½ cup, 100 gm.	.05	.50	.053	.026	NA	.162	0
Cowpeas (blackeye peas only), frozen, cooked, boiled, drained—1 cup, 165 gm.	.11	1.47	.15675	---	NA	---	0
Cowpeas, young pods w/seeds, cooked, boiled, drained—1 cup, 140 gm.	.12	1.12	NA	NA	NA	NA	0
Cowpeas, mature seeds, dry, cooked— ½ cup, 125 gm.	.05	.50	.702	.548	NA	1.312	0
Cress, garden, raw—6 sprigs, 10 gm.	.02	.10	NA	NA	NA	NA	0

* Yellow varieties; white varieties contain only trace amounts.

Vitamin C mg.	Vitamin D IU	Vitamin E IU	Calcium mg.	Iodine mg.	Iron mg.	Magnesium mg.	Phosphorus mg.	Potassium mg.	Sodium mg.
47	NA	NA	20	NA	.57	15	43.7	238	11.5
78	NA	NA	25	.012	1.1	24	56	295	13
4	NA	.15	16	.00049 Ohio	.1	9	11.2	136	50
9	NA	.38	39	.00123 Ohio	.3	22	28	341	126
5.4	NA	NA	---	NA	---	NA	---	---	---
---	NA	NA	150	NA	6.9	NA	331	797	26
---	NA	.05	4.5	NA	.12	3.25	5.25	45.5	1.75
21	NA	NA	81.7	NA	.85	12.35	38	399	---
5.6	NA	NA	6.9	NA	.17	3.2	4.4	25	---
31.8	NA	NA	46.1	NA	.44	NA	28.08	221.4	289.44
31.9	NA	NA	46.2	NA	.44	NA	27.5	216.7	144.1
34.8	NA	NA	52.8	NA	.48	NA	34.8	238.8	144
34.8	NA	NA	51.6	NA	.48	NA	33.6	230	148.8
87	NA	NA	289	NA	1.1	NA	74.1	445	47.5
6.25	NA	.06	3.75	NA	.75	23	70	121	295
12.1	NA	.12	7.26	NA	1.21	45	176.66	234.74	571.12
13	NA	.12	10	NA	1.0	48.64	123	248	604
7	NA	---	2	.00073 Ohio	.5	NA	125	274	trace
4.5	NA	.17	2.7	NA	.72	19.8	66	166	.90
5.95	NA	.16	2.55	NA	.68	18.7	81.6	196.35	.85
28	NA	NA	38	NA	3.4	88	234	606	1.6
3	NA	NA	18	NA	1.5	---	112	352	236
9.45	NA	NA	26	NA	2.94	90.75	176	353	41
23.8	NA	NA	77	NA	.98	---	68	274	4.2
---	NA	NA	21	NA	1.62	287	119	286	10
6.9	NA	NA	8.1	NA	.13	NA	7.6	61	1.4

Food and Amount	Calories	Carbo-hydrate gm.	Protein gm.	Sat. Fatty Acids gm.	Unsat. Fatty Acids gm.	Vitamin A IU	Thiamin B₁ mg.
Cucumber, raw, pared—1 cucumber, 7½" x 2", 207 gm.	30	7	1	---	---	trace	.07
Cucumber, raw, pared—1 slice, approx. 2" x ⅛", 8 gm.	1.12	.25	.04	---	---	trace	.002
Cucumber, raw, not pared—1 cucumber, 7" x 2", 219 gm.	33	7.44	1.97	---	---	547	.06
Cucumber, raw, not pared—1 slice, approx. 2" x ⅛", 9 gm.	1.35	.3	.08	---	---	22.5	.002
Dandelion greens, cooked, boiled, drained—1 cup, 180 gm.	60	12	4	---	---	21,060	.24
Dandelion greens, raw—1 cup, 100 gm.	45	9.2	2.7			14,000	.19
Eggplant, cooked, boiled, drained—½ cup diced, 100 gm.	19	4.1	1	---	---	10	.05
Endive (curly endive and escarole), raw —1 cup, shredded, 70 gm.	14	2.87	1.19	---	---	2,310	.04
Escarole—see Endive							
Fennel, common, leaves, raw—⅓ of vegetable, 3" diam., 50 gm.	14	2.55	1.4	NA	NA	1,750	---
Garbanzos—see Chickpeas							
Garlic, cloves, raw—1 clove (¾" x ½"), 7 gm.	9.59	2.15	.43	NA	NA	trace	.01
Jerusalem-artichoke, raw—1 small, 1½" diam., 25 gm.	10	4.17	.57	NA	NA	5	.05
Kale, cooked, boiled, drained, leaves including stems—1 cup, 110 gm.	30	4	4	---	---	8,140	---
Kale, frozen, cooked, boiled, drained— ½ cup, 90 gm.	28	4.86	2.7	---	---	7,380	.05
Kale, raw, leaves including stems— 1 cup, 100 gm.	38	6	4.2	NA	NA	8,900	---
Leeks, bulb and lower leaf portion, raw —1 cup, 110 gm.	57	12	2.4	NA	NA	44	.12
Lentils, mature seeds, raw, dry, whole —½ cup, 100 gm.	340	60.1	24.7	---	---	60	.37
Lentils, mature seeds, dry, drained, cooked—1 cup, 135 gm.	466	83.4	33.3	---	---	81	.49
Lettuce, raw, butterhead types, Boston or Bibb—1 head, 4" diam., 220 gm.	30	6	3	---	---	2,130	.14
Lettuce, raw, butterhead types, Boston or Bibb—6 leaves, 40 gm.	5.6	1	.48	---	---	388	.02
Lettuce, raw, Romaine—2 leaves, 45 gm.	8.1	1.57	.58	---	---	855	.02
Lettuce, raw, crisp head, e.g., Iceberg— 1 head, 4¾" diam., 454 gm.	60	13	4	---	---	1,500	.29
Lettuce, raw, crisp head, e.g., Iceberg— 5 leaves, 38 gm.	5	1.10	.34	---	---	125	.02
Lettuce, raw, looseleaf or bunching varieties, e.g., Grand Rapids, Salad Bowl—2 large leaves, 50 gm.	10	2	1	---	---	950	.03
Mixed Vegetables, frozen—see Vegetables, mixed, frozen							
Mushrooms, canned, solids and liquid —1 cup, 244 gm.	40	6	5	---	---	trace	.04
Mushrooms, raw—½ cup, slices, 35 gm.	9.8	1.54	.94	---	---	trace	.03
Mustard greens, cooked, boiled, drained —1 cup, 140 gm.	35	6	3	---	---	8,120	.11

Riboflavin B_2 mg.	Niacin mg.	B_6 mg.	Folic Acid mg.	PABA mg.	Pantothenic Acid mg.	B_{12} mcg.	Vitamin C mg.	Vitamin D IU	Vitamin E IU	Calcium mg.	Iodine mg.
.09	.4	NA	NA	NA	NA	0	23	NA	NA	35	NA
.003	.016	NA	NA	NA	NA	0	.88	NA	NA	1.36	NA
.08	.43	.092	.015	NA	.547	0	24	NA	NA	54.75	NA
.003	.01	.000	.0006	NA	.022	0	.99	NA	NA	2.25	NA
.29	---	NA	NA	NA	NA	0	32	NA	---	252	NA
.26	---	NA	NA	NA	NA	0	35	NA	---	187	NA
.04	.5	NA	.010	NA	NA	0	3.0	NA	NA	11	NA
.09	.35	NA	.033	NA	NA	0	7.0	NA	1.4	56.7	NA
---	---	NA	NA	NA	NA	0	15.5	NA	NA	50	NA
.0056	.035	NA	NA	NA	NA	0	1.05	NA	NA	2.03	NA
.01	.32	NA	NA	NA	NA	0	1.0	NA	NA	3.5	NA
---	---	---	.077	NA	---	0	68	NA	8.80	147	NA
.13	.63	.166	---	NA	.338	0	34.2	NA	---	109	NA
---	---	.185	.07	NA	1.29	0	125	NA	8	179	NA
.06	.55	NA	NA	NA	NA	0	18	NA	2.09	57	NA
.22	2	---	---	NA	---	0	---	NA	NA	79	NA
.29	2.7	.6615	.14445	NA	2.02	0	---	NA	NA	62	NA
.13	.6	---	.055	NA	---	0	18	.27	---	77	NA
.02	.12	---	.01	NA	---	0	3.2	---	---	14	NA
.03	.18	---	---	NA	---	0	8	NA	---	30.6	NA
.27	1.3	.249	.095	NA	.908	0	29	NA	.27	91	.00191 Ohio
.02	.11	.0209	.00798	NA	.076	0	2.28	NA	.02	7.6	NA
.04	.2	---	.022	NA	---	0	9	NA	---	34	NA
.60	4.8	.146	.0097	NA	2.44	0	4	NA	NA	15	NA
.16	1.47	.044	.0084	.29	.770	0	1.05	15.05	NA	2.1	.007
.19	.9	---	.084	NA	---	0	68	NA	---	193	NA

Food and Amount	Iron mg.	Mag- nesium mg.	Phos- phorus mg.	Potas- sium mg.	Sodium mg.
Cucumber, raw, pared—1 cucumber, 7½" x 2", 207 gm.	.6	22.7	37	331	12
Cucumber, raw, pared—1 slice, approx. 2" x ⅛", 8 gm.	.02	.88	1.44	12.8	.48
Cucumber, raw, not pared—1 cucumber, 7" x 2", 219 gm.	2.4	24	59.13	350	13
Cucumber, raw, not pared—1 slice, approx. 2" x ⅛", 9 gm.	.09	.99	2.43	14.4	.54
Dandelion greens, cooked, boiled, drained—1 cup, 180 gm.	3.2	65	75	417	79
Dandelion greens, raw—1 cup, 100 gm.	3.1	36	66	397	76
Eggplant, cooked, boiled, drained— ½ cup diced, 100 gm.	.6	NA	21	150	1
Endive (curly endive and escarole), raw —1 cup, shredded, 70 gm.	1.19	7	37.8	206	9.8
Escarole—see Endive					
Fennel, common, leaves, raw—⅓ of vegetable, 3" diam., 50 gm.	1.35	NA	25.5	198	---
Garbanzos—see Chickpeas					
Garlic, cloves, raw—1 clove (¾" x ½"), 7 gm.	.1	2.52	14.14	37.03	1.33
Jerusalem-artichoke, raw—1 small, 1½" diam., 25 gm.	.85	2.75	19.5	---	---
Kale, cooked, boiled, drained, leaves including stems—1 cup, 110 gm.	1.3	---	51	243	47.3
Kale, frozen, cooked, boiled, drained— ½ cup, 90 gm.	.90	27.9	43	174	18.9
Kale, raw, leaves including stems— 1 cup, 100 gm.	2.2	37	73	378	75
Leeks, bulb and lower leaf portion, raw —1 cup, 110 gm.	1.2	25.3	55	381	5.5
Lentils, mature seeds, raw, dry, whole —½ cup, 100 gm.	6.8	80	377	790	30
Lentils, mature seeds, dry, drained, cooked—1 cup, 135 gm.	9.18	---	351	---	---
Lettuce, raw, butterhead types, Boston or Bibb—1 head, 4" diam., 220 gm.	4.4	---	57	581	19.8
Lettuce, raw, butterhead types, Boston or Bibb—6 leaves, 40 gm.	.80	---	10	105	3.6
Lettuce, raw, Romaine—2 leaves, 45 gm.	.63	NA	11.25	119	4.05
Lettuce, raw, crisp head, e.g., Iceberg— 1 head, 4¾" diam., 454 gm.	2.3	50	100	795	41
Lettuce, raw, crisp head, e.g., Iceberg— 5 leaves, 38 gm.	.19	4.18	8.36	66	3.42
Lettuce, raw, looseleaf or bunching varieties, e.g., Grand Rapids, Salad Bowl—2 large leaves, 50 gm.	.7	---	12.5	132	4.5
Mixed Vegetables, frozen—see Vegetables, mixed, frozen					
Mushrooms, canned, solids and liquid —1 cup, 244 gm.	1.2	19	166	481	976
Mushrooms, raw—½ cup, slices, 35 gm.	.28	---	40.6	145	5.25
Mustard greens, cooked, boiled, drained —1 cup, 140 gm.	2.5	---	44.8	308	25.2

Food and Amount	Calories	Carbo-hydrate gm.	Protein gm.	Sat. Fatty Acids gm.	Unsat. Fatty Acids gm.	Vitamin A IU	Thiamin B₁ mg.
Mustard greens, raw—1 cup, 100 gm.	31	5.6	3	---	---	7,000	.11
Okra, cooked, boiled, drained—1 pod, 3" x ⅝", 10 gm.	2.9	.60	.20	---	---	49	.01
Okra, frozen, cuts and pods, cooked, boiled, drained—½ cup, 90 gm.	34.2	7.92	1.98	---	---	432	.12
Okra, raw—one pod, 2½", 7 gm.	2.52	.53	.16	---	---	36	.01
Onions, mature, dry, cooked—1 cup, 210 gm.	60	14	3	---	---	80	.06
Onions, mature, dry, dehydrated, flaked —1 tablespoon, 1 gm.	3.5	.821	.087	---	---	2.0	.0025
Onions, mature, dry, raw—1 onion, 2½" diam., 110 gm.	40	10	2	---	---	40	.04
Onions, mature, dry, raw—1 slice, 2¼" diam., 25 gm.	9.5	2.17	.37	---	---	10	.01
Onions, young green, raw, bulb and entire top—18" long, ½" diam., 25 gm.	9	2.05	.37	---	---	500	.01
Onions, young green, raw, bulb and white portion of top—6 small (4" long), 50 gm.	20	5	1	---	---	trace	.02
Onions, young green, raw, tops only (green portion)—12" long, 10 gm.	2.7	.55	.16	---	---	400	.007
Parsley, raw, chopped—1 tablespoon, 4 gm.	trace	trace	trace	---	---	340	trace
Parsnips, cooked—1 cup, 155 gm.	100	23	2	---	---	50	.11
Parsnips, raw—1 cup diced, 160 gm.	121	28	2.72	---	---	48	.12
Peas, edible-podded, raw—1 pod, 4" x ¼", 2 gm.	1.06	.24	.06	---	---	13.6	.008
Peas, edible-podded, cooked, boiled, drained—4" x ¼", 4 gm.	1.72	.38	.11	---	---	24.4	.009
Peas, green (reg. peas), immature, raw —1 cup, 135 gm.	113	19.4	8.5	---	---	864	47.2
Peas, green (reg. peas), immature, cooked—1 cup, 160 gm.	115	19	9	---	---	860	.44
Peas, green, immature, early or first canned, solids and liquid—1 cup, 249 gm.	165	31	9	---	---	1,120	.23
Peas, green, immature, sweet (sugar peas), canned, solids and liquid— 1 cup, 150 gm.	85	15.6	5.1	---	---	675	.16
Peas, green, immature, frozen, cooked, boiled, drained—1 cup, 80 gm.	54	9.4	4.08	---	---	480	.21
Peas, mature seeds, dry, whole, raw— 1 cup, 200 gm.	680	120.6	48.2	---	---	240	1.48
Peas, mature seeds, dry, split, without seed coat, raw—1 cup, 205 gm.	713	128.5	49.6	---	---	246	1.51
Peas, mature seeds, dry, split, without seed coat, cooked—1 cup, 190 gm.	219	39.5	15.2	---	---	76	.28
Peas and carrots, frozen, cooked, boiled, drained—1 cup, 85 gm.	45	8.58	2.7	---	---	7,900	.16
Peppers, hot, chili, immature, green, raw, pods, excl. seeds—2" x ½", 14 gm.	5.18	1.27	.18	---	---	107.8	.01
Peppers, hot, chili, immature, green, canned, pods, excl. seeds, solids and liquid—1½" x ¾", 12 gm.	3	.73	.1	---	---	73.2	.004

Food and Amount	Ribo-flavin B₂ mg.	Niacin mg.	B₆ mg.	Folic Acid mg.	PABA mg.	Panto-thenic Acid mg.	B₁₂ mcg.
Mustard greens, raw—1 cup, 100 gm.	.22	.8	.133	.06	NA	.25	0
Okra, cooked, boiled, drained—1 pod, 3″ x ⅝″, 10 gm.	.01	.09	---	.002	NA	---	0
Okra, frozen, cuts and pods, cooked, boiled, drained—½ cup, 90 gm.	.15	.90	.040	---	NA	.193	0
Okra, raw—one pod, 2½″, 7 gm.	.01	.07	---	---	NA	---	0
Onions, mature, dry, cooked—1 cup, 210 gm.	.06	.4	---	.021	NA	---	0
Onions, mature, dry, dehydrated, flaked —1 tablespoon, 1 gm.	.0018	.014	---	---	NA	---	0
Onions, mature, dry, raw—1 onion, 2½″ diam., 110 gm.	.04	.2	.143	.012	NA	.143	0
Onions, mature, dry, raw—1 slice, 2¼″ diam., 25 gm.	.01	.05	.032	.002	NA	.032	0
Onions, young green, raw, bulb and entire top—18″ long, ½″ diam., 25 gm.	.01	.1	---	---	NA	---	0
Onions, young green, raw, bulb and white portion of top—6 small (4″ long), 50 gm.	.02	2	---	.007	NA	.072	0
Onions, young green, raw, tops only (green portion)—12″ long, 10 gm.	.01	.06	---	---	NA	---	0
Parsley, raw, chopped—1 tablespoon, 4 gm.	.01	trace	.006	.0015	NA	.012	0
Parsnips, cooked—1 cup, 155 gm.	.12	.2	.139	.036	NA	.93	0
Parsnips, raw—1 cup diced, 160 gm.	.14	.32	---	---	NA	---	0
Peas, edible-podded, raw—1 pod, 4″ x ¾″, 2 gm.	.004	---	---	---	NA	---	0
Peas, edible-podded, cooked, boiled, drained—4″ x ¾″, 4 gm.	.004	---	---	---	NA	---	0
Peas, green (reg. peas), immature, raw —1 cup, 135 gm.	.18	3.91	.2025	.03375	NA	1.1	0
Peas, green (reg. peas), immature, cooked—1 cup, 160 gm.	.17	3.7	---	.040	NA	---	0
Peas, green, immature, early or first canned, solids and liquid—1 cup, 249 gm.	.13	2.2	.10956	.024	NA	.373	0
Peas, green, immature, sweet (sugar peas), canned, solids and liquid— 1 cup, 150 gm.	.09	1.5	---	---	NA	---	0
Peas, green, immature, frozen, cooked, boiled, drained—1 cup, 80 gm.	.07	1.36	.124	NA	NA	NA	0
Peas, mature seeds, dry, whole, raw— 1 cup, 200 gm.	.58	6.0	NA	NA	NA	NA	0
Peas, mature seeds, dry, split, without seed coat, raw—1 cup, 205 gm.	.59	6.15	.6266	.104	NA	4.1	0
Peas, mature seeds, dry, split, without seed coat, cooked—1 cup, 190 gm.	.17	1.71	.6232	.0969	NA	4.14	0
Peas and carrots, frozen, cooked, boiled, drained—1 cup, 85 gm.	.05	1.10	---	---	NA	---	0
Peppers, hot, chili, immature, green, raw, pods, excl. seeds—2″ x ½″, 14 gm.	.008	.23	NA	NA	NA	NA	0
Peppers, hot, chili, immature, green, canned, pods, excl. seeds, solids and liquid—1½″ x ¾″, 12 gm.	.007	.09	NA	NA	NA	NA	0

Vitamin C mg.	Vitamin D IU	Vitamin E IU	Calcium mg.	Iodine mg.	Iron mg.	Magnesium mg.	Phosphorus mg.	Potassium mg.	Sodium mg.
97	NA	1.75	183	NA	3	27	50	377	32
2	NA	NA	9.2	NA	.05	---	4.1	17.4	.20
10.8	NA	NA	84.6	NA	.45	47.7	38.7	148	1.8
2.17	NA	NA	6.44	NA	.04	2.87	3.57	17	.21
14	NA	NA	50	NA	.8	---	61	231	14.7
.35	NA	NA	1.66	NA	.029	1.06	2.73	13.83	.88
11	NA	.24	30	.00230 Fla.	.60	13	39.6	173	11
---	NA	.05	6.75	.00052 Fla.	.12	3	9	39	2.5
8	NA	---	12.75	NA	.02	---	9.75	57.75	1.25
12	NA	.10	20	NA	.3	---	19.5	116	2.5
5.1	NA	---	5.6	NA	.22	---	3.9	23.1	.5
7	---	.22	8	NA	.2	1.64	2.5	29	1.8
16	NA	NA	70	NA	.9	49.6	96	587	12.4
25.6	NA	NA	80	NA	1.12	51.2	123	865	19.2
.42	NA	---	1.24	NA	.01	---	1.8	3.4	---
.56	NA	--.-	2.24	NA	.02	---	3.04	4.76	---
36.45	NA	.74	35	.031	2.56	47.25	157	427	2.7
33	NA	---	37	NA	2.9	56	158	314	1.6
22	NA	.04	50	NA	4.2	50	164	239	588
13.5	NA	---	28	NA	2.25	---	87	144	354
10.4	NA	.04	15	NA	1.52	19	69	108	92
---	NA	NA	128	.00018 Calif.	10.2	360	680	2,010	70
---	NA	NA	68	NA	10.4	369	426	1,835	82
---	NA	NA	21	.00124 Penn.	3.23	---	169	562	25
6.8	NA	NA	21	NA	.93	16.15	48	133	71
32.9	NA	NA	1.4	NA	.09	NA	3.5	---	---
8.16	NA	NA	.84	NA	.06	NA	2.04	---	---

Food and Amount	Calories	Carbo-hydrate gm.	Protein gm.	Sat. Fatty Acids gm.	Unsat. Fatty Acids gm.	Vitamin A IU	Thiamin B₁ mg.
Peppers, hot, chili, immature, green, canned Chili Sauce—1 tbsp., 20 gm.	4	1	.14	NA	NA	122	.009
Peppers, hot, chili, mature, red, raw, pods incl. seeds—1 pod, 2½" x 1" diam., 28 gm.	26.04	5.06	1.03	---	---	6,048	.06
Peppers, hot, chili, mature, red, canned, Chili Sauce—1 tbsp., 20 gm.	4.2	.78	.18	---	---	1,918	.003
Peppers, hot, chili, mature, red, dried, pods—3" x 1" diam., 2 gm.	6.42	1.19	.25	---	---	1,540	.008
Peppers, hot, chili, mature, red, dried, Chili powder w/added seasoning—1 tbsp., 15 gm.	50	8	2	---	---	9,750	.03
Peppers, sweet, immature green, raw—1 pod, 2½" diam., 74 gm.	15	4	1	---	---	310	.06
Peppers, sweet, immature green, cooked, boiled, drained—1 pod, 2½" diam., 73 gm.	15	3	1	---	---	310	.05
Peppers, sweet, mature, red, raw—3" piece, 25 gm.	7.75	1.77	.35	NA	NA	1,112	.02
Pimentos, canned, solids and liquid—1 medium, 40 gm.	11	2.3	.36	NA	NA	920	.008
Potato chips—1 chip, 2" diam., 2 gm.	11	1.0	.10	---	---	trace	.004
Potato salad, home recipe, cooked dressing and seasoning—½ cup, 100 gm.	99	16.3	2.7	---	---	140	.08
Potato salad, home recipe, mayonnaise and French dressing, hard-cooked eggs, seasonings—½ cup, 100 gm.	145	13.4	3	---	---	180	.07
Potato sticks—1 cup, 35 gm.	190	17.78	2.24	---	---	trace	.07
Potatoes, baked in skin—1 potato, 3¼" diam., 152 gm.	141	32	1.95	---	---	trace	.15
Potatoes, boiled in skin—1 potato, 3" diam., 145 gm.	110.2	24.79	3.04	---	---	trace	.13
Potatoes, boiled, pared before cooking—1 potato, 2¼" diam., 100 gm.	65	14.5	1.9	---	---	trace	.09
Potatoes, canned, solids and liquid—1 cup, 250 gm.	110	24.5	2.75	---	---	trace	.10
Potatoes, dehydrated, mashed flakes without milk, prepared w/water, milk, and table fat—½ cup, 105 gm.	98	15.2	1.99	---	---	137	.04
Potatoes, dehydrated, mashed granules without milk, prepared w/water, milk, and table fat—½ cup, 105 gm.	101	15.1	2.10	---	---	116	.04
Potatoes, dehydrated, mashed granules with milk, prepared with water and table fat—½ cup, 105 gm.	83	13.75	2.10	---	---	95	.03
Potatoes, French-fried from raw—10 pieces, each 2" x ½" x ½", 57 gm.	155	20	2	2	6	trace	.07
Potatoes, French-fried, frozen, heated—10 pieces, each 2" x ½" x ½", 57 gm.	125	19	2	1	3	trace	.08
Potatoes, frozen, diced for hash-browning, cooked—1 cup, 190 gm.	425	55	3.8	---	---	trace	.13
Potatoes, frozen, mashed, heated—1 cup, 200 gm.	186	31.4	3.6	---	---	280	.12
Potatoes, hash-browned—1 cup, 200 gm.	458	58	6.2	---	---	trace	.16

Ribo-flavin B_2 mg.	Niacin mg.	B_6 mg.	Folic Acid mg.	PABA mg.	Panto-thenic Acid mg.	B_{12} mcg.	Vitamin C mg.	Vitamin D IU	Vitamin E IU	Calcium mg.	Iodine mg.
.009	.14	NA	NA	NA	NA	0	13.6	NA	NA	1	NA
.1	1.23	NA	NA	NA	NA	0	103.32	NA	NA	8.12	NA
.01	.12	NA	NA	NA	NA	0	6	NA	NA	1.8	NA
.02	.21.	NA	NA	NA	NA	0	.24	NA	NA	2.6	NA
.17	1.3	NA	NA	NA	NA	0	2	NA	NA	40	NA
.06	.4	.1924	.00518	NA	.170	0	94	NA	NA	7	NA
.05	.4	---	---	NA	---	0	70	NA	NA	7	NA
.02	.12	NA	NA	NA	NA	0	51	NA	NA	3.25	NA
.02	.16	NA	NA	NA	NA	0	38	NA	NA	2.8	NA
.001	.09	.0036	NA	NA	---	0	.32	NA	.12	.80	NA
.07	1.1	---	NA	NA	---	0	11	NA	•••	32	NA
.06	.9	---	NA	NA	---	0	11	NA	•••	19	NA
.02	1.68	---	NA	NA	---	0	14	NA	•••	15	NA
.06	2.58	NA	NA	---	---	0	30	NA	.041	13.7	NA
.05	2.17	NA	NA	NA	NA	NA	23.2	NA	NA	10.15	NA
.03	1.2	.174	.007	---	---	0	16.	NA	.04	6	.0034 Ohio
.05	1.5	---	---	NA	---	0	32.5	NA	•••	10	NA
.04	.94	---	---	NA	---	0	5.25	NA	•••	33	NA
.05	.73	---	---	NA	---	0	3.15	NA	•••	34	NA
.05	.84	---	---	NA	---	0	3.15	NA	•••	33	NA
.04	1.8	---	---	NA	---	0	12	NA	.15	9	NA
.01	1.5	.1026	---	NA	.3078	0	12	NA	.15	5	NA
.03	1.9	---	---	NA	•••	0	15.2	NA	•••	34	NA
.08	1.4	---	---	NA	---	0	8	NA	•••	50	NA
.10	4.2	---	---	NA	---	0	18	NA	•••	24	NA

Food and Amount	Iron mg.	Magnesium mg.	Phosphorus mg.	Potassium mg.	Sodium mg.
Peppers, hot, chili, immature, green, canned Chili Sauce—1 tbsp., 20 gm.	.08	NA	2.8	---	---
Peppers, hot, chili, mature, red, raw, pods incl. seeds—1 pod, 2½″ x 1″ diam., 28 gm.	.33	---	21.84	---	---
Peppers, hot, chili, mature, red, canned, Chili Sauce—1 tbsp., 20 gm.	.1	---	3.2	---	---
Peppers, hot, chili, mature, red, dried, pods—3″ x 1″ diam., 2 gm.	.15	---	4.8	24.02	7.46
Peppers, hot, chili, mature, red, dried, Chili powder w/added seasoning— 1 tbsp., 15 gm.	2.3	25.35	31	150	236
Peppers, sweet, immature green, raw— 1 pod, 2½″ diam., 74 gm.	.5	13.32	16	158	9.6
Peppers, sweet, immature green, cooked, boiled, drained—1 pod, 2½″ diam., 73 gm.	.4	NA	12	109	6.6
Peppers, sweet, mature, red, raw— 3″ piece, 25 gm.	.15	NA	7.5	---	---
Pimentos, canned, solids and liquid— 1 medium, 40 gm.	.60	NA	6.8	---	---
Potato chips—1 chip, 2″ diam., 2 gm.	.03	---	2.78	23	20
Potato salad, home recipe, cooked dressing and seasoning—½ cup, 100 gm.	.6	---	64	319	528
Potato salad, home recipe, mayonnaise and French dressing, hard-cooked eggs, seasonings—½ cup, 100 gm.	.8	---	63	296	480
Potato sticks—1 cup, 35 gm.	.63	---	49	396	350
Potatoes, baked in skin—1 potato, 3¼″ diam., 152 gm.	1.06	---	98	764	6
Potatoes, boiled in skin—1 potato, 3″ diam., 145 gm.	.87	---	76.85	590.15	4.35
Potatoes, boiled, pared before cooking —1 potato, 2¼″ diam., 100 gm.	.5	---	42	285	2
Potatoes, canned, solids and liquid— 1 cup, 250 gm.	.75	---	75	625	2.5
Potatoes, dehydrated, mashed flakes without milk, prepared w/water, milk, and table fat—½ cup, 105 gm.	.31	---	49	300	243
Potatoes, dehydrated, mashed granules without milk, prepared w/water, milk, and table fat—½ cup, 105 gm.	.52	---	55	305	269
Potatoes, dehydrated, mashed granules with milk, prepared with water and table fat—½ cup, 105 gm.	.63	---	46	352	246
Potatoes, French-fried from raw—10 pieces, each 2″ x ½″ x ½″, 57 gm.	.7	---	63	486	3.4
Potatoes, French-fried, frozen, heated— 10 pieces, each 2″ x ½″ x ½″, 57 gm.	1	---	49	372	2.3
Potatoes, frozen, diced for hash-browning, cooked—1 cup, 190 gm.	2.28	---	95	537	568
Potatoes, frozen, mashed, heated— 1 cup, 200 gm.	1.2	---	84	430	718
Potatoes, hash-browned—1 cup, 200 gm.	1.8	---	158	950	576

Food and Amount	Calories	Carbohydrate gm.	Protein gm.	Sat. Fatty Acids gm.	Unsat. Fatty Acids gm.	Vitamin A IU	Thiamin B₁ mg.
Potatoes, mashed, milk added—1 cup, 195 gm.	125	25	4	•••	•••	50	.16
Potatoes, mashed, milk and table fat added—1 cup, 195 gm.	185	24	4	4	3	330	.16
Potatoes, raw—1 potato, 2¼" diam., 100 gm.	76	17.1	2.1	•••	•••	trace	.10
Potatoes, scalloped and au gratin with cheese—1 cup, 180 gm.	261	24.48	9.54	7.2	5.4	576	.1
Potatoes, scalloped and au gratin without cheese—1 cup, 185 gm.	192.4	27.19	5.55	•••	•••	296	.11
Pumpkin, canned—1 cup, 228 gm.	75	18	2	•••	•••	14,590	.07
Pumpkin, raw—1 cup, 160 gm.	41.6	10.4	1.6	•••	•••	2,560	.08
Radishes, common, raw—1 small, 1" diam., 10 gm.	1.7	.36	.10	NA	NA	1.0	.003
Rutabagas, cooked, boiled, drained— ½ cup cubed, 100 gm.	35	8.2	.9	•••	•••	550	.06
Rutabagas, raw—½ cup diced, 68 gm.	31	7.48	.74	NA	NA	394	.04
Salsify, cooked, boiled, drained— 1 cup, 160 gm.	66	24.16	4.16	NA	NA	16	.04
Salsify, raw—1 salsify, 6" long, 50 gm.	24	7.55	1.3	NA	NA	5	.015
Sauerkraut, canned, solids and liquid —1 cup, 235 gm.	45	9	2	•••	•••	120	.07
Sauerkraut juice, canned—1 cup, 249 gm.	25	5.72	1.74	•••	•••	•••	.07
Seaweed, raw, Agar—1 tbsp., 10 gm.	•••	•••	•••	NA	NA	•••	•••
Seaweed, raw, Dulse—1 tbsp., 10 gm.	•••	•••	•••	NA	NA	•••	•••
Seaweed, raw, Irish moss—1 tbsp., 10 gm.	•••	•••	•••	NA	NA	•••	•••
Seaweed, raw, Kelp—1 tbsp., 10 gm.	•••	•••	•••	NA	NA	•••	•••
Seaweed, raw, Laver—1 tbsp., 10 gm.	•••	•••	•••	NA	NA	•••	•••
Shallot bulbs, raw—1 bulb, ¾" diam., 10 gm.	7.2	1.68	.25	NA	NA	trace	.006
Spinach, raw—1 cup, 50 gm.	13	2.15	1.6	•••	•••	4,050	.05
Spinach, cooked, boiled, drained— 1 cup, 180 gm.	40	6	5	•••	•••	14,580	.13
Spinach, canned, drained solids— 1 cup, 180 gm.	45	6	5	•••	•••	14,400	.03
Spinach, frozen, chopped, cooked, boiled, drained—½ cup, 100 gm.	23	3.7	3	•••	•••	7,900	.07
Spinach, frozen, leaf, cooked, boiled, drained—½ cup, 100 gm.	24	3.9	2.9	•••	•••	8,100	.08
Squash, raw, summer, all varieties**— 6½" x 2" diam., 155 gm.	29	6.5	1.7	•••	•••	635	.07
Squash, raw, Zucchini and Cocozelle (green)—7½" x 1½" diam., 168 gm.	28	6.04	2.01	•••	•••	537	.08
Squash, raw, winter, all varieties†— 1 cup diced, 144 gm.	72	17.8	2.01	•••	•••	5,328	.07
Squash, all summer varieties,** cooked, boiled, drained—1 cup, diced, 210 gm.	30	7	2	•••	•••	820	.10

** Yellow, crookneck, and straightneck, white and pale green—scallop varieties; summer varieties.
† Acorn, butternut, and hubbard; winter varieties.

Food and Amount	Riboflavin B₂ mg.	Niacin mg.	B₆ mg.	Folic Acid mg.	PABA mg.	Pantothenic Acid mg.	B₁₂ mcg.
Potatoes, mashed, milk added—1 cup, 195 gm.	.10	2.0	---	---	NA	---	0
Potatoes, mashed, milk and table fat added—1 cup, 195 gm.	.10	1.9	---	---	NA	---	0
Potatoes, raw—1 potato, 2¼" diam., 100 gm.	.04	1.5	---	---	.4	---	0
Potatoes, scalloped and au gratin with cheese—1 cup, 180 gm.	.21	1.62	---	---	NA	---	0
Potatoes, scalloped and au gratin without cheese—1 cup, 185 gm.	.16	1.85	---	---	NA	---	0
Pumpkin, canned—1 cup, 228 gm.	.12	1.3	.1276	.018	NA	.912	0
Pumpkin, raw—1 cup, 160 gm.	.17	.96	NA	NA	NA	NA	0
Radishes, common, raw—1 small, 1" diam., 10 gm.	.003	.03	.0075	.007	NA	.0184	0
Rutabagas, cooked, boiled, drained— ½ cup cubed, 100 gm.	.06	.8	.100	.005	NA	.160	0
Rutabagas, raw—½ cup diced, 68 gm.	.04	.74	---	---	NA	---	0
Salsify, cooked, boiled, drained— 1 cup, 160 gm.	.06	.32	NA	NA	NA	NA	0
Salsify, raw—1 salsify, 6" long, 50 gm.	.02	.1	NA	NA	NA	NA	0
Sauerkraut, canned, solids and liquid —1 cup, 235 gm.	.09	.47	.3055	NA	NA	.2185	0
Sauerkraut juice, canned—1 cup, 249 gm.	.09	.49	NA	NA	NA	NA	0
Seaweed, raw, Agar—1 tbsp., 10 gm.	---	---	NA	NA	NA	NA	0
Seaweed, raw, Dulse—1 tbsp., 10 gm.	---	---	NA	NA	NA	NA	0
Seaweed, raw, Irish moss—1 tbsp., 10 gm.	---	---	NA	NA	NA	NA	0
Seaweed, raw, Kelp—1 tbsp., 10 gm.	---	---	NA	NA	NA	NA	0
Seaweed, raw, Laver—1 tbsp., 10 gm.	---	---	NA	NA	NA	NA	0
Shallot bulbs, raw—1 bulb, ¾" diam., 10 gm.	.002	.02	NA	NA	NA	NA	0
Spinach, raw—1 cup, 50 gm.	.10	.3	.14	.0385	.4	.15	0
Spinach, cooked, boiled, drained— 1 cup, 180 gm.	.25	1.0	.234	.135	---	.135	0
Spinach, canned, drained solids— 1 cup, 180 gm.	.21	.6	.126	.0882	NA	.117	0
Spinach, frozen, chopped, cooked, boiled, drained—½ cup, 100 gm.	.15	.4	---	---	NA	---	0
Spinach, frozen, leaf, cooked, boiled, drained—½ cup, 100 gm.	.14	.5·	---	---	NA	---	0
Squash, raw, summer, all varieties**— 6½" x 2" diam., 155 gm.	.13	1.55	.09765	.02635	NA	.6	0
Squash, raw, Zucchini and Cocozelle (green)—7½" x 1½" diam., 168 gm.	.15	1.68	NA	NA	NA	NA	0
Squash, raw, winter, all varieties†— 1 cup diced, 144 gm.	.15	.86	.13104	.01728	NA	.7	0
Squash, all summer varieties,** cooked, boiled, drained—1 cup, diced, 210 gm.	.16	1.6	.132	.023	NA	.363	0

** Yellow, crookneck, and straightneck, white and pale green—scallop varieties; summer varieties.

† Acorn, butternut, and hubbard; winter varieties.

Vitamin C mg.	Vitamin D IU	Vitamin E IU	Calcium mg.	Iodine mg.	Iron mg.	Magnesium mg.	Phosphorus mg.	Potassium mg.	Sodium mg.
19	NA	---	47	.00080 (w/o milk) Ohio	.8	---	96	509	587
18	NA	---	47	NA	.8	---	94	488	645
20	NA	.1	7	.00061 Penn.	.6	34	53	407	3
18	NA	---	228.6	NA	.9	---	219.6	550.8	804.6
20.35	NA	---	99.9	NA	.74	---	136.9	604.95	656.75
12	NA	NA	57	NA	.9	---	59	547	4.6
14	NA	NA	33	NA	1.28	19.2	70	544	1.6
2.6	NA	NA	3	NA	.10	1.5	3.1	32	1.8
26	NA	NA	59	NA	.3	15	31	167	4
29	NA	NA	45	NA	.27	10.2	27	163	.40
11.2	NA	NA	67	NA	2.08	NA	85	425	---
3.5	NA	NA	21	NA	.65	NA	27	133	---
33	NA	NA	85	NA	1.2	---	42	329	1,755
45	NA	NA	92	NA	2.73	---	35	---	1,960
---	NA	NA	56.7	NA	.63	NA	2.2	---	---
---	NA	NA	29.6	NA	---	NA	26.7	806	208.5
---	NA	NA	88.5	NA	.89	NA	15.7	284	289
---	NA	NA	109.3	NA	---	NA	24	527.3	300.7
---	NA	NA	---	NA	---	NA	---	---	---
.8	NA	NA	3.7	NA	.12	NA	6	33.4	1.2
25.5	NA	1.7	47	NA	1.55	44	25.5	235	36
50	NA	3.06	167	.0009 Ohio	4.0	---	68	583	90
24	NA	.03	212	NA	4.7	63	47	450	425
19	NA	---	113	NA	2.1	---	44	333	52
28	NA	---	105	NA	2.5	---	44	362	49
34	NA	NA	43	NA	.62	---	45	313	1.5
32	NA	NA	47	NA	.67	---	48	339	1.68
19	NA	NA	31	NA	.86	24.48	54	531	1.44
21	NA	NA	52	NA	.8	16	53	296	2.1

Food and Amount	Calories	Carbo-hydrate gm.	Protein gm.	Sat. Fatty Acids gm.	Unsat. Fatty Acids gm.	Vitamin A IU	Thiamin B₁ mg.
Squash, Zucchini and Cocozelle, cooked, boiled, drained—½ cup, 76 gm.	9.1	1.9	.76	---	---	228	.03
Squash, all winter varieties,† cooked, baked—1 cup (mashed), 205 gm.	130	32	4	---	---	8,610	.10
Squash, all winter varieties,† cooked, boiled, mashed—1 cup, 250 gm.	95	23	2.75	---	---	8,750	.10
Squash, frozen, summer, Yellow Crookneck, cooked, boiled, drained —½ cup, 100 gm.	21	4.7	1.4	---	---	140	.06
Squash, frozen, winter varieties,† heated—½ cup, 100 gm.	38	9.2	1.2	---	---	3,900	.03
Succotash (corn and lima beans), frozen, cooked, boiled, drained— ½ cup, 96 gm.	89	19.7	4.03	---	---	288	.08
Sweet potatoes, canned, in syrup, solids and liquid—1 cup, 240 gm.	273.6	66	2.4	---	---	12,000	.07
Sweet potatoes, canned, vacuum or solid pack—1 cup, 218 gm.	235	54	4	---	---	17,000	.10
Sweet potatoes, dehydrated flakes, prepared w/water—½ cup, 125 gm.	119	28	1.25	---	---	15,000	.02
Sweet potatoes, cooked, baked, peeled after baking—1 potato, 5″ x 2″, 110 gm.	155	36	2	---	---	8,910	.10
Sweet potatoes, cooked, boiled, peeled after boiling—1 potato, 5″ x 2″, 147 gm.	170	39	2	---	---	11,610	.13
Sweet potatoes, cooked, candied— 1 potato, 3½″ x 2¼″, 175 gm.	295	60	2	2	4	11,030	.10
Sweet potatoes, raw, all varieties— 1 potato, 5″ x 2″, 170 gm.	194	44.7	2.9	---	---	14,960	.17
Swiss chard, cooked, boiled, drained— ½ cup, 95 gm.	17	3.1	1.7	---	---	5,130	.03
Swiss chard, raw leaves and stalks— 1 cup, 100 gm.	25	4.6	2.4	---	---	6,500	.06
Tomato catsup, bottled—1 cup, 273 gm.	290	69	6	---	---	3,820	.25
Tomato catsup, bottled—1 tablespoon, 15 gm.	15	4	trace	---	---	210	.01
Tomato juice, bottled or canned— 1 cup, 243 gm.	45	10	2	---	---	1,940	.12
Tomato juice, bottled or canned— 1 glass (6 oz.), 182 gm.	35	8	2	---	---	1,460	.09
Tomato juice, canned concentrate, diluted w/3 pts. water—1 cup, 245 gm.	49	11	2	---	---	2,205	.12
Tomato juice, dehydrated, prepared w/water, 1 lb. = 1¾ gals.—1 cup, 244 gm.	49	11	2	---	---	2,098	.07
Tomato juice cocktail, canned or bottled—1 cup, 240 gm.	50.4	12	1.68	---	---	1,920	.12
Tomato paste, canned—1 avg. can, 6 oz., 170 gm.	139	31	6	---	---	5,610	.34
Tomato purée, canned, regular pack— 1 cup, 249 gm.	97	22	4	---	---	3,984	.22
Tomatoes, green, raw—1 tomato, 2¼″ diam., 125 gm.	30	6.37	1.5	---	---	337.5	.07

† Acorn, butternut, and hubbard; winter varieties.

Riboflavin B_2 mg.	Niacin mg.	B_6 mg.	Folic Acid mg.	PABA mg.	Pantothenic Acid mg.	B_{12} mcg.	Vitamin C mg.	Vitamin D IU	Vitamin E IU	Calcium mg.	Iodine mg.
.06	.6	NA	NA	NA	NA	0	6.8	NA	NA	19	NA
.27	1.4	NA	NA	NA	NA	0	27	NA	NA	57	NA
.25	1.0	NA	.030	NA	NA	0	20	NA	NA	50	NA
.04	.4	.063	---	NA	.173	0	8	NA	NA	14	NA
.07	.5	.091	---	NA	.282	0	8	NA	NA	25	NA
.04	1.24	NA	NA	NA	NA	0	5.7	NA	NA	12	NA
.07	1.44	---	---	NA	---	0	19.2	NA	NA	31.2	NA
.10	1.4	---	---	NA	---	0	30	NA	NA	54	NA
.03	.37	---	---	NA	---	0	13.75	NA	NA	19	NA
.07	.7	---	.0132	---	---	0	24	NA	NA	44	NA
.09	.9	---	---	---	---	0	25	NA	NA	47	NA
.08	.8	---	---	NA	---	0	17	NA	NA	65	NA
.10	1.02	.3706	.0204	.17	1.394	0	35.7	NA	NA	54	NA
.10	.38	---	.04	NA	.163	0	15	NA	---	69	NA
.17	.5	---	---	NA	.172	0	32	NA	---	88	.0992 (dried) Ohio
.19	4.4	.292	NA	NA	---	0	41	NA	NA	60	NA
.01	.2	.01605	NA	NA	---	0	2	NA	NA	3	NA
.07	1.9	.466	.017	NA	.607	0	39	NA	.53	17	.00114 Ohio
.05	1.5	.34944	.01274	NA	.455	0	29	NA	.4	13	.00086 Ohio
.07	1.9	---	---	NA	---	0	32	NA	---	17	NA
.07	2.2	---	---	NA	---	0	39	NA	---	15	NA
.04	1.44	NA	NA	NA	NA	0	38.4	NA	NA	24	NA
.20	5.27	NA	NA	NA	NA	0	83	NA	NA	46	NA
.12	3.48	NA	NA	NA	NA	0	82	NA	NA	32	NA
.05	.62	NA	NA	NA	NA	0	25	NA	NA	16.25	NA

Food and Amount	Iron mg.	Mag- nesium mg.	Phos- phorus mg.	Potas- sium mg.	Sodium mg.
Squash, Zucchini and Cocozelle, cooked, boiled, drained—½ cup, 76 gm.	.3	---	19	107	.76
Squash, all winter varieties,† cooked, baked—1 cup (mashed), 205 gm.	1.6	---	98	945	2.05
Squash, all winter varieties,† cooked, boiled, mashed—1 cup, 250 gm.	1.25	---	80	645	2.5
Squash, frozen, summer, Yellow Crookneck, cooked, boiled, drained —½ cup, 100 gm.	.7	---	32	167	3
Squash, frozen, winter varieties,† heated—½ cup, 100 gm.	1.0	---	32	207	1
Succotash (corn and lima beans), frozen, cooked, boiled, drained— ½ cup, 96 gm.	.96	NA	82	236	36
Sweet potatoes, canned, in syrup, solids and liquid—1 cup, 240 gm.	1.68	---	69.6	288	115.2
Sweet potatoes, canned, vacuum or solid pack—1 cup, 218 gm.	1.7	---	89	436	105
Sweet potatoes, dehydrated flakes, prepared w/water—½ cup, 125 gm.	.75	---	25	175	56
Sweet potatoes, cooked, baked, peeled after baking—1 potato, 5″ x 2″, 110 gm.	1.0	---	61.8	310	13.2
Sweet potatoes, cooked, boiled, peeled after boiling—1 potato, 5″ x 2″, 147 gm.	1.0	---	68	354	14.7
Sweet potatoes, cooked, candied— 1 potato, 3½″ x 2¼″, 175 gm.	1.6	---	75	333	74
Sweet potatoes, raw, all varieties— 1 potato, 5″ x 2″, 170 gm.	1.19	52.7	80	413	17
Swiss chard, cooked, boiled, drained— ½ cup, 95 gm.	1.7	61	23	305	81
Swiss chard, raw leaves and stalks— 1 cup, 100 gm.	3.2	65	39	550	147
Tomato catsup, bottled—1 cup, 273 gm.	2.2	57.33	137	991	2,845
Tomato catsup, bottled—1 tablespoon, 15 gm.	.1	3.15	7.5	54	156
Tomato juice, bottled or canned— 1 cup, 243 gm.	2.2	24.3	44	552	486
Tomato juice, bottled or canned— 1 glass (6 oz.), 182 gm.	1.6	18.2	33	413	364
Tomato juice, canned concentrate, diluted w/3 pts. water—1 cup, 245 gm.	2.2	---	47	576	512
Tomato juice, dehydrated, prepared w/water, 1 lb. = 1¾ gals.—1 cup, 244 gm.	1.2	---	44	564	630
Tomato juice cocktail, canned or bottled—1 cup, 240 gm.	2.16	---	43.2	530.4	480
Tomato paste, canned—1 avg. can, 6 oz., 170 gm.	5.95	---	119	1,509	64
Tomato purée, canned, regular pack— 1 cup, 249 gm.	4.2	49.8	84	1,060	993
Tomatoes, green, raw—1 tomato, 2¼″ diam., 125 gm.	.62	---	33.75	305	3.75

† Acorn, butternut, and hubbard; winter varieties.

Food and Amount	Calories	Carbo-hydrate gm.	Protein gm.	Sat. Fatty Acids gm.	Unsat. Fatty Acids gm.	Vitamin A IU	Thiamin B₁ mg.
Tomatoes, ripe, raw—1 tomato, 3" x 2½", 200 gm.	40	9	2	---	---	1,640	.11
Tomatoes, ripe, cooked, boiled—½ cup, 100 gm.	26	5.5	1.3	---	---	1,000	.07
Tomatoes, ripe, canned, solids and liquid—1 cup, 241 gm.	50	10	2	---	---	2,170	.12
Turnip greens, leaves and stems, canned, solids and liquid—½ cup, 100 gm.	18	3.2	1.5	---	---	4,700	.02
Turnip greens, leaves and stems, cooked, boiled, drained—1 cup, 145 gm.	30	5	3	---	---	8,270	.15
Turnip greens, leaves and stems, frozen, cooked, boiled, drained—½ cup, 78 gm.	18	3	1.95	---	---	5,382	.03
Turnip greens, leaves and stems, raw—1 cup, 100 gm.	28	5	3	---	---	7,600	.21
Turnips, cooked, boiled, drained—1 cup, diced, 155 gm.	35	8	1	---	---	trace	.06
Turnips, raw—1 cup diced, 130 gm.	39	8	1.3	---	---	trace	.05
Vegetable juice cocktail, canned—1 cup, 250 gm.	42	9	2.25	---	---	1,750	.12
Vegetables, mixed (carrots, corn, peas, green snap beans, lima beans), frozen, cooked, boiled, drained—½ cup, 90 gm.	57	12	2.9	---	---	4,455	.10
Water chestnuts, raw—4 chestnuts, 25 gm.	20	4.7	.35	---	---	0	.03
Watercress, leaves and stems, raw—1 sprig, 1 gm.	.19	.03	.02	---	---	49	.0008
Yam, cooked in skin—1 cup, 200 gm.	210	48.2	4.8	---	---	trace	.18
Yam, tuber, raw—1 tuber, 5½" x 1½", 125 gm.	126.25	29	2.62	---	---	trace	.12
VEGETABLE JUICES							
Carrot juice—1 cup, 240 gm.	70	14.4	.8	NA	NA	NA	NA
Celery tonic—1 cup, 242 gm.	NA	NA	NA	NA	NA	NA	NA

Food and Amount	Ribo-flavin B_2 mg.	Niacin mg.	B_6 mg.	Folic Acid mg.	PABA mg.	Panto-thenic Acid mg.	B_{12} mcg.
Tomatoes, ripe, raw—1 tomato, 3" x 2½", 200 gm.	.07	1.3	.200	.016	NA	.660	0
Tomatoes, ripe, cooked, boiled— ½ cup, 100 gm.	.05	.8	---	---	NA	---	0
Tomatoes, ripe, canned, solids and liquid—1 cup, 241 gm.	.07	1.7	.2169	.0096	NA	.554	0
Turnip greens, leaves and stems, canned, solids and liquid—½ cup, 100 gm.	.09	.6	---	.042	NA	.068	0
Turnip greens, leaves and stems, cooked, boiled, drained—1 cup, 145 gm.	.33	.7	---	---	NA	---	0
Turnip greens, leaves and stems, frozen, cooked, boiled, drained—½ cup, 78 gm.	.07	.31	---	---	NA	---	0
Turnip greens, leaves and stems, raw— 1 cup, 100 gm.	.39	.8	.098	.042	NA	.38	0
Turnips, cooked, boiled, drained— 1 cup, diced, 155 gm.	.08	.5	.139	006	NA	.310	0
Turnips, raw—1 cup diced, 130 gm.	.09	.78	.117	NA	NA	.260	0
Vegetable juice cocktail, canned— 1 cup, 250 gm.	.07	2	NA	NA	NA	NA	0
Vegetables, mixed (carrots, corn, peas, green snap beans, lima beans), frozen, cooked, boiled, drained—½ cup, 90 gm.	.06	.99	.1098	.0144	NA	.27	0
Water chestnuts, raw—4 chestnuts, 25 gm.	.05	.25	NA	NA	NA	NA	0
Watercress, leaves and stems, raw— 1 sprig, 1 gm.	.001	.009	NA	NA	NA	NA	0
Yam, cooked in skin—1 cup, 200 gm.	.08	1.2	NA	NA	NA	NA	0
Yam, tuber, raw—1 tuber, 5½" x 1½", 125 gm.	.05	.62	NA	NA	NA	NA	0

VEGETABLE JUICES

Carrot juice—1 cup, 240 gm.	NA	NA	NA	NA	NA	NA	0
Celery tonic—1 cup, 242 gm.	NA	NA	NA	NA	NA	NA	NA

Vitamin C mg.	Vitamin D IU	Vitamin E IU	Calcium mg.	Iodine mg.	Iron mg.	Magnesium mg.	Phosphorus mg.	Potassium mg.	Sodium mg.
42	NA	.80	24	.00052 Ohio	.9	28	54	488	6
24	NA	---	15	NA	.6	---	32	287	4
41	NA	.96	14	NA	1.2	28.92	46	523	313
19	NA	NA	100	NA	1.6	58	30	243	236
68	NA	---	252	NA	1.5	---	53	---	---
15	NA	NA	92	NA	1.2	---	30	116	13
139	NA	---	246	NA	1.8	58	58	---	---
34	NA	.03	54	NA	.6	31	37	291	52
46	NA	.02	50	.052	.65	26	39	348	63
22	NA	NA	30	NA	1.25	---	55	552	500
7	NA	NA	22	NA	1.17	---	56	172	48
1	NA	NA	1.0	NA	.15	3	16	125	5
.79	NA	NA	1.5	NA	.01	.2	.54	2.8	.52
18	NA	NA	8	NA	1.2	NA	100	NA	NA
11.25	NA	NA	25	NA	.75	NA	86.25	750	---
NA	NA	NA	NA	NA	NA	NA	NA	NA	NA
NA	NA	NA	NA	NA	NA	NA	NA	NA	NA

Index